Homes That Heal

The depth of knowledge and solid information in this book is truly impressive.
Homes That Heal is a must for homeowners and renters of all ages.
You'll refer to this book again and again: it has it all!
— ROBYN GRIGGS LAWRENCE, Editor-in-Chief, *Natural Home* magazine

Athena Thompson has done something that should have been done long ago: she
has taken the complicated domains of public health and the built environment and has
made them clear and accessible to those who need it most — families. *Homes that Heal*, with
its easy-to-understand language, features, and solutions-oriented focus, bridges an essential,
but often overlooked, gap. It should be required reading for all homeowners.
— ROBERT K. MUSIL, PhD, MPH, Executive Director and CEO,
Physicians for Social Responsibility

Smart, compelling and timely, Athena Thompson's *Homes That Heal* is full of practical,
and often eye-opening, information. It should be on every homeowner's bookshelf.
— BOB FEEMAN, Managing Editor, *Smart HomeOwner* magazine

Athena Thompson's cast of fictional characters vividly illustrate the true facts....
We must all become informed and proactive homeowners in order for our homes
to nurture our families' optimum health. This book is thorough, provocative,
informative and, on top of all that, it is fun to read!
— PAULA BAKER-LAPORTE, architect, author, *Prescriptions for a Healthy House*

A masterpiece of "knowledge translation" of complex information on a vital topic for all
of us, with plenty of resources provided for further learning. A riveting read that makes a
passionate plea for prudent purchasing and the precautionary principle in public health policy.
— LYNN M. MARSHALL MD, Fellow of the American Academy of Environmental Medicine,
Fellow of the Royal Society of Medicine (Great Britain)

Homes that Heal is an exciting and informative book. I thought that I'd just thumb through it
to see if there was an easy step I can take to make my house healthier. I found myself reading
every page! It's simple and most suggestions are very doable even on a tight budget.
— LOIS MARIE GIBBS, Executive Director, Center For Health, Environment and Justice
Community leader winning the evacuation of families from the
Love Canal toxic dumpsite in Niagara Falls

If after cleaning your house, a question lingers: "it smells clean, but is it safe?" — then stop right here. This is the book for you! *Homes That Heal* is filled to the rafters with sensible and simple ways to create a safe and healthy home for you and your family.

— WENDY GORDON, Executive Director, The Green Guide Institute

Homes that Heal is an extremely important resource covering all aspects of environmental health for the home. Athena Thompson is an expert in this field and she has presented the information in a way that is accessible and entertaining.

— MEGAN KEMPLE, Public Education Coordinator, Northwest Coalition for Alternatives to Pesticides

Homes that Heal is the ideal book. Through the use of simple stories to illustrate a variety of situations, Athena Thompson conveys the problems and provides solutions that everyone can apply. The awareness gained will result in actions that will benefit the entire family. This is knowledge that everyone can use to create healthy living and working spaces.

— HELMUT ZIEHE, Director, International Institute for Baubiologie and Ecology

This book offers timely, practical and entertaining reading on a most important subject, the health of our homes and those who live in them. It shows us that what we don't know can hurt us and that there is always a natural and least toxic choice to each of our building and remodeling decisions. Choose wisely.

— WILL SPATES, President, Indoor Environmental Technologies, Inc.

The information contained in this book is a long leap forward in our efforts to change the way we create our individual spaces. In creating healthy environments that comfort our souls and heal our bodies we can begin to step more lightly on our planet. *Homes That Heal* gives step-by-step assistance, a must read before buying or remodeling.

— CONNIE MENUEY MCCULLAH, Co-owner of Odin's Hammer, Certified Green Remodeling Professionals

Athena Thompson follows in the steps of Florence Nightingale, who said that "the connection between health and the dwelling of the population is one of the most important that exists."

— RUTH A. ETZEL, MD, PhD, Children's Environmental Health Network

Athena Thompson has applied her extensive knowledge as a health professional and Building Biologist to creating healthy spaces to live, learn and work in. It is the toxicity of our world that creates most illnesses that kill us or reduces our quality of life. *Homes that Heal* is a must read!

— SATYA AMBROSE. L.Ac., N.D., Founder of the Oregon College of Oriental Medicine, Clinician, National College of Naturopathic Medicine.

Homes That Heal provides a new blueprint for living healthier through Building Biology. It's well worth the read!

— NANCY CHUDA, President and co-founder, Children's Health Environmental Coalition

ATHENA THOMPSON

HOMES *that* HEAL

and
those
that
don't

How your home may be
harming your family's health

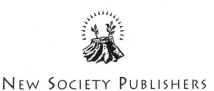

NEW SOCIETY PUBLISHERS

Cataloguing in Publication Data:
A catalog record for this publication is available from the National Library of Canada.

Cover design by Diane McIntosh. Cover image: Wane Fuday.

Printed in Canada.

Paperback ISBN: 0-86571-511-4

This book is not intended to provide medical or legal advice. The services of a competent professional should be obtained whenever medical, legal, or other specific advice is needed

Inquiries regarding requests to reprint all or part of *Homes That Heal* should be addressed to New Society Publishers at the address below.

To order directly from the publishers, please add $4.50 shipping to the price of the first copy, and $1.00 for each additional copy (plus GST in Canada). Send check or money order to:

New Society Publishers
P.O. Box 189, Gabriola Island, BC V0R 1X0, Canada
1-800-567-6772

New Society Publishers' mission is to publish books that contribute in fundamental ways to building an ecologically sustainable and just society, and to do so with the least possible impact on the environment, in a manner that models this vision. We are committed to doing this not just through education, but through action. We are acting on our commitment to the world's remaining ancient forests by phasing out our paper supply from ancient forests worldwide. This book is one step towards ending global deforestation and climate change. It is printed on acid-free paper that is **100% old growth forest-free** (100% post-consumer recycled), processed chlorine free, and printed with vegetable based, low VOC inks. For further information, or to browse our full list of books and purchase securely, visit our website at:
www.newsociety.com

NEW SOCIETY PUBLISHERS   www.newsociety.com

To Wane and Sean, my inspirations.

and

To all our children and future generations, may we be worthy of their trust.

Table of Contents

Acknowledgments

Homes that Heal was shaped and formed by a cast of many characters, both on the written page and in real time. First and foremost, I would like to thank my husband, Wane, and my son, Sean, for their love, patience, and support during the process of writing this book. It is a challenge to the best of families to have a wife and mother preoccupied for so many months. In addition to cooking many great meals, Wane was an invaluable proofreader of the text in all its incarnations, while Sean helped specifically in the creation of the children's characters and offered input on all the cartoons.

Cris Hammond deserves great praise for his exceptional talent as an artist. His memorable cartoons will keep us all chuckling as we embrace the more serious task of making our homes safe places in which our families can thrive.

Allan Lieberman M.D., has done a great service by writing the foreword to this book. With 44 years experience as a dedicated and caring physician his words offer both encouragement to everyday families as well as an authoratative perspective to family physicians not yet familiar with the effects our home environment can have on our health.

Special thanks go to various colleagues and friends who reviewed chapters and provided valuable suggestions: Paula Baker-Laporte, Helmut Ziehe, Lynn Marshall M.D., Ruth Etzel M.D. PhD, Will Spates, and Houston Tomasz.

I would also like to thank the whole team at New Society Publishers for a truly collaborative effort and the forging of many friendships.

Many other individuals and organizations, too numerous to mention here, have provided encouragement, information, and direct support over the years that have been vital to writing this book. I thank them all.

Foreword

By Allan Lieberman, M.D.

This is one incredible book. It is, in my opinion, the sequel to Rachel Carson's *Silent Spring*, which was the first book of its kind to warn the public in 1962 about the dangers of pesticides. But whereas Ms. Carson wrote about an "outside world", Athena Thompson is writing about our indoor world — our homes and buildings — building biology.

Prior to the last 25 years spent in the medical practice of environmental medicine, I was a pediatrician seeing 25-40 sick children a day and it never dawned on me to ask why these children were sick. It was only after falling under the spell of Dr. Theron Randolph, the father of environmental medicine in America, that I learned we don't just get sick, we are being made sick.

Dr. Randolph taught us the principle of individual susceptibility influenced by our genetics, but even more importantly by our environment. The air we breath, the food we eat, the water we drink and the chemicals that pollute them, often play the dominant role in a person's deteriorating health. The good news was and still is today, that these environmental causes of illness can be changed, often purely by avoidance.

As an environmental physician I am always looking for the cause of illness. I almost always find it in the air, food or water someone is being exposed to. Even though we live in a world full of all kinds of microorganisms, the great scientists Pasteur and Metchnikoff were right when they said, "It's not the germ, but the turf." When we live in a toxic environment we become susceptible to life-threatening organisms.

As I see it now, after 44 years of medical practice, our survival is a race between our ignorance and learning about the hazards of our environment. Athena Thompson has done a remarkable job creating a book that is enjoyable, easy to understand, and comprehensive while showing us the hazards existing in our homes and buildings. Most importantly she tells us what we can do about them.

Most of us have lived the majority of our lives oblivious to these hazards, and many of us have begun to feel the effect. We have an obligation not only to ourselves, but to our children and grandchildren to heed this warning.

This book is a must read for everyone.

— Allan D. Lieberman, M.D., FAAEM, Medical Director,
Center for Occupational & Environmental Medicine North Charleston, SC

Introduction

Our modern world is full of multiple-pollution challenges. Everything from the air we breathe, to the water we drink, to the food we eat, and the personal care products we use, now contains low-level amounts of toxic chemicals. At the same time our children's health is declining in epidemic proportions. Could there be a connection between the two? What if I told you that your own home could be a major contributor in both these scenarios? Would you know if your home is helping or harming your family's health?

Unfortunately today we all seem to know someone with depression, fatigue, insomnia, frequent headaches, muscle and joint pains, irritability, immune problems, or cancer. Or we know a child with asthma, allergies, autism, or a behavior or learning problem. Many of us are faced with these challenges in our own family and want to know the causes for these problems and better solutions. But left to your own devices, where do you begin to look for answers that make sense? Where are the solutions that will allow you to get involved and help your family and yourself? Well, right here in this book, is one good place to start!

Homes that Heal was researched and written to empower mothers and family members to keep or take back their health on a daily basis. We are about to embark on a revolutionary journey together in the most personal of domains — your own home. "But wait a minute," some of you are already saying, "there's no problem with MY home, there couldn't be, it's:

❒   Brand new;   ❒   Perfectly clean;

❒   Just remodeled;   ❒   MINE!

(Check the appropriate box for your answer.)

I know, I know. We all assume our homes are safe and healthy places. After all, look how much we spend on them! Our home is often the single largest investment we make in a lifetime; what more could there be to it than that? Actually, there's quite a bit more to it and you're about to find out.

So here are a couple of thoughts to ponder to set this process in motion:

1. How is it that your cereal box can tell you more about its ingredients and what it does for your health than the building materials your home is made from?

1

Is it too much to ask that your new home or remodel has its own health and safety label so that you can compare one house to another and evaluate the health benefits or the possible health risks imposed upon your family?

2. How can common household products and personal care products be so easily available when they contain known toxic chemicals?

It's time for us to ask a lot more questions when it comes to our homes. But first we must educate ourselves so that we know the right questions to ask. Once we have the right information under our belt, we must persist with our questions until we find the true answers and solutions. How do we know if we've found the right answer? We simply ask, "Does this ... (product, material, service) add to the amount of toxic chemicals or pollution in my home or not?" If it does, choose a safer alternative.

Our goal is to reduce the chemical and pollution load on all of us while at the same time helping to create natural, ecologically sound living environments that nurture our families' health.

Not knowing how to get started is a major factor in peoples' failed attempts to make positive changes in their lives. With this in mind, every chapter in *Homes that Heal* identifies a variety of places to get started transforming your home. Whether you want to do something grand or something subtle, you will find something you can begin today. Even those with zero budget can start by getting rid of toxic products lining the darker recesses of kitchen and bathroom cabinets, and if all else fails you can at least open a window in your bedroom and air it out!

For ease of use, this book is divided into two parts. Part one focuses on the physical structure of your home and explains how a conventionally built new home is different from a healthfully built new home. Remodels are also discussed. Part two focuses on how we live in our homes and the many ways we ourselves pollute them. Take the *Healthy Home Quiz* to find out how healthy your home is. Then, with detective-like curiosity, we will explore your home room by room looking for any health hazards, and discuss ways to remedy these situations. Each chapter ends with a list of the most immediate gains you can begin working on to upgrade the health of your home. The back of the book has a glossary of terminology and a resource section of different organizations, newsletters, books, and product suppliers to help you explore all of this further.

If you find any of this information helpful, please do spread the word. The "mothers' grapevine" is a powerful communication tool that allows everyone to participate and contribute. Together we are a powerful force to reckon with! Our children and future generations are depending on us to safeguard their health and their future. Everyone who reads this book gets the chance to become a true hero or heroine in a child's life. How extraordinary! Won't you do your part and help?

Thank you in advance for any of your efforts. *Athena*

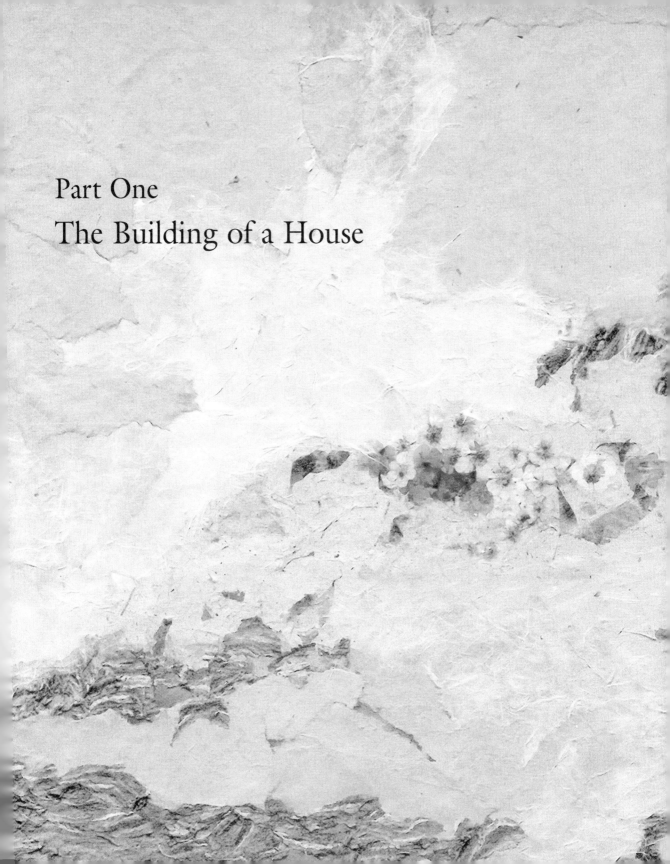

Part One

The Building of a House

CHAPTER 1

The Basics

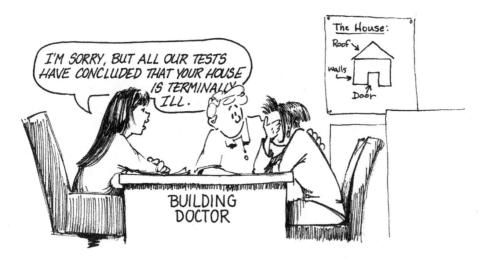

So how exactly does your home affect your health? There are two main ways. The first is the building itself and the second is how you, the occupants, live in and maintain your homes. Through the course of this book, we will examine both.

But before we get started let's discuss some of the basic concepts that I will refer to throughout the book.

Environmental Health

For the sake of simplicity, the total environment can be divided into two connected but separate fields, the inside and the outside. We are all familiar with the larger, outside environment and

> "The test of the morality of a society is what it does for its children."
> — Dietrich Bonhoeffer

its corresponding health concerns such as global warming, emissions from coal burning industries, the use of pesticides on food, polluted water sources, and the detrimental effects of diesel exhaust fumes. However, there is also a smaller, more personal environment that affects our health dramatically. This is the inside environment found within our own homes.

In this book we will be paying particular attention to children's environmental health at home. But do remember, what affects our children's health also affects us. While the

CHILDREN'S HEALTH IN AMERICA

1. Asthma, afflicting nearly 4.8 million US children, is the primary cause of absenteeism and hospital admission among chronic conditions (American Lung Association 1999)

2. Cancer is the number one disease-related cause of death in children (National Cancer Institute, 1998). Approximately 8,500 US children – new-borns to age 15 – are diagnosed with cancer annually.

The most recent cancer statistics on children from the National Cancer Institute (1998) show that the percentage of cancer increased in children 0 – 4 years old between 1973 and 1995:

- 53% rise in brain and other nervous system cancers
- 37% rise in soft tissue cancer
- 32% rise in kidney and renal pelvis cancers
- 18% rise in acute lymphoid leukemia

They reveal increased cancer in teenagers ages 15 - 19 during the same period:

- 128% rise in non-Hodgkin's lymphoma
- 78% rise in ovarian cancer
- 65% rise in testicular cancer
- 30% rise in bone and joint cancer
- 29% rise in thyroid cancer

3. Childhood learning disabilities, hyperactive behavior, and inability to maintain attention have also soared nationwide. The number of children in special education programs increased 191% from 1977 – 1994 (Greater Boston Physicians for Social Responsibility, 2000)

4. Autism appears to be skyrocketing. In California, childhood autism is thought to have risen over 200% between 1987 and 1998 (California Health and Human Services Agency, 1999)

Courtesy of Center for Health, Environment and Justice[1]

government and industries continue their convoluted quest to establish safe levels of toxic chemicals and pollutants in our everyday environment, ultimately we are the ones responsible for raising our children and safeguarding their health. We must become our own Environmental Protection Agency and take back our decision-making power. At the very least, we can control what we are exposed to within our own homes.

Let's look more closely at some current children's health statistics and think this through.

These statistics speak for themselves, loud and clear! What does the future hold for these youngsters? Numerous scientists believe many of these diseases and learning problems may be related to children's exposure to environmental chemicals in the womb or in their everyday environment. Children's everyday environments include their homes, schools, daycare facilities, and their babysitters. Think about it. How much do you really know about these environments? How healthy are they?

It's important to study children's health for a variety of reasons:

- Concern for our children's well-being cuts through skepticism, doubt, blame, politics, and the moneyed interests of industry. Protecting our children's health should be the common platform on which we can all stand together.
- Young children represent the closest thing to a baseline or a control group in our society to which we can compare our own health. After all, they don't hold stressful jobs smoke, or drink alcohol. Children do, however, receive greater doses of whatever chemicals are present in the air they breathe, the water they drink or bathe in, and the food they eat because, pound for pound, they breathe, drink, and eat more than adults do. Looking closely at our children's

health reveals what we all are being exposed to on a daily basis, namely massive amounts of low-level, chemical toxins on every front.

- Children have special vulnerabilities. Their growing bodies do not have fully developed musculature, skeletal, nervous, or immune systems. Therefore they cannot withstand the same exposures to chemicals and pollution as adults. Most safety levels for exposure to toxic chemicals have been set based on a 155 pound white male in the work place not a 20 pound toddler at home.
- If environmental toxins interfere with children's growth and development during critical time periods, this can lead to structural and functional losses that result in lifelong disabilities. In the future, if a large percentage of society has disabilities, what will be the resulting costs and who will pay for the necessary care? Also, the longer life expectancy of children carries the potential for accumulating higher levels of exposures and more time to develop delayed adverse health outcomes. We truly have no idea what our children's health will look like in the future or what devastating costs we may have passed along to them.

Our children are our greatest resource, so let's make sure we are at least protecting them at home.

The Barrel Effect and the Total Body Burden

So what exactly are safe levels of these toxic chemicals and pollution? Official levels vary depending on which country you live in. As a basic guideline I offer the following suggestion for us all to adopt: the only safe level is zero.

> The only safe level is zero

It can be argued that some toxic substances occur in nature and are therefore natural, such as radon gas, so how can they be bad for us in our home? Well, nature has a much better system in place than we currently do in our homes. Radon levels outside your home are easily dissipated by the elements and therefore diluted. Radon in your basement or crawl space can accumulate over time in these tight spaces and concentrate to the dangerous levels associated with lung cancer and other health problems.

But what if you are only being exposed to "low-level" amounts of toxic chemicals in your home? Let me explain what's called the "barrel effect." Picture if you will an empty rain barrel. This empty rain barrel represents your body, completely free of any toxic chemicals or substances. In daily life you are exposed to a rising tide of synthetic chemicals. If your body could metabolize all these chemicals into completely benign breakdown products and excrete them, they would pose less of a health hazard. But unfortunately our bodies, and especially our children's, are not equipped to cope with a daily onslaught of these chemicals in ever more complex combinations. Instead, many of these substances accumulate inside your body and your rain barrel begins to fill. As this process of filling continues, you may or may not start to get some messages (symptoms) from your body such as fatigue, headaches, or allergies. In addition to getting these symptoms, children may become hyperactive or have problems concentrating, complain

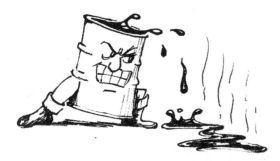

of "tummy aches", get sleepy, or just behave "differently" and "not feel like themselves". Does any of this sound familiar to you?

At this point many people respond by having an extra cup of coffee or a soda for an energy boost, or take a pill for their headache, allergies or concentration/ behavior problem. This might bring some temporary relief but invariably these tactics only add more chemicals to the barrel. You see, we tend to operate with an "addition" mentality. If we don't feel well we usually look to add something such as a pill instead of thinking with a "subtraction" mentality, which would look at what we could take away. Instead of taking a pill for a headache, we could open a window and let out the strong smell of a co-worker's perfume.

This accumulation of toxins can also be called "increasing the total body burden" or the "toxic chemical load." Eventually the barrel becomes full and this is where more serious health problems such as asthma, crippling immune system problems, or even cancer start to show up. Your barrel may be quietly and invisibly filling for several years then — wham! Seemingly overnight your health, and often your life, somehow fall apart.

What we are describing here are chronic, low-level, daily exposures. But exposures can also be sudden and acute, such as a massive dose of pesticides received while spraying your own lawn without using personal protective gear. In either situation, many people become sensitized to specific chemicals or pollutants from these kinds of exposures and will experience symptoms whenever they are re-exposed to them.

Once set in motion, this process can lead to additional sensitivities to an ever-widening range of other, often dissimilar, chemicals that cause similar symptoms. This characteristic is known as the "spreading phenomenon" and this condition is called multiple chemical sensitivity (MCS). For example, headaches that were originally caused by formaldehyde exposure from new kitchen cabinets could progress to headaches that are triggered by fragranced products, progressing to headaches provoked by diesel exhaust fumes. Eventually, almost everything can seem to cause headaches. This can become a very serious and debilitating illness. Because symptoms can be so varied or so erratic, it can be hard to properly diagnose them, which unfortunately leads to a lot of misdiagnoses and therefore inappropriate care.

Rachel Carson in her book *Silent Spring* pointed out that the innumerable small-scale exposures to which we are subjected day by day, year after year, are "like the constant dripping of water that in turn wears away the stone, this birth-to-death contact with dangerous chemicals may in the end prove disastrous. Lulled by the soft sell and the hidden persuader, the average citizen is seldom aware of the deadly materials with which he is surrounding himself; indeed he may not realize he is using them at all."[3] It continues to amaze me that Rachel Carson so eloquently identified a health problem that has vastly increased in magnitude since she wrote these words in 1962.

The sad truth about today's children is that many of them are being born with barrels already dangerously full. How else can we explain the increase in childhood cancer in the 0-4 year age group? Previously, it has been thought that cancer develops over extended years of time: as much as 20-30 years. It would seem likely that the total body burden of the parents at the time of conception and the quality of their genes, combined with chemical exposures the mother receives while pregnant are critical factors in this outcome. As more and more synthetic chemicals and pollution are introduced into the environment, larger numbers of children and adults are likely becoming affected.

But how do you know how full your barrel is? There are now health professionals who specialize in what's called Environmental Medicine. They can give us a clear glimpse. The American Academy of Environmental Medicine (AAEM) and the American Academy of Pediatrics (AAP) can provide you with further information and referrals if you are interested to pursue this further (see Appendix C). When asking for a referral be sure to specify whether it is a child or an adult who needs help. Environmental hazards may pose different risks for children than for adults because children are not simply miniature adults. Environmental pediatricians are especially aware of this; they are experts at tailoring guidance and treatment to the unique, complex, and changing needs of each developing child. I wholeheartedly encourage you to let your intuition guide you in these matters. Sometimes we get in our own way with our feelings of intimidation, skepticism, doubt, and busy lifestyles and all the while keep ourselves from getting the help we really need.

Another good source of information if you are interested in doing a little self-diagnosis is: *Is This Your Child? Discovering and Treating Unrecognized Allergies in Children and Adults,* by Doris Rapp M.D. Dr. Rapp is also a member of the AAEM. This information is not difficult to understand. Always remember — you know more about your health or your child's health than anybody else because you experience it on a daily basis.

I would also like to clarify why I usually refer to "toxic chemicals" in conjunction with the general term "pollution". This is because we need to recognize that there are other forms of pollution that can affect our health that are not chemical in origin. Electromagnetic radiation (EMR) from the multitutde of electrical appliances we use is one such source of daily pollution with which we are all bombarded.

In a study led by Mount Sinai School of Medicine in New York, in collaboration with the Environmental Working Group and Commonweal, researchers at two major laboratories found an average of 91 industrial compounds, pollutants, and other chemicals in the blood and urine of nine volunteers, with a total of 167 chemicals found in the group. Like most of us, the people tested do not work with chemicals on the job and do not live near an industrial facility.

Scientists refer to this contamination as a person's "body burden." Of the 167 chemicals found, 76 cause cancer in humans or animals, 94 are toxic to the brain and nervous system, and 79 cause birth defects or abnormal development. The dangers of exposure to these chemicals in combination has never been studied.[2]

In the meantime, I believe that the precautionary principle offers us some important guidelines.

The Precautionary Principle

The definition of the Precautionary Principle is: "When an activity raises threats of harm to human health or the environment, precautionary measures should be taken even if some cause and effect relationships are not fully established scientifically."[4] The precautionary principle means taking preventive action in the face of uncertainty. In order to do this we must shift the burden of proof from those who might be harmed to those who create the risks, and choose safer alternatives to potentially harmful activities or substances.

Instead of asking what level of harm is acceptable, a precautionary approach asks: How much contamination can be avoided? What are the alternatives to this product or activity, and are they safer? Is this activity even necessary? Taking a precautionary approach means not only considering risks, but looking for better options and solutions.

Remember what happened with lead and asbestos? First we were told these substances were safe and then later we were told they were hazardous. Actually, we've known about lead poisoning since the 1930s; we just didn't act on it. As our knowledge about the toxicity of chemicals increases, the "safe" thresholds of exposure have been continuously revised down. The safe level of exposure to the toxic chemical formaldehyde (which is found in high concentrations inside many newly constructed homes) was set by the American Conference of Governmental Industrial Hygienists (ACGIH) at 10 parts per million (ppm) in 1946. By 1992 the safe level had dropped to 0.3 ppm, further qualified as a level not to be exceeded at any time.[5] We must use our voices and our buying power and insist that government and industries alike adopt precautionary measures in their thinking. The only really safe amount of any toxic chemical is zero.

> "Unless our governmental monitoring agencies begin to protect the people rather than big business, we and future generations are truly in jeopardy."
> — Doris Rapp, M.D.
> *Is This Your Child's World?*

I believe we must now adopt the precautionary principle in the building of our homes too.

Bau-biologie (Building Biology)

The German term "Bau-biologie" (pronounced "bow" or "bough" -biology) translates into English as "Building Biology". These terms can be used interchangeably, although I prefer to use the English translation, as it is easier for most people to pronounce. Building Biology is the science that studies how buildings affect our health, and the application of this knowledge in the design and construction of new buildings, renovations, or remediation (fixing sick buildings).

It began in post-war Germany when there was a great demand for reconstruction. Many new buildings were built quickly and cheaply. This had a devastating effect on the health of a large portion of the population and placed an enormous burden on their health care system. It was discovered that commonly used building materials and certain methods of construction were causing these problems. Today we call this sick building syndrome (SBS) and the resulting human health problems associated include multiple chemical sensitivity (MCS), environmentally triggered illness (ETI), asthma, and allergies, to name but a few.

In light of this, many Germans realized it was better, and ultimately much less expensive, to construct buildings in a healthy manner. As a result, the study of Bau-biologie began and was developed by people such as Anton Schneider, Ph.D., Hubert Palm, M.D., and Alfred Hornig. Over the years guidelines for healthy homes and workplaces were established to ensure the health of buildings. (See Appendix D.)

Although well known to architects and health professionals in Europe, this specialized science, or way of building and living, is still relatively unknown in the U.S.A. I believe it is a science whose time has come.

> "We shape our buildings and afterwards our buildings shape us."
> — Winston Churchill

On average, we spend 90 percent of our time indoors. Shouldn't we make sure that the buildings that house us are built with health, nature, and good business practice in mind? Changing the way we build following Building Biology principles is an effective and sustainable way to positively impact the health and wellbeing of the greatest number of people. The following chapters describe how Building Biology works in our homes.

Now let's continue with the rest of the book. You may want to refer back to this chapter from time to time to remember these basic concepts.

CHAPTER 2

The Healthy Versus The Unhealthy Home

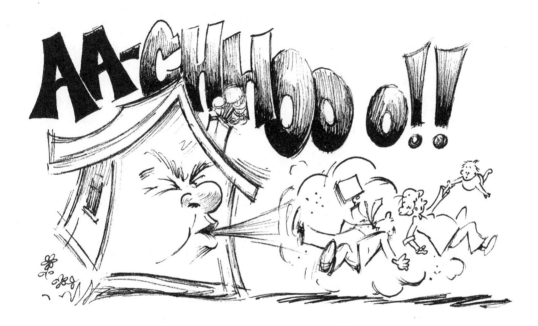

At first glance the title of this chapter may bring to mind ideas of dirty, germ-ridden, bug-infested homes versus sparkling clean, beautifully decorated, well-maintained homes. There are many obvious health problems associated with the first home: cockroaches make most people cringe and they create all kinds of problems. But what I want to talk about is a whole other arena in which what may look new or clean and beautiful is actually highly toxic and dangerous to your health.

Let me start by saying that many people live in the kind of homes we're about to discuss. I call these homes "conventional" because this is the standard way most homes are built in North America. So, if you live in one of these homes and you find the following information disturbing, know that you are not alone.

We all make the best choices we can based upon the information we have. The problem is that a lot of vital information has been kept from us making our choices

According to the American Lung Association "Eighty-five percent of Americans don't realize the air in their homes may be a health hazard."[1]

inherently limited. Through a combination of clever marketing, industries that resist change because of their moneyed interests, and a plain old dose of ignorance, it has become very difficult to know what a modern-day healthy home is. Our thinking on this subject is becoming obsolete.

What you need to know

To rectify this situation you need to know, in common sense language, *how* your house is built and *what* it's built from. I'm guessing that about 90 percent of you reading this book (like myself once) have never had these basic principles explained to you in a way that made sense or was interesting. Until you have this very basic understanding you cannot explore what your house does and does not do *for* you and also what your house may or may not be doing *to* you. Herein lie many important clues to improving your family's health and well-being. So let's set the record straight and then you can decide for yourself what's true.

What is happening?

For thousands of years people have built homes that were in harmony with nature and healthy for their inhabitants. Today however we are hearing more and more about sick buildings, about people who have become sensitized to all kinds of everyday chemicals, and about the part environmental factors play in some of our most common acute and chronic illnesses such as asthma and allergies. Some newly constructed homes are even sick before anyone has moved in. Many more homes are developing health problems such as poor Indoor Air Quality (IAQ) and mold problems to the point that all of these hazards are becoming part of our everyday terminology. You may even know someone who has been or is currently faced with such problems.

History of the problem

Let's take a brief look at what is behind many of these problems. As a result of the energy crisis in the early 1970s, construction techniques began to focus more on sealing buildings tightly to conserve energy. Unfortunately, this solution overlooked the occupants' need for fresh air and the vital role it plays in our overall health and well-being. In solving one problem, we inadvertently created another.

At the same time the petrochemical industry underwent explosive growth, resulting in thousands of chemicals finding their way into all kinds of everyday products including building materials. "There are now more than four million registered man-made chemicals, 70,000-80,000 of which are in common use. We know very little about the health effects of most of these chemicals and even less about what happens when they interact with one another in an enclosed environment. We do know that many chemicals found in building products, and once thought to be safe, are making people ill."[2]

This combined effect has created an unnatural world that has been undermining our health. Years later we are finally beginning to understand the real price we have paid.

Visualize if you will a home, tightly sealed so that no air (energy) can escape and on the inside the chemical residues of building construction and of everyday living are accumulating day in day out. It's rather like living in a pressure cooker and being bathed in a kind of chemical soup all day long. The impact on our indoor air quality is huge. When you consider that the average American spends up to 90 percent of their time indoors, is this what we should be breathing? I don't think so.

How homes get sick

A home can become sick before occupancy as a result of the building materials selected and how the house has been designed. A home can also become sick after occupancy as a result of faulty workmanship and from the activities of the very people who have moved in

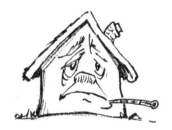

Your home is a living organism

The best way to prevent problems from happening in the first place is to design a house with health in mind. An architect may spend a lot of time designing the proportions and the look of a house, how many rooms, where to put the refrigerator, and so on, but you'd be surprised how few architects know anything about how to design a healthy house or about the health impact the building materials they specify have on the occupants. Aesthetics are no guarantee of health.

Whatever we do to our home we do to ourselves.

I am no architect, but when I discovered Building Biology and how the health of a building affects the health of its occupants, I began to understand buildings from a completely new perspective that I found fascinating. Anyone with an ounce of intuitive sense can grasp these basic concepts easily. Women and mothers in particular do very well; I think it's because of our nurturing tendencies. Building biology is a very nurture-oriented science. It all begins with considering your home as a living organism — rather like having another member of the family. After all, doesn't a home require a certain amount of time, energy, and care, just like everyone else?

From a Building Biology perspective your home is your "third skin," your outermost layer. Your physical skin is the first layer and your clothes are the second layer or second skin. As you start thinking of your home this way, and how it interacts with you and your family, you realize it's all interconnected. Everything from the

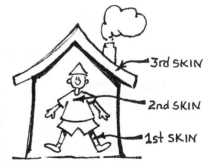

materials used to build your home, to the furnishings inside, to how we care for it, need to be considered in an overall plan for health. You have to think holistically and you have to think in terms of systems. When everything works together to support everything else in this way an optimally healthy environment is achieved. To use an anatomical example, if you were attempting to build yourself a healthy body from scratch, and you could choose each major organ and any supporting systems, wouldn't you choose the healthiest, strongest organs you could? After all, your body has to last you a lifetime. It would be no use choosing a really healthy heart but then using really flimsy veins and arteries: that system would break down sooner or later with catastrophic results. This is one of the key differences between the conventionally designed homes we see everywhere today and the healthy design that we are talking about in this book.

Let me give you some more analogies to take this idea further. In order for a home to be healthy it needs to be able to facilitate a balanced exchange of air and humidity, just like our physical lungs do. This process is a form of breathing. A breathing home needs to be able to allow humidity and air to move in and out of its walls. Homes need to be able to keep warm or stay cool, just like we do.

Thinking this way creates a whole new relationship to how things are supposed to function within our homes. It makes it more personal and easier to understand once you have got the basics. And guess what? You've already got most of the basics because you have your own body as a study guide! For example, don't you feel better when you get some fresh air and sunshine? Well, so does your home. Doesn't high humidity or low humidity affect how comfortable you feel? Well, it affects your house this way too.

This is how I propose we learn about our homes, how to live in them, and how to take care of them. You may even discover some intriguing things about your own health along the way. In fact you might find it an interesting experiment to use a personal health problem you may be currently challenged by and identify the parallel in your home and see if it needs fixing.

What do we mean by faulty workmanship?

Once an architect has designed your home and all the specifications have been made (which building materials and systems are to be used), then it's ready to be built. Now your home passes into the hands of the general contractor, the builder, and the sub-contractors. What they physically do or do not do when building, often determines if a home will be healthy or sick.

For instance, the average home often contains multiple tubes of commercial adhesives. But have you ever read the label on a tube of adhesive? Builders and sub-contractors use these products on a daily basis without giving a thought to the impact on their health or the future health of the soon-to-be owners of the house they are building.

The use of toxic substances in construction is standard. The average person (builder or homeowner) lacks a background in chemistry and operates under the false assumption that in order for building products to be allowed on the market, they must be reasonably safe. This form of faulty workmanship falls under the category of ignorance. Try walking down the aisle of your local home improvement store where the adhesives or paints are and turn the containers around so you can read the warnings on the back of the label. Don't be surprised to see warnings such as, "This product contains a chemical known to the State of California to cause cancer, birth defects, or other reproductive harm." Does this sound reasonably safe to you?

Other forms of faulty workmanship can result when general contractors and builders are trying to save money or time. It's not unheard of that one specified building material gets traded out for a cheaper one that's poorer quality and won't last as long. They know, but you don't! Or the sub-contractor runs out of glue and goes down to the local home improvement store and grabs any old commercial glue off the shelf without reading what's in it and then uses that in your new home. Often these problems arise from a workman being rushed to finish his job and get on to the next one. Someone higher up the food chain wants to make their profit quickly. We are the ones shortchanged and left with what can be dire consequences down the road.

But what about building codes, aren't they supposed to protect us? Building codes are basic guidelines to ensure a home is sound, but that does not necessarily mean that it's safe for human health. Code is mostly about making sure the structure isn't going to fall down or that the wiring will not set the house on fire. Building inspectors are often very busy and only give visual inspections. For example, electrical inspectors don't usually use equipment such as a multimeter (an electrical measuring device) to check if the electricity is actually flowing where it's supposed to, i.e., inside the wires. A poorly wired house can lead to all kinds of health problems from headaches to heart palpitations. Most of us, who are not electricians by profession, have no idea our home may be sick in this way because these things are invisible.

How do we pollute our own homes?

Then there are the many ways we pollute our own homes simply by living in them. Part two of *Homes that Heal* covers this in more detail. There was a study done in Canada where the Indoor Air Quality of six newly constructed homes was checked before the occupants moved in, and then again at one month and then six months later. As would be expected, at first there were very high levels of volatile organic chemical (VOCs — see Appendix A for definition) from the building materials used, such as the toxic chemical formaldehyde. But one of the most significant findings was that at six months the occupant related sources of VOCs were predominant.[3] The

> "The journey of a thousand miles begins with a single step."
> — Lao Tzu

occupants themselves became the primary source of pollution! It's ironic that so many of our attempts to keep our homes clean or to have them look a certain way, actually make things much worse because of the type of products and furnishings we are using. Fortunately, much of this is easily resolved with the right information.

A Word of Encouragement

Turning your home into a health haven is a process, just like raising a child or caring for a family member. It takes time and effort and no one may ever pat you on the back or say thanks, but you will know you did your best, and that goes a long way when you have some of life's most important responsibilities on your hands, such as raising your children and shaping the face of the future.

Since World War II the production of synthetic chemicals has increased significantly. In 1945, the estimated worldwide production of these chemicals was fewer than 10 million tons. Today it is over 110 million tons.[4]

According to the American Academy of Environmental Medicine, nearly half of all Americans suffer from at least one chronic disease and one fifth have two or more chronic illnesses. The annual medical costs of treating chronic diseases are expected to double to almost $1.07 trillion dollars by 2020.

According to *Asthma in America,* there are currently 14.6 million Americans with asthma, of whom 4.8 million are children under the age of 18. In 1994, 5.8 percent of children under age 5 had asthma (as reported by a family member), a 160 percent increase since 1980![5]

The American Cancer Society estimates that in 2000, 1,220,100 people were diagnosed with cancer for the first time and 563,100 died from it. It is estimated that environmental factors account for 72% of cancers.

Indoor pollution is estimated to cause thousands of cancer deaths and hundreds of thousands of respiratory health problems each year. In addition, hundreds of thousands of children have experienced elevated blood lead levels resulting from their exposure to indoor pollutants.[6]

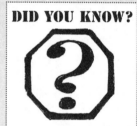

DID YOU KNOW?

CHAPTER 3

The Conventionally Built New Home

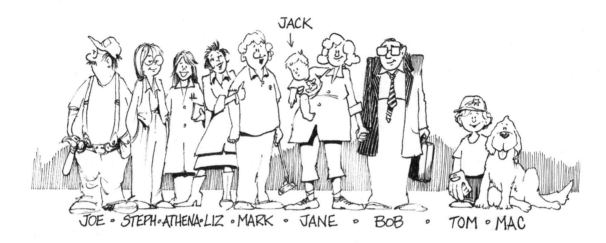

JOE • STEPH • ATHENA • LIZ • MARK • JANE • BOB • TOM • MAC

Introducing Jane and Liz

In the spirit of "a picture tells a thousand words," a cast of imaginary characters has been conjured to further illuminate the basic concepts in this book. These fictitious characters represent all of us at different times, on our evolutionary path towards health, happiness, and the regeneration of our planet. Hopefully you will find the combination of cartoons and stories a welcome break from the rigors of daily life. One of the best-known tonics in life is smiling and laughing and they cost nothing!

Jane and Liz are sisters who live in the same town but in different neighborhoods. Jane is a lady in her late thirties-early forties. She is married to Bob and they have two sons, a six-year-old boy called Tom and a two-year-old boy named Jack. Jane is currently pregnant with their third child and having her house remodeled in anticipation of the birth of the new baby. Jane has an adorable mongrel dog called Mac that everyone loves.

Liz is in her early thirties and is a career woman. She is married to Mark and they have just moved into their newly constructed dream home.

Liz's friend Steph has just moved into her new healthy home. She is a Gen-X'er, raised on recycling, and on the ball when it comes to her own and her family's health.

Uncle Joe is Jane and Liz's uncle. He's in his 60s, retired, and loves an opportunity to fix things around the home, even though he invariably botches everything he touches!

I act as a commentator (with my own cartoon caricature) at the end of each story shedding light on how things in our home affect our health.

Our story begins early one Saturday morning ....

The front doorbell rings. The sound seems to echo around the house as though it were a racket ball court. Liz is laying in bed basking in the delight of her lovely new home. All those decisions she had to make about carpeting, kitchen tiles, curtains, and all the new furniture — it was really stressful there for a while but it all seems to have paid off now as she looks around her "designer" bedroom. "I should take some photographs and send them to one of those beautiful home magazines," Liz thinks.

The doorbell rings again and startles Liz from her dreamy reverie. She leaps out of bed and runs to the front door. Upon opening the door Liz finds a huge spider plant with what looks like a rather pregnant belly behind it.

"Morning," says the voice behind the plant. It's Liz's older sister Jane who is eight months pregnant and looks like she could burst at any moment.

Liz unloads the plant from Jane's arms and gives her sister a hug. Jane is here to get the "grand tour" of Liz's new house. She wishes she and Bob could afford a new home but they can't, and so have opted to have their existing home remodeled instead.

Liz's new home looks like an immaculate showroom home: lots of attention-to-detail; lots of matching, pale colors; thick, wall-to-wall carpet. "This house wouldn't last five minutes with my family!" Jane thinks to herself, visualizing

her two sons, the dog, and her husband Bob who she can't seem to train to take off his dirty shoes before coming into the house.

Jane's questions begin immediately. One of her hobbies is looking through better housekeeping and new home magazines. She's even learned a little bit about construction and interior design along the way.

"Wow! This is beautiful" enthuses Jane. "I want to know everything about this place. What kind of heating system do you have?"

"I thought there was only one kind of heating," Liz answers, looking puzzled.

"What kind of hot water heater do you have? Have you got one of those energy-efficient ones?"

"I have no idea, that's Mark's department! You sound like a builder," says Liz scrutinizing her sister.

Jane uses her older-sister tone of voice. "Oh, I've been reading up on some of this stuff. I find it interesting in a strange sort of way. Most people have no idea how their house is built or what kind of systems their house runs on. I started out just wanting to learn more so I would know what my options were for our remodel. I didn't want some fly-by-night builder charging me a fortune and selling me a bunch of cheap rubbish. You have to watch out for that kind of stuff you know."

They pass through a very large sitting area and formal dining room into the kitchen.

"Everything smells so ... *new*" Jane says, scrunching her nose up.

"Thanks." Liz takes that as a compliment.

The kitchen has a small breakfast nook by the window that looks out onto the deck and then the garden and beyond to the neighbors' house next door, which is still being built.

"Oh, I love your little breakfast nook!" Jane exclaims.

Liz smiles with pride. "Isn't it cute? We've been eating all our meals there so far. With only the two of us it doesn't make sense to eat in the big dining room. We don't want to mess it up. We're saving it for when we have friends over and entertain."

Jane begins to feel light-headed and sits down for a minute. "Don't you ever open any windows in this place?"

"We don't need to. We just use the thermostat to heat up or cool the house down. We were told when we bought the house that we'd save money if we kept the house closed up and after what this place cost us to buy, I'm all for saving some money wherever we can," replies Liz.

"Don't you feel claustrophobic though, not opening any windows?" Jane persists.

Liz reluctantly opens a kitchen window, just a crack.

Jane looks around the kitchen. "What a great kitchen, I love those cabinets."

"Aren't they great? We have so much storage space. I'm going to have to buy a ton more stuff to fill them up," laughs Liz. "They do smell strongly though, I'm not sure what to do about that."

"Oh, that won't last long, its just that 'new' smell," Jane says reassuringly.

Off the side of the kitchen is a small sitting area with a sofa, large TV, DVD player, VCR, stereo and all kinds of technical looking stuff. Jane has no idea what most of it is.

"This is where we spend most of our time in the evening," Liz says, casually waving her hand as she walks through the room.

The downstairs bathroom is like a hotel bathroom with no windows. Everything matches and looks pristine. Jane notices this room smells differently from the other rooms. It smells new but there's something else too.

"What's that smell in here?"

"Yes, I've noticed that. I'm not sure. It might be the plastic in the shower curtain. Mark's the only one who uses this bathroom. For some reason he likes to shower in here after he's played golf," Liz replies.

Jane scrutinizes the bathroom. "No, it's something else, I can't put my finger on it. Oh, it's probably me, everything smells more when I'm pregnant."

"Want to see the basement?" Liz asks enthusiastically. "It's huge. We plan to finish it and put another bedroom and family room or an office down there."

Liz is right. The basement is huge and full of empty boxes from all the new furniture they've bought.

"What's that wet patch over there on the wall?" asks Jane heading off towards the far corner of the basement.

"What wet patch?"

In the far corner of the basement the sisters stare at a large wet patch on the wall.

"I've never noticed that before. That must be new. Where's it coming from?" Liz says with a hint of concern in her voice.

"It looks like it's coming from above. What's the room directly above this wall?" questions Jane.

"You know what, it's that bathroom with the funny smell. Something must be leaking.

It can't be possible, this is a new house!" Liz exclaims. "I'd better get the builder back over here to check it out. God, isn't anything built to last anymore?"

"Well, something's not been done right, that's for sure," Jane emphasizes.

The girls continue their tour. Upstairs there are three bedrooms and two bathrooms. Liz has gone to town on the large master bedroom with ensuite bathroom. It has everything from designer fabrics to every conceivable electrical gadget you can think of. A computer and printer, TV, DVD, VCR, stereo, electric clock radio, coffee maker, bedside lamps, electric blanket …. and so on.

"This is my favorite room in the whole house!" delights Liz.

"I like the colors," Jane says, while under her breath she adds quietly, "but it looks like an office." Jane goes over to the window and opens it for some fresh air. "At least keep a window open in your bedroom."

"You're starting to sound like Mother!" Liz teases as she rolls her eyes.

"Well, the older I get the more I realize how right she was about a lot of that 'old-fashioned' stuff. You know … like how she used to clean the house and air it out. Remember how great our beds used to smell when she would dry our sheets outside all day long?" Jane says in a reverie.

Liz folds her arms across her chest. "Yes, well I get my 'fresh air smell' from my convenient little fabric sheets that I use in my very convenient clothes dryer as I run out the door to my very busy job, thank you very much."

"It's not the same and you know it," Jane concludes.

The last stops on the tour are the laundry room, which doesn't look like it's ever been used, the garage which contains all Mark's "guy things," and finally the yard which has just had a lawn put in with a few shrubs.

Jane begins to rub her aching back. "What do you plan to do with your yard?"

"Who, me? I don't know a thing about gardening and besides I'm too busy. We found a service that comes by each week and mows the lawn, gardens a bit, puts down stuff to stop any weeds growing. Mark's a fanatic when it comes to killing weeds. They're doing most of the gardens in the neighborhood so they should be pretty good. I just want to be able to sit in the hot tub and have something nice to look at," says Liz.

"Well, you have a lovely new home. You'll have to come over to my house and give me some of your designer ideas for our remodel."

With her sister's official "seal of approval" Liz smiles. "I'd love to, between the two of us we'll make it look really great. Have they started yet?"

Jane groans. "They started last week, knocking walls down and ripping things out, but I need a cup of tea if we're going to talk about that!"

Introduction to "Commentaries"

Whenever a Jane and Liz story is told it will be followed by a commentary where I review parts of the story, focusing in on health. Obvious things will be pointed out and sometimes several invisible or less obvious factors will be identified. Wherever possible, solutions and suggestions will be offered so that you can implement and experiment with them immediately. This strategy helps to save time by learning as we go along. I encourage you to jot down any personal "aha's" or ideas you may have as you read. I find that if I don't write these kinds of ideas down immediately they often get lost or it takes forever to find them again because a mother's life is full of ongoing family distractions. Even if you only implement one suggestion from each commentary section, over time the health gains will be huge.

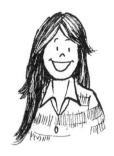

Commentary

So, in the above story let's review Liz's new home in terms of what's healthy about it and what's not.

First let's look at how Liz's house was built. It's shocking to discover how so much has literally been set in stone before we even move into a new home. Modern construction techniques use many products and practices that are polluting, toxic, and can endanger not only the health of the future occupants but the builders themselves as they build the home.

As a brief overview, the products and practices listed below are the most common sources of pollution and potential health problems in new construction:

1. Insecticides, mildewcides, herbicides and other biocides are found in many building materials and are sometimes applied on-site to the ground before it is built upon. Pesticides are designed to kill (see Chapter 14). Saying that a pesticide is "approved" by the Environmental Protection Agency (EPA) is no guarantee of human safety. In fact, according to the EPA, companies are not supposed to use the word "approved" on their products and instead are allowed only to say "registered." There's a huge difference between these two terms. The EPA does not approve any of these pesticides as being safe for human health.

   A 1981 Polish study of 106 seemingly healthy workers in contact with organic solvents in paints and varnishes found immune-system suppression (depressed levels of T cells, part of the body's protective mechanism) which it was thought could predispose the workers to allergies and cancer.[1]

2. Composite wood products including oriented strand board (OSB), particleboard, chipboard, plywood, sill plates, and manufactured sheathing are used extensively to frame a house. Each contains varying amounts of toxic chemicals such as formaldehyde. The EPA classifies formaldehyde as a "probable human carcinogen." These chemicals can accumulate to high levels in your home and significantly pollute your indoor air quality.

3. Many other standard building products contain synthetic chemicals. At room temperature these products can release vapors called volatile organic compounds (VOCs). This process is called offgassing or outgassing and it can last from days to years. We are then exposed to these chemical intruders in the air we breathe, creating serious health hazards. Many of these chemicals are known to cause cancer, damage the nervous system, and suppress the immune system. Some of the

more common VOCs you may have heard of are toluene, benzene, formaldehyde, acetone, and solvents commonly found in solvent-based paints, sealants, finishes, and adhesives. If you put carpeting in your home the carpet will act as a sink or reservoir for these chemicals.

4. Asphalt and products containing asphalt, including impregnated sheathing, roofing tars, and asphalt driveways are highly toxic.

5. Building materials may already contain mold due to water damage and poor storage on site. Also, certain building practices, such as the improper use of vapor barriers that can trap moisture on the inside of the building, can create environments friendly to mold growth.

6. Toxic cleaning products and solvents used to mop up spills and accidents while building can impregnate the structure and continue to release VOCs for some time.

7. Heaters used during construction create pollutants from combustion by-products, which can impregnate other building materials, challenging future indoor air quality in yet another way.

All of this could have taken place in building Liz's house and visually she would never know. But you can't fool your health! Problems can quickly arise after people move in, especially if they are already sensitive or have health challenges such as asthma or allergies. The tricky thing most people face with these kinds of "beginning" health problems is that people don't realize they are being triggered by their home. Even if they do suspect it's their home, it can be difficult to pinpoint the main source, as all these chemicals interact with each other and you start to live in a sort of chemical soup which leaves you feeling generally unwell.

You are probably wondering by now "How can this be? Why do we build this way?" Well, the truth is, it wasn't always like this.

A Short History of Buildings

Historically, our first buildings were made from natural materials. Whatever was around and close-by was used to build with, including rock, sticks, and mud. Even good old manure was put to good use as a binder, and despite its pungent smell was much safer than our modern day synthetic counterparts like formaldehyde. Buildings had lots of natural ventilation and these dwellings reflected a close connection with nature.

It was the Industrial Revolution that finally ended thousands of years of the timeless way. We moved away from craftsman-built homes clustered in small villages, towards what we consider normal today, which are anonymous, over-populated urban dwellings, often packed like sardines in a can around industries such as power plants and factories that heavily pollute the environment.

Wait a minute though! Hasn't modern technology benefited us tremendously? I mean, we don't have the bubonic plague going around anymore right? Yes, and no. You could say we've traded plagues.

Back to Liz

If we asked Liz if she thought her home was healthy, especially now that she's in a new home, she would probably answer "yes." But her answer is based on an assumption: that homes are automatically built healthfully. Unfortunately, "new" does not guarantee "healthy."

Liz thought they were doing a good thing in her new home by keeping their windows closed. It saves energy and keeps their bills down. That's a good "environmental" or "sustainable" choice right? Yes, it is a good thing to save on energy costs. It's personally beneficial from a financial standpoint and it's good for conserving the planet's resources. But here's what Liz doesn't understand: if a house is built right in the first place the savings magnify across the board. You save in energy costs; you save in health costs; you save due to less absenteeism for you from work and your children from school; you help save the planet; and ultimately you save your sanity. How's that for a great deal! When you figure in all these additional costs you begin to realize how much depends on the choices we make and the health of our homes.

Now let's look at the individual key building components of Liz's new home with more detailed explanations. As Liz lives on the West Coast, the construction methods used represent the way many conventional new homes are currently built in North America. Depending on where you live, slight differences may be found in construction techniques because of climate demands.

1. Scary crawl spaces

Liz's house has a crawl space. A crawl space is the gap underneath your house between the earth and the under-floor of your home. Sometimes these spaces are big enough to walk into and sometimes they are so small there is only enough room to crawl into them. Hence the name. Either way they are notorious for being dark, dirty, and rather scary.

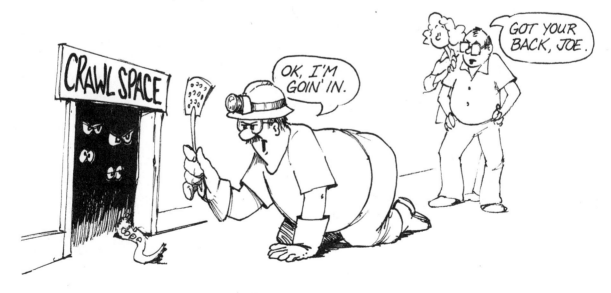

A colleague of mine was once conducting an environmental inspection of someone's home, which required that he go under the house to check for any mold problems. The crawl space was dark and very narrow. As he crawled carefully along with his little flashlight he suddenly came face to face with a rather large snake! Unable to turn around, he carefully and very quickly had to crawl backwards to get out of the space and avoid a nasty experience.

As this story indicates, your crawl space may be home to a whole host of extended family members you know nothing about. This is a prime place for rodents and pests of all kinds to set up their own home and potentially cause all kinds of building damage as well as health problems for the occupants upstairs. Crawl spaces can also contain lots of residual building scraps that were not disposed of properly. Some people even use the space to store excess cans of paint, stains, and other products, all of which can contain toxic chemicals which will steadily offgas into the space and may find their way into your home. Definitely not something you want to be living on top of.

The alternative to these kinds of crawl spaces is to either build your house on what's called "slab on grade" (see Chapter 5) or build a "conditioned" crawl space, where there is a concrete floor instead of dirt and the space is completely sealed.

Radon

Another thing to be aware of when it comes to the lower levels of your home is radon. Radioactive contaminants such as radium and uranium occur naturally within the earth's crust. During the decay or breakdown of uranium, radon gas is produced. This gas can quite easily find its way from the earth beneath your house into an unconditional crawl space, and even through cracks in concrete slabs into your home. See Chapter 5 for how to prevent radon from entering your home.

> The US Surgeon General has stated that radon exposure is second only to tobacco smoke as a cause of lung cancer.

It has been estimated that as many as one in fifteen homes in the United States contain elevated radon levels. If you are curious about your own home, there are inexpensive radon test kits for homeowners that are very simple to use (see Appendix C). Radon levels can differ from room to room in your home so always test all bedrooms if they are on the ground floor; this is where you spend a third of your life and so are liable to get the greatest exposure. Levels can also differ depending on the time of year. In winter months, when homes are generally kept closed up to stay warm, radon levels can increase. The EPA recommends remediation (doing something about it) at levels higher than 4.0 pCi/L (pico-curies of radon per liter of air). Even at 4.0 pCi/L there is an increased risk of lung cancer.[2] From a Building Biology standpoint we recommend reducing radon to levels of 0.5-1.5 pCi/L[3] which is similar to the levels found outdoors in nature.

Crawl spaces can also have moisture problems. Water vapor can exist as a soil gas and infiltrate into building materials causing damage and mold growth. High water tables, poor site drainage, improper grading that slopes towards the building, underground springs, hardpan soils that cause excess moisture to remain at the surface, and soils that have a tendency to hold moisture rather than let it percolate through can contribute to this problem.

2. Attics that can give you an attack

Attics come in all shapes, sizes and designs. Liz would never think to get to know her attic. Attics are for storing things, and as she has such a large basement she will probably never even open her attic door. If she did, she would see lots of thick, pink, fluffy material between the ceiling rafters. It's important to know what kind of insulation you have. Your attic should be completely sealed from the rest of the house in order to prevent the passage of contaminated air into the living spaces. If your attic is not sealed properly and you have bare insulation like fiberglass or vermiculite containing asbestos, this can migrate as tiny particles into adjoining spaces such as bedrooms, creating health problems.

Look for any ventilation pipes that enter the attic and do not continue on and out through the roof. In Liz's house the range hood over her stove vents into the attic and terminates there. Liz has no idea of this and even if she did climb up there and notice this protruding open-ended piece of pipe she probably would not think twice about it. This means that the attic gets a direct dose of high moisture and odors every time she uses the range hood. This is a mold problem waiting to happen. Ventilation pipes should extend all the way to the outside of the building, but sometimes in efforts to save time or money a builder or a sub may make a decision like this, assuming that no one will be any the wiser. Obviously a builder or sub would have to be clueless when it comes to the long-term consequences to the integrity of the building and the health of the occupants. So, do check your attic.

3. Exterior walls built from light-weight stick frame construction

Liz's home has been constructed using light-weight stick frame construction. To Liz, all she sees are walls, doors, windows: the finished product. But if you were to strip away her house's exterior siding or finish, and strip away the interior sheet rock wall surface, you would actually see a framework — rather like peeling back our own skin to see the bones underneath. Most conventional homes in North America are built this way. The walls are constructed out of light-weight pieces of two-by-four or two-by-six lumber assembled into a framework which is stuffed full of insulation. The outside of the building is then covered with oriented strand board (OSB) or plywood, a layer of building wrap followed by siding. The interior side of the framed wall may include a vapor barrier followed by a layer of sheetrock. It's rather like a big sandwich.

The insulation commonly used is spun fiberglass, which looks like cotton candy, but unfortunately it's not so innocent. The fiberglass itself and the formaldehyde binder, which is usually used to hold it together, are both problematic to health. Then there is the use of vapor barriers. These are large sheets of thin material air cannot pass through.

They are attached to the frame and cover the entire surface area of the walls. They are supposed to keep moisture out of the building but actually restrict ventilation and the breathing quality we talked about earlier, which can impair the drying-out process all new houses go through. Vapor barriers can easily trap moisture in the walls.

Building this way can create a mold breeding ground. All mold needs to grow is moisture and food (see Chapter 4). Trapped moisture in the building envelope, combined with food sources such as wood and the paper on sheet rock, create the perfect environment for mold to run rampant. Across the country health problems with mold, and subsequent litigation, have become massive problems.

Additionally, stick frame walls are not nearly as energy efficient as high mass walls. ("High mass" refers to the density of the building materials used. See Chapter 5.) Liz will spend a lot of time and money trying to figure out how to keep her house comfortable, whether that's keeping it warm in the winter or cool in the summer.

And finally, conventional stick frame construction is not built to last. Primarily, it's an easy way to build fast that has been kept artificially cheap due to industry subsidies that are paid for with your own tax dollars. Add to this the additional environmental costs of continuing to log massive areas of woodlands to support these practices and the real price tag proves astronomical. It is time to consider better options. High mass homes last decades longer. Let's save trees and use lumber more efficiently. The interior of our home and the last inch of finish work is the best place to use wood so we can all enjoy its benefits and appreciate its beauty.

4. Forced air heating

This system is where some of the greatest building and design atrocities occur. Right from the start, unless the installed ducting is completely sealed during construction, all kinds of dirt and debris will find their way into the ducting where they can remain for a long time, affecting your indoor air quality in innumerable ways whenever the system is used. Sometimes this kind of heating system makes me feel like I'm taking part in some grand scale laboratory experiment, and I'm the lab mouse being tested!

Throughout most of the U.S., forced air is the most common form of heating and cooling in new, conventional construction. Many people like Liz don't even know there are other ways to heat or cool your home. Unless you keep the ducting impeccably clean and the furnace well maintained, it becomes a "merry-go-round" transportation system for dust, pollen, pet dander, mold spores, and germs. People with asthma, allergies, or weakened immune systems can be especially affected by forced air heating. Most ducting systems immediately lose 30 percent of their energy efficiency due to leaky ductwork. Filters need to be good quality High-Efficiency Particulate Arrestance (HEPA) pleated media filters and replaced regularly (every two months in heavy use periods). Most people forget to replace them regularly or try to save money by making them "last" as long as possible. The bottom line is, they are incredibly inefficient, noisy systems to operate, that can have a negative impact on health.

I once visited a very expensive house that was under construction. It was being built with no expense spared using conventional construction methods. This house had a forced-air system that had been "upgraded" with extra insulation on the inside of the ducting at great cost. What was it insulated with? An asphalt-covered paper. In the NIOSH *Pocket Guide to Chemical Hazards,* "asphalt fumes" are classified as carcinogenic.[4] So these people paid extra to have asphalt fumes blown around their home — at what cost to their health?

If you notice unusual or chemical smells in your new home it's important to identify the source of them. This is something that needs to be done in the early days of moving in because people usually become accustomed to these smells. Actually, your smell receptors can become incapacitated if you are exposed to the same smell over and over again. So beware if you have stopped smelling it, and a guest comes over and politely asks, "What's that smell?" The smell is still there and you should definitely find what's causing it.

5. Floor coverings

Every home contains a floor, on that much we can all agree. However, did you know that what you cover your floors *with* directly affects your health too.

Carpet

Liz's house has wall-to-wall carpet. We're going to assume here that Liz chose carpet for the same reasons many other people choose to put carpeting in their homes. Carpet feels cushy and soft underfoot. It offers some sound insulation. When you have young children running up and down stairs all day long, this can reduce some of the cacophony of daily life. Lots of people want it just because they are used to it, or as a decorative feature, or because it can be one of the cheapest floor coverings. However, there is another side to this coin that many people don't know about and which definitely needs to be discussed. Here are some important questions to ask when considering installing carpet:

- What is the carpet made from?
- How is the carpet installed?
- What's the effect on our health from the carpet, the backing, and any adhesives used?
- How is it maintained?
- If cleaning products are recommended, what is their effect on health?
- Does it add to our overall chemical load?
- How long will it last?
- How is it disposed of?

Toxic emissions from carpets can include fumes from formaldehyde, benzene, xylene, toluene, butadiene, styrene, and 4-phenyl-cyclo-hexene (4PC). These chemicals can

The two best-selling carpet fibers, nylon and olefin, are both synthetics derived from petroleum, a non-renewable resource. The EPA estimates that in 2000 over 2.2 million tons of carpeting were dumped.[6]

potentially cause cancer, birth defects, reproductive disorders, respiratory problems, and neurological damage such as anxiety, depression, inability to concentrate, confusion, short-term memory loss, and seizures.[5] Is this something you want your baby crawling around on, or your toddler getting on his hands which he then puts in his mouth? Is this what you want for your pets? All of these problems are magnified in proportion to the amount or surface area of carpet installed in any given home.

In 1992, in response to growing consumer concern about the chemicals used in carpets and their effects on human health, the Carpet and Rug Institute (CRI), a trade association created by the carpet and rug industry, created a standard called the Green Tag Label. Today it is called the CRI Indoor Air Quality Testing Program. According to CRI this label on a carpet provides "assurance that the product is a responsible, low-emitting carpet."[7] However, this program has been criticized for having set arbitrary maximums for total VOCs rather than basing them on risk-assessment data. It could be said that an industry that creates its own voluntary safety standards might have a conflict of interest!

In 1991 New York Attorney General Robert Abrams published a consumer alert warning people about the adverse health affects associated with carpet. He also said, "The carpet industry has mounted a massively deceptive merchandising campaign to intentionally mislead the public by implying that all carpets with the green tag have met safety standards. First of all, there are no such recognized standards of safety. Secondly, CRI's testing program is completely inadequate because it measures only a small percentage of the chemicals emitted from carpets. Finally, a manufacturer can get a green tag for an entire product line simply by having one small piece of carpet tested."[8]

If you are still not convinced, Anderson Laboratories (an independent commercial testing lab) has done some of the most extensive testing on carpets. Visit their website or order some of their published research reports to learn for yourself the extent of what they have found in carpets and their subsequent health effects. You can send samples of your own carpet to them for testing (see Appendix C).

I'm not advocating we all go back to dirt floors or just throw some extra straw down on the floor occasionally! But do make sure you have the whole picture so that you can make truly informed choices when it comes to carpet. As a general rule, if carpet is absolutely an essential part of your home, then choose carpet made from natural fibers such as pure wool, cotton, hemp, jute, ramie, sisal, coir, or seagrass. Undyed is safest, as many dyes and fixatives give off unhealthy VOC fumes. Opt for carpet with as few chemical treatments as possible because many fabric finishes, including stain, moth, and flame repellants, can offgas their own VOCs. Don't forget to choose non-toxic carpet backing and adhesives too.

The good news is that today we have more choices than ever before. There are a handful of companies that now specialize in natural floor coverings. Choose a company that really knows what they are talking about and have been in business for some time (see Appendix C).

Carpets serve as reservoirs for dirt, dust, mold, bacterial growth, flea eggs, pesticide residues, and various toxins tracked in from the outside, making them resemble more of a biology project than a home furnishing! Regular vacuuming and careful shampooing is essential. A HEPA vacuum cleaner works best, as other vacuums cleaners on average re-release about 70 percent of what they vacuum up. Another choice is a whole house vacuum cleaner (see Chapter 5).

Carpet cleaning products themselves often contain harmful ingredients such as perfumes, chemical soil removers, brighteners, and antibacterial and antimicrobial chemicals. Do your research before you have a professional company come in and clean your carpet. Find out what method of cleaning they use, what chemical products they use and if their products contain fragrance. You are perfectly within your rights to ask them to send you the Material Safety Data Sheet (MSDS) on their cleaning products. A variety of healthy carpet cleaning products are available. You can arrange for your carpet cleaning professional to use the products you provide. Be sure to let carpet dry out thoroughly after any cleaning, otherwise mold will happily grow in these moist environments.

Vinyl

The only other flooring in Liz's house is in the kitchen and laundry room. Sheet vinyl has been installed here for its ease of cleaning and because it's economical. But vinyl flooring has its own health hazards. Vinyl chloride fumes, emitted from the flooring, are a known carcinogen.[9] In a hot or humid environment the vinyl will trap moisture, which can promote delamination of sub-floors and mold growth or rot. The manufacture and disposal (incineration) of vinyl products also has a significant detrimental effect on the outdoor environment, producing toxic byproducts such as carcinogenic dioxins.[10] Clearly not a great choice for you or the planet! Healthier flooring suggestions will be covered in Chapter 5.

Manufacturers of toxic products are not required by law to list all their ingredients. If you contact the manufacturer directly, you can ask for the Material Safety Data Sheet for their product. An MSDS will typically list the manufacturer, certain ingredients, hazards to safety and health, and precautions to follow when using the product. Unfortunately, manufacturers are only required to report hazardous ingredients when they are present at levels of 1% or greater. The threshold for carcinogens is 0.1%. Some ingredients can be omitted because they are classified as "trade secrets." Information about neurotoxic, reproductive, developmental, or long-term exposure effects or any reference to effects on children's health is often omitted. Neither will it contain any studies showing the health effects of all the ingredients when combined. MSDS's provide only basic information, but usually this is more than you will find on a product label.

6. Recycled modern designs that never worked in the first place

Liz's new home is way too big for just her and her husband. They actually use only a third of their house. Her favorite parts of the house are the cozy parts like the kitchen nook.

Polyvinyl chloride, commonly known as "PVC" or "vinyl," is one of the most common synthetic materials. Over 14 billion pounds of PVC are currently produced per year in North America. Approximately 75% of all PVC manufactured is used in construction materials. ...

Dioxin (the most potent carcinogen known), ethylene dichloride, hydrochloric acid and vinyl chloride are unavoidably created in the production of PVC and can cause severe health problems, including:

DID YOU KNOW?

- Cancer
- Endometriosis
- Neurological damage
- Birth defects and impaired child development
- Reproductive and immune system damage.

The dioxin exposure of the average American already poses a calculated risk of cancer of greater than 1 in 1,000, thousands of times greater than the usual standard for acceptable risk. Most poignantly, dioxins concentrate in breast milk to the point that human infants now receive high doses, orders of magnitude greater than those of the average adult.[11]

Yes, it might be useful to have more space to entertain. But how often do they really have that need? And it might be useful to have more space if they want to start a family. But that might not be for a while, if at all. Liz's home could house a family of six easily. How many people are raising families of that size today? Are people really buying homes and planning to stay there or has it all become an economic game like Monopoly? Do people really want monstrous entryways and massive great rooms that they use three times a year? I wonder if this design strategy is based on the public's demand or on a developer's personal preference for big and impressive homes to boost his own ego and income!

If you really want a large-square-footage home that's affordable by mainstream America's current standards, there's a strong probability that cheaper, mass-produced building materials and short-cut measures will be used, with little to no consideration for the healthiness of those materials or the health of the occupants.

I believe it's worth living in a slightly smaller home in order to have better quality, healthy materials and systems installed. Built this way, your home will last longer too. There are many ways of using innovative design to incorporate the outdoors and the land surrounding your home — even on a tight lot in a large development — to create a feeling of greater space within your home. This is the Building Biology way of building with nature.

Don't think big, think healthy!

In truth, smaller homes are often more comfortable. They are easier to manage and keep clean. People often comment on how they enjoy feeling like they use all parts of their home as opposed to living only in a third of it as Liz and Mark do.

7. SAD homes: where did all the sunshine go?

There is a medical condition known as Seasonal Affective Disorder (SAD), which results when people are deprived of of adequate natural light. Symptoms include depression and a lack of vitality. An abundance of natural light helps create a sense of well being and happiness and lifts the spirits. Depending on where you live you may have more or less sunshine. When it comes to your home, this is an important consideration.

So where does natural light come from in your home? Windows! In a lot of modern-day homes the placement, size, and functionality of windows has changed drastically. Most people don't realize what a negative impact this can have on them. Liz has huge windows at the front of her house; they face north and do not open. She has lots of windows in her kitchen, which faces west, some of which open. Her laundry room and downstairs bathrooms have no windows at all.

Window areas can account for up to 40 percent of the entire floor WALL area in modern houses and subsequently can account for up to 80 percent of total heat loss.[12] Liz's large windows on the north side will be a huge energy drain in the winter and probably will feel cold and uninviting most of the time. As these windows do not open she will not be able to get fresh air into this part of the house or create cross ventilation between windows to move fresh air through. VOC levels in this part of the house will probably remain higher than the rest of the house because of this. Even large windows are no guarantee of good quality natural light. They can be blocked by trees or constantly in a shadow.

On the other hand, some windows have been omitted from other parts of her house, such as bathrooms and laundry rooms, where they actually serve a function. These rooms are particularly prone to high moisture levels from showering, bathing, and laundry. If they're not adequately ventilated, through using exhaust fans or opening windows, you will have moisture build up which creates ideal conditions for mold to grow. A laundry room or an extra bathroom without windows can also feel very claustrophobic.

Liz has already noticed a strange smell in her downstairs bathroom, which is one sign that she has a mold problem in that room. In actual fact, what Liz does not know is that her husband regularly forgets to run the ventilation fan when he showers (a user error) and the shower drain pipe is not sealed properly and is leaking (a plumbing error). Hence the big wet patch in the basement underneath this room.

The multitude of west-facing windows in Liz's kitchen will make the kitchen uncomfortably hot on summer afternoons. She will have to find ways of creating some shade, such as installing an awning or planting a tree or two. Good window design can greatly reduce dependence on mechanical heating and cooling. If windows are placed so they prevent overheating and allow cross ventilation and solar gain when needed, the result will be energy savings and a higher level of comfort. Proper window placement and the right type of window design, used in conjunction with overhangs and trellises, are all part of a healthy, comfortable home design.

An additional health consideration is Ultra-Violet light rays (UV). UV light has had a lot of bad press in recent years, and as the ozone layer in the atmosphere continues to diminish we do need to take some health precautions. However, it's important to remember that a certain amount of the right kind of UV light is beneficial to our health. UV rays stimulate the production of Vitamin D and affect melatonin levels.[13]

8. Wiring that will leave you wired too!

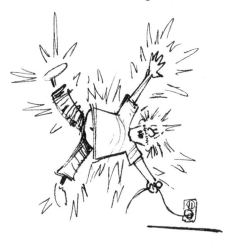

What you are about to read may be shocking to your health — pun intended! Have you ever heard of Electrobiology? It's the study of the effects that electricity has on the human body. You may have heard of EMF, which stands for Electromagnetic Fields. A more accurate term when discussing these phenomena is Electromagnetic Radiation, or EMR. When people say "EMF" they are usually only referring to AC magnetic fields, whereas EMR refers to both AC magnetic and AC electric fields, both of which can affect our health. In Building Biology we use the term EMR.

Electromagnetic radiation is the subject of much debate. I'm no electrical engineer or electrician, but I have to say that from studying electrobiology with some of the best teachers in the country and abroad, having read research and studied books, having performed many experiments in my own home, and having heard the personal stories of many people, I am convinced that electricity does affect our health.

In the next couple of paragraphs we are going to take a mini-course on electrobiology. I promise that you will learn some interesting things!

Let's start out by clarifying some terminology. First, there are two kinds of electrical current. One is called Direct Current (DC), which flows in one direction, and the other is called Alternating Current (AC), which, as its name implies, flows in alternating directions back and forth. We are interested here in the man-made AC current found in our homes that alternates 60 times a second (60Hertz).

Next, AC current generates both electric and magnetic fields that are actually two distinctly different phenomena even though they are interconnected. I will refer to them individually as AC electric fields and AC magnetic fields.

Let's compare the two:

A 1996 study by the Ontario Hydroelectric Company indicated asevenfold increase in cancers among workers exposed simultaneously to AC magnetic and AC electric fields.[14]

AC Electric Fields	AC Magnetic Fields
1. Flow in straight lines in all directions from the source unless conductors attract them. Humans act as conductors.	1. Radiate out from the source, flowing in hoops.
2. Can be easily shielded.	2. Are difficult and expensive to shield. (Even lead is not effective).
3. Are attracted by conductors such as metal or salt-water bodies, or people.	3. Penetrate all normal building materials.
4. Are present whether switches for machinery or appliances are off or on.	4. Only occur when appliances are switched on and current is flowing.
5. Reportedly affect the nervous system and can cause insomnia, anxiety, depression, and aggressive behavior. Recently they have been associated with a higher risk of leukemia.[15]	5. Reportedly affect cellular function and have been statistically linked in some studies with increased cancer cell growth rate, Alzheimer's, miscarriage, and birth defects. Some sensitive individuals report physical reactions when in elevated magnetic fields.[16]
6. Electrical code permits but does not mandate reduced electric field wiring.	6. Electrical code offers protection against exposure to magnetic fields produced by wiring in the structure, with some exceptions.
7. Requires expertise with electrical field meters to measure properly.	7. Are easily measured with a Gaussmeter.

Like the average person without any electrical engineering background, Liz has no idea about the EMRs in her home. For a system that is so essential to the functioning of our homes, and present in every room, it is one of the most elusive systems to consider because it is essentially invisible. The only indications of a problem may be subtle health effects like having difficulty falling asleep at night or waking up tired in the morning, both of which could be attributed to dozens of other reasons.

In Liz's case she would probably only question the presence of EMRs in her house if something drew her attention to it, like an article in the news (which would probably call it EMF), a book like this one, or if a friend told her something about them. For some people it takes a debilitating, mysterious illness that leads them to an Environmental Health doctor or a Building Biologist for answers.

If this topic sparks your curiosity, an inexpensive and safe way to do some personal detective work in your own home is to purchase a tool called a Gaussmeter. You will learn how to use this, and how to take a Body Voltage reading in Chapter 7.

So where do all these invisible electric and magnetic fields come from? AC electrical fields can result from a variety of things including unshielded and ungrounded wiring in walls, faulty wiring, faulty installation by the electrician, and unshielded and ungrounded electrical appliances. AC magnetic fields can result from net current on water pipes or gas pipes and certain appliances. In general, electrical appliances that remain plugged into the wall, even when not in use, will still create an AC electric field. Magnetic fields can also enter your home from the outside if you live near a high-voltage power line. As you cannot shield yourself from these fields the only way to prudently avoid them is to live away from such locations.

Three factors determine how harmful an EMR exposure is:
- the strength of the field,
- your distance from the field,
- how long you are exposed to the field.

A more in depth discussion of EMRs in homes is beyond the scope of this book. For further information consult *Prescriptions for a Healthy Home* by Paula Baker-Laporte, Erica Elliot, and John Banta or the online study course offered by the International Institute for Bau-Biologie and Ecology.

9. Seriously ... are you really going to drink that water?

This might sound a little ridiculous, but when you buy your new home don't you expect that it to come fully equipped with running water and that the water is available in several key rooms in the house like the kitchen and bathrooms? Then is it not equally important to expect the water to be safe for consumption and other household uses? Yet, how many people ask this when shopping for a new house? Unfortunately, not many.

Let's discuss Liz's house and what she bought without knowing it. The water to Liz's house is fed by the local municipality, which means the water supply at the plant is checked for basic contaminants like lead, arsenic, nitrates, and microorganisms. But then her municipality adds chlorine to kill bacteria and fluoride, ostensibly to strengthen teeth. The water then gets pumped from the plant in large concrete pipes, picking up on reintroduced contaminants the entire way, and when it arrives at Liz's house is distributed via PVC pipes. As far as Liz is concerned, she turns the tap on and water comes out, end of story, no questions asked.

However, Liz does not know that her municipality is rather antiquated and checks only for the same basic water contaminants that it has for years. This system is not adequate to really test for the more than 2,100 synthetic organic chemicals (SOCs) now polluting our water sources, with more than a hundred new ones added every year. These include pesticide residues, herbicides, and industrial byproducts such as solvents. The chlorine added will react with naturally occurring organic compounds such as bacteria, viruses, hair, and anything else that was once living, creating potentially harmful organochlorides and trihalomethanes (THMs). Some parts of the country also add fluoride to drinking water. See Chapter 9 for some startling information on fluoridating water.

Then there are the old concrete pipes, which also contain small amounts of asbestos, which, as the pipes erode, is released into her water. And finally, the PVC pipes that distribute water within her home release their own chemicals into the water too. PVC is useless without the addition of a plethora of toxic chemical stabilizers such as lead, cadmium, and phthalate plasticizers. These leach, flake, or outgas from the PVC over time raising risks from asthma to lead poisoning to cancer.[17]

Do you really feel safe drinking this kind of water or bathing your children in it?

Water purification is not yet standard in conventional, new home construction. Unless you specify that water testing and purification is required, it will not be included. As the water quality on our planet continues to decline it is now a necessity to install whole-house water filtration systems. Choosing a system depends on several factors including location, budget, water use, and taste preference. No single filtration medium can remove all contaminants from all water. It is best to choose a system in the design phase of your home to reduce installation costs and then install it during construction. For a further discussion of water filtration see Chapter 5.

10. Built-ins you could do without

Other things your house comes equipped with are doors, trim, built-in closets, pantry shelving, and kitchen cabinets. Once again, there is more to consider that just style and color. Unless you

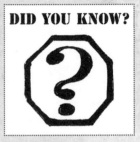

DID YOU KNOW?

A study done in June 2003 by the National Resource Defense Council (NRDC) found rocket fuel, lead, germs, and arsenic in the drinking water systems of 19 cities in the U.S. The study revealed that periodic spikes in contaminant levels are on the rise, a sign that aging pipes and water-treatment facilities often can't handle today's contaminant loads (for example, after a major storm or an industrial spill).[18]

The EPA's standard for tolerable arsenic levels dates from 1942 — before it was known to cause cancer! The Safe Drinking Water Act (SDWA) Amendments of 1996 required the EPA to propose a revised arsenic standard by January 2000, a deadline the agency has missed. This is the third time the EPA has violated a statutory mandate to update the arsenic standard.[19]

Despite pressure from dentists, 99 percent of Western Europe has rejected, banned, or stopped fluoridation due to environmental, health, legal, or ethical concerns. The World Health Organization (WHO) may endorse fluoridation, BUT MANY COUNTRIES DO NOT PRACTISE FLUORIDATION BECAUSE OF HEALTH CONCERNS. [20]

have requested non-toxic materials you can assume that all of these fixtures and fittings contain formaldehyde and other toxic chemicals that will continue to offgass for some indefinite amount of time.

This is what Liz smells in her kitchen and passes off as the "new" smell. This "new" smell represents a low level daily toxic exposure. People who develop permanent health problems associated with formaldehyde exposure often report it starting out with a flu-like illness, which is often wrongly diagnosed as a viral infection. Other symptoms can include rashes, eye irritation, frequent sore throats, hoarse voice, repeated sinus infections, nasal congestion, chronic cough, chest pains, palpitations, muscle spasms and joint

The EPA maintains a list of permitted chemical releases in your community. You can find out about these releases by consulting the EPA's Toxic Release Inventory at <www.scorecard.com>, a website created by Environmental Defense. Under the community Right-to-Know Act, you have a right to know what sorts of chemicals industrial sources are releasing into the air and water of your community

pains, numbness and tingling of the extremities, colitis and other digestive disorders, severe headaches, dizziness, loss of memory, inability to recall words and names, and disorientation. Formaldehyde is an immune system sensitizer, which means that chronic exposure can lead to multiple allergies and sensitivities to substances that are entirely unrelated to formaldehyde.[21]

When you remember the precautionary principle, we should definitely be choosing safer alternatives when it comes to chemicals like formaldehyde.

11. Attached Garages

My husband and I sometimes joke that if aliens were to visit our modern-day neighborhoods and study the outside of our homes, they would probably assume that humans were very tall and very wide. What's one of the most striking features at the front of our homes? Huge boxes with massive doors. We call them garages.

Attached garages have become synonymous with our modern-day home. We have come to expect that when we get out of our car we are already inside our home. Often it's only a matter of strides from our car door to our kitchen table. But this everyday convenience has silently brought along with it many forms of serious pollution such as carbon monoxide, sulfur dioxides, nitrogen oxides and particulates (see Chapter 13).

In Liz's case, she is in the habit of letting her car engine warm up on cool mornings whilst still parked in her garage. Only a poorly sealed door separates a whole host of toxic exhaust fumes from her kitchen and the rest of her home. The carbon monoxide (CO) levels alone that quickly build while a car idles in a garage can have serious health effects, particularly on young children with asthma and allergies.

When Liz returns home from work and parks her car in her garage, she promptly closes the garage door thereby trapping in more exhaust fumes to contaminate her home as soon as she opens the connecting door into her kitchen. Liz's garage also contains a varied assortment of other products such as pesticides, car maintenance products, cleaning products, and fuel powered lawn mower, all of which can release their own toxic fumes.

Emissions from diesel-fueled engines are composed of thousands of substances including more than 40 air toxics that are known or suspected human carcinogens.[22]

12. Miscellaneous "other stuff"

The interior of Liz's home should also be mentioned. The last eighth of an inch on many surfaces is often coated with paints, stains, and sealers. These products usually cover a large surface area of any home. As these products dry out or "cure" they will release high amounts of VOCs, which will pollute the indoor air quality of her home and can be quite noxious. Once cured there should be no further VOCs emitted, but this takes time, anything from a few days to a few months.

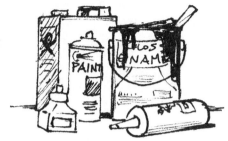

In Liz's home, the builders failed to ventilate the space while they were applying these "wet" products. Neither did they use low or no VOC products. Consequently, when her wall-to-wall carpet was installed the high levels of VOCs being emitted were absorbed into the carpet. Now whenever the temperature or humidity in her house rises, the carpet springs to life re-emitting these same VOCs and polluting the indoor air Liz and Mark breathe. This is made worse by the fact that Liz's carpet covers such a vast amount of surface area.

VOCs are not the only problem to consider. Many of these wet products used in conventional, new construction also contain synthetic binders and additives such as biocides (pesticides), which can cause additional health problems.

It's hard to find what you don't know to look for

Having said all of this, you may by now be feeling bewildered if not outraged. All of these materials in Liz's home (and maybe yours) contain toxic chemicals to greater or lesser degrees. We have looked at some chemicals such as formaldehyde in isolation and seen the devastating health consequences that can result from exposure to just one chemical. The unfortunate truth is, we are not being exposed to just one chemical in isolation, we are being exposed to a multitude of chemicals all at once on a daily basis.

Many of these chemicals interact with each other and currently there is no testing available to find out what the outcome of such chemical concoctions might be. This lack of scientific proof allows ignorance to prevail and much harm to be done.

Environmental Medicine teaches us to "prudently avoid" toxic substances. How can you avoid these chemicals when they impregnate the very materials your home is built from? And by the same token, how can we be expected to live in homes that pose potentially life-threatening health consequences to our loved ones and where no one assumes responsibility?

It's hard to find what you don't know to look for. Fortunately, you are already well on your way to having a much clearer picture of how homes affect health. Change begins with awareness and from that comes power. Let's use that power to protect our family's health.

CHAPTER 4

The Remodeled Home

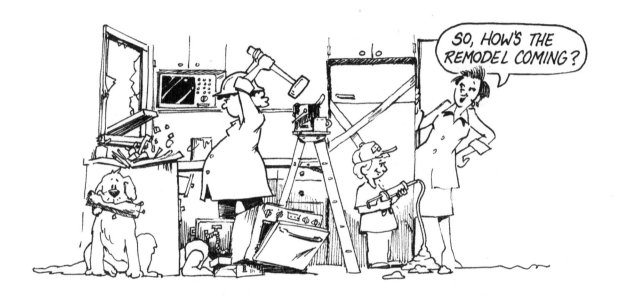

It's 4 p.m. on a Friday afternoon. Liz decides to pop in and see her sister Jane on the way home from her doctor's visit about her allergies. It's the first chance she's had to visit since Jane's remodel began two weeks ago.

In Jane's driveway stands a huge dumpster overflowing with all kinds of construction and demolition debris, pieces of wood, drywall, and shreds of wallpaper. Something catches Liz's eye: what are those dark patches of stuff on those pieces of drywall? She gets out of her car and carefully picks her way through scattered pieces of debris, noticing more pieces of drywall and wood with dark stuff on them and a couple of pieces that even have mold growing on them. "Where's that stuff come from?" she wonders.

Liz goes around the back of the house to enter through the kitchen door, the way all friends and family enter Jane's house. They call it "the tradesman's entrance."

Even before she enters the kitchen she can hear her two-year-old nephew Jack crying. Liz is not prepared for the scene she walks in on. Jane's lovely, cozy family kitchen has been ransacked! The appliances are gone, the cupboards are ripped out, the walls and ceiling have been stripped down to their barest structure and oh dear…she can see patches of light coming through the rafters. The floor is bare plywood and around the edges of the kitchen are collections of debris, which have been swept aside to make little pathways from one doorway to another.

Jane is standing by the kitchen sink, bulging with pregnancy. She looks harrowed and tired, holding a kettle in her hand, trying to figure out why the water is not flowing from her tap. Jack is on the floor crying at her feet. Fragments of animal crackers and smears of apple sauce camouflage his face, and he clasps a stray piece of shredded wallpaper in his frustrated little fist.

In a split second Liz affirms her resolve to not have kids anywhere in her near future, as she charges across the kitchen just in time to stop Jack from stuffing the dirty piece of wallpaper into his mouth.

"Oh, hello," says Jane in an exhausted and resigned tone of voice.

"What the heck's going on?" Liz demands. "What have they done to your lovely little kitchen?"

"Don't ask!" was Jane's simple reply. "I don't think the builder turned my water back on."

Jane begins to cry. "I can't cope with this; I'm supposed to be having a baby in two weeks and all I want is to clean my house and get things organized. Instead I'm living in 'The Remodel From HELL!'" More sobs.

"I thought they were supposed to be finished by now," Liz says, feeling ready to do battle with anyone who dares to try and stress her sister out one more wit.

"That's what they told us before they started; now they're not sure if they can get it

all finished before the baby comes."

"Where's Bob?" Liz demands.

"He has to work late today."

Liz begins to fume. "Where's the contractor then? I'll have a word with him. I'll get things sorted out, don't you worry."

"They all left early because it's the weekend."

"What! You're supposed to cope like this till Monday? You haven't even got any water." Liz's voice has now risen to a yell.

Fortunately, Jack has stopped crying and is now looking from his mother to his aunt with tremendous curiosity. He sneezes so loudly that both Jane and Liz jump.

Jack's older brother Tom momentarily appears from behind a pile of rubble hiding a glue gun behind his back to say, "Bless you!" then disappears again.

"He's having an awful time of it." Jane scoops Jack up in her arms to wipe his runny, snotty-green nose.

Liz cringes; she finds children's snotty-green noses particularly gross. "So why have they turned your water off?"

"Well, when they went to take the old kitchen cabinets out, they took the old dishwasher out too. We've bought a new one, one of those that conserve water and are super quiet. The old one made such a racket! Anyway, when they pulled the dishwasher out, part of the wall behind it literally fell down! It had rotted! Apparently we've had a slow water leak from the dishwasher for some time. I had no idea. I mean, I have to admit there's been a funny smell in this kitchen for a while, but I always thought it was just the trash that needed to be taken out or Jack's poopy diaper," explains Jane.

"Well, can't they just patch it up a bit and turn your water back on?" Liz asks.

Jane gives up and puts the kettle down. "Oh no! The builder said we need to bring in a mold remediator to fix it. Some mold's toxic you know. Haven't you seen it on the news lately? People can get really sick from having mold in their home."

"What's a mold remedi-whatsit? Sounds like an undertaker!" Liz says with a sarcastic laugh.

"A mold remediator is someone who specializes in fixing mold problems from water damage in buildings. There'll be an investigation and everything."

Liz begins to warm to her own sarcasm. "What, like they visit the scene of the crime, interrogate the suspects?"

"Stop it! It's serious stuff. First someone has to come here with all these gadgets and check how much damage has been done and measure things." Jane continues to explain, "Then someone has to come and fix it. It can take days."

"And how much does all this cost? And who has to pay for it?" Liz asks.

"I don't know how much it's going to cost yet, but the builder says it can get very expensive," Jane says with a sigh.

Liz persists. "Who has to pay for it?"

Jane begins to pace back and forth between piles of debris. "Well, I've called the insurance company and they say our policy's changed and they don't cover water damage problems any more. In fact they say they may have to cancel our policy altogether because we have this mold problem. So that leaves us with the bill and I've no idea what we're going to do for insurance now. It seems no one wants you if you've had a mold problem any more. It's bad enough this remodel is taking forever, but now I've no idea what our final bill's going to be or how we're going to pay

for it." Jane starts to cry again.

Liz puts her arm around her sister to comfort her. She wonders about the mold in the kitchen where they are sitting; her mind becomes slightly paranoid as she wonders if the mold is only in the wall. What if it's been mobilized by all this bashing around that's been going on? What if tiny bits of it are floating around in the air they are breathing right now? What if they are all being exposed to toxic mold right now? How would they know? How sick would they get? What would be the first signs? She notices she has a slightly sore throat. When did that start?

All these racing thoughts push Liz to her feet and without saying a word she drags Jane, Jack, and Tom out of the house, bundles them into her car and drives off towards her house.

Jack squashes his runny-nosed face against the car window and says enthusiastically, "Bye, bye."

A short time later Jane is relaxing with her feet up drinking a cup of tea in her sister's home. Liz appears with a freshly bathed, clean Jack wearing one of Liz's t-shirts that looks like a rather bad toga on him. She deposits Jack on the sofa next to Tom who is already engrossed in a cartoon on TV.

Liz sits down next to Jane.

"So what's the plan? Hire a mold detective, get him to fix the problem, give him a nice fat check, put your kitchen back together, have a baby some time in the midst of all this, and get your life back?" Liz says being sarcastic again. "Is that it? Did we cover everything?"

"Actually, no."

"You mean there's more?" Liz says incredulously.

Jane sighs. "Yes. The builder says even when the mold problem has been taken care of he can't put my new ceiling up until I get the roof fixed. It's got holes in it and if I don't get it fixed it's just going to ruin all his work when it starts to rain, and guess what? We'll probably have more mold problems."

Liz reaches her limit. "Is the world going mad? Does everything cause mold now?"

"Yes. I read a really disturbing article this week in a magazine. It was called 'The New Baby's Bedroom.' I thought I'd read it and get some ideas for the baby's room, you know, where to get cute bedding and stuff like that. But they said that new babies' bedrooms are full of toxic chemicals! They're in everything, the paint, the carpet, the bedding, the toys. I mean, what is the point of having kids any more! Here I am having a new room built onto the side of the kitchen as part of this remodel, I have the carpet paid for, the paints waiting in the garage. Just last week I went out and bought a new mattress for the crib and it's all toxic! How can people be allowed to sell this stuff if it's so dangerous?" yells Jane.

"Surely it can't be that bad, weren't they exaggerating?" Liz asks.

"I don't think so. Some doctor who specializes in pediatrics wrote the article. He helps children who've been exposed to toxic chemicals like pesticides and all these other things. I'm thinking of taking Jack to see him about his asthma."

Liz notices Jane looks exhausted. "How is Jack's asthma?"

"Well, it's been awful since we started this stupid remodel. He's up a lot in the night and he's wheezing a lot in the day. It's so exhausting for everyone. I'm wondering if it's all due to mold," Jane says.

Liz goes over to the sink and fills the kettle. Momentarily she appreciates the convenience of having running water. "It does make you start to wonder doesn't it? So what are you going to do about the new baby's room?"

"I'm not sure. I think I'll do some research on the Internet. See if there are some organizations that know more about this kind of thing. The doctor who wrote this article is part of some organization called the American Academy of Environmental Medicine. They should know something. And I'm just going to start asking around to see if any friends know anything. Worst case scenario I'll just put the baby in our bedroom until I know more."

"Hey, I know someone we should talk to. My friend Steph at work. She has allergies. She did tons of research because she wanted to build a house that wouldn't aggravate her allergies. Her house is supposed to have zero-chemical anything! I wonder if she'd let us come over and see her new place. I've been dying to go over there. Let me give her a call." Liz disappears into another room.

As Jane leans back in her chair the baby begins to kick and wriggle in her belly. "Don't you worry little one, I'm not going to let anything harm you" and with that Jane dozes off.

Commentary

Stories like this are occurring all around the country. Jane represents a growing number of people who are deciding to invest back into their homes and remodel them rather than buy a new one. Having read the last chapter about the "Conventional New Home" and all the problems associated with the chemicals in new building materials, you might be thinking that remodeling is a safer way to go. What we are about to discuss are considerations specific to remodels that can also affect your family's health.

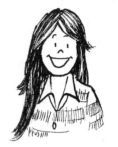

The basic idea behind a remodel is to expand or improve your existing home structure in some way. This often involves such things as taking down some of the current structure and adding on new structure. People change walls, windows, kitchen cabinets, and just about anything else you can think of. But from a Building Biology point of view, any change to the structure or surfaces of a building has the ability to impact the inhabitant's health, either positively or negatively. Let's look closer.

Toxic building materials revisited.

I spoke with a builder recently who specializes in remodels. He said he's seeing mold problems in just about every job he does these days. His concern is that if the house got this way from the original construction and materials used, it didn't make sense to remodel using the same problematic materials. Would it not just lead to the same rotten results somewhere in the future? This builder had thought this through and realized he needed to find better building materials and systems that would be resistant to mold problems. He is ahead of the learning curve and definitely the kind of builder to look for if you are planning to remodel. Replace the old, rotten parts with healthy materials that will last. It's really that simple.

Jane had an architect draw up some plans and specifications, found a builder, and got underway. Sound familiar? Isn't that what most people do? But unless your architect or builder knows about healthy building materials, they are probably going to use the same standard materials that we just discussed

> "Problems cannot be solved at the same level of awareness that created them." — Albert Einstein

in great detail in the previous chapter. Namely, building materials that contain toxic chemicals and systems that can be problematic to health. It's also important to keep in mind that builders are not trained mold remediators.

If you're contemplating a remodel, treat it as though you're adding a new home and follow the guidelines in the next chapter about healthy homes. Ask for healthy building materials before you contract with someone, choose non-toxic products, and get involved. It's your home and it's your family's health that's at stake. If your requests for a healthy remodel fall on deaf ears, keep talking to builders until you find the right one. If you do this in the planning stage, your remodel will be much easier and more affordable.

Mold and Remediation

If your home is several years old, a lot of the problematic synthetic chemical VOCs from the new construction will have offgassed by now. That's a good thing. However, when you start opening up or taking down walls, taking out windows, or pulling up old carpet you may well find that problems like mold have been quietly festering without your knowledge for some time.

Mold will only grow where there is sufficient moisture. Typical sources of elevated moisture content in buildings include windows, roof leaks (the exterior building envelope), plumbing, appliance leaks, and construction errors when installing showers. Jane had no idea her dishwasher had a slow leak. Even though she had noticed a strange smell in the kitchen, it never registered that water damage was going on. Again, it's hard to find what you don't know to look for.

So what is mold?

Molds are part of the natural environment and can be found outdoors and indoors. Outdoors, molds play a part in nature by breaking down dead organic matter such as fallen leaves and dead trees, but indoors we don't need these services, so mold growth should be avoided.

Molds are a group of organisms that belong to the fungi kingdom. "Fungi" and "mold" are often used interchangeably. There are reported to be over 100,000 species of mold. Fungi are neither animals nor plants and are classified in a kingdom of their own. Fungi include molds, yeasts, mushrooms, and puffballs.[1] It is estimated that more than 1.5 million species of fungi exist. Some molds are very toxic just as some mushrooms are very poisonous. During active microbial growth, molds produce microbial Volatile Organic Compounds (mVOCs) as part of their metabolic process of breaking down their nutrient source. These mVOC chemicals are volatile, are released directly into the air, and have a moldy or musty odor. If you have musty odors in your home, it is possible that mold is growing somewhere.

Some molds can produce toxic substances called *mycotoxins*. Some mycotoxins cling to the surface of mold spores; others may be found within spores. More than 200 mycotoxins have been identified from common molds, and many more remain to be identified.[2] According to Will Spates, who is an experienced mold remediator and

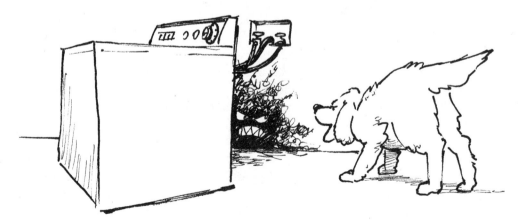

Building Biologist, "Mycotoxins are produced by some molds some of the time. They are usually produced when a mold colony is in competition for a nutrient source or when the colony is stressed by environmental conditions. Mycotoxins may be stimulated by the application of biocides and antimicrobials. There are anecdotal references to very high mycotoxin concentrations in molds that have been exposed to ozone. Mycotoxins are present whether the spore is viable (alive) or not viable (dead)." Mycotoxins are not usually odorous but can be very problematic to health.

How does mold grow and spread?

Molds reproduce by means of tiny spores; the spores are invisible to the naked eye and are able to float through outdoor and indoor air. Mold may begin growing indoors when spores land on moist surfaces and find food. "Food" means virtually any organic substance, such as wood, paper, carpet, human food, and insulation.

It's important to understand that when someone says they have a mold problem what they actually have is a *moisture problem*. In today's modern homes moisture can accumulate for a variety of reasons and hence the proliferation of mold problems we are hearing so much about.

Let's identify some of the most common sources of excess moisture:

1. Unforeseen accidents, such as a water pipe bursting. This needs to be addressed within 48 hours, otherwise a mold problem can really get out of hand and cause extensive damage.
2. Maintenance problems, such as slow leaks, constant drips, a window that hasn't been sealed properly, a shower or bath that hasn't been caulked adequately, or leaky roofs. These hidden defects are usually not obvious until you have a larger problem, as in Jane's home.
3. Condensation. Many activities of modern day living produce huge amounts of moisture. It's not uncommon to have all family members take showers or baths on a daily basis. Then there's cooking and laundry. Bathrooms and kitchens need vents with fans that will extract excess moisture to the outside of the house. If all the water vapor released into the air of a home could escape somewhere, condensation would not occur. When homes were draughtier and open fires were common, this water mainly went up chimneys. Now that chimneys are mostly closed and draughts prevented (by sealing homes up tightly), condensation problems result.
4. Building materials. If the materials used to build your home do not dry out thoroughly after the manufacturing process they can have high moisture content.

MOLD BASICS

1. The key to mold control is moisture control.
2. If mold is a problem in your home, you should promptly fix the water problem *and* clean up the mold.
3. It is important to dry water-damaged areas and items within 24-48 hours to prevent mold growth.[3]

One example of this is "green lumber," which is still wet, as opposed to kiln dry lumber, which has been dried. Mold may already be growing on such materials when it arrives at the construction site. Many builders use these materials. Another concern is green cement that has not properly cured before floors and walls are installed.

5. Construction. Builders unfortunately do not control the weather. I'm sure many of them wish they could! They can, however, keep building materials dry and protect the building itself during construction. If this kind of protection is not provided and the building materials are allowed to get wet and are then used or sealed up into the building envelope, you can have a massive mold problem just waiting to happen.

6. Poor ventilation can also cause molds to grow. Molds are often most severe in the corners of rooms that are external walls. This is mainly because insufficient ventilation creates pockets of stagnant air in these corners. Built-in cupboards, particularly when located against external walls, suffer from the same disadvantage.[4] Closets, basements, and storerooms are prone to mold growth for the same reasons.

7. Yet another source of mold growth are appliances that have standing water in them such as air conditioners, drip pans under refrigerators, humidifiers, and dehumidifiers.

8. Two last sources that are worth mentioning here are plants that are over-watered and food left out in the open. Even a moldy orange in the fruit bowl can result in a significant release of spores.

As you can see some of these mold problems are building-related and some are to do with proper housekeeping. For information on healthy housekeeping see Part Two of this book.

In Jane's situation, when the dishwasher was removed, it was very obvious there was a problem because part of the wall collapsed. But sometimes these problems are not so obvious; sometimes there is only a slight amount of visible mold on the surface of the wall, representing the tip of the iceberg, and much more will be inside the wall cavity itself. Once mold is set in motion it will spread to the extent that the moisture migrates. As a result of a prolonged leak, there could be many species of molds, which have colonized over time. In these situations, where there is a multicultural environment, there is a greater likelihood of mycotoxins being present. Many molds associated with water-damaged buildings produce mycotoxins.[5]

If you do discover a mold problem, it is important to understand that mold spores can travel in several ways: they may be passively moved (by a breeze or waterdrop), mechanically disturbed (by a person or animal passing by), or actively discharged by the mold itself as part of its normal life cycle (usually under moist conditions or high humidity).

When mold spores land on a damp spot indoors, they usually start digesting whatever they are growing on in order to survive. Molds gradually destroy the things they grow on. In Jane's situation, some of the mold in her kitchen was dislodged when the wall fell down and also because the builders did not put the moldy pieces of wood and drywall into bags before taking them outside to the dumpster. Mold spores are minute and even carrying a contaminated piece of wood through the kitchen is enough to distribute countless mold spores to new locations — all ready to do their thing as soon as conditions are right. In Jane's house, some of these mold spores have found their way into the forced air ducting and so will be blown around and travel to all parts of Jane's house. What a thought! Jack already has asthma; how will this mass dispersal of mold spores impact his health?

It is important to understand that settled spores will remain dormant until sufficient moisture is present to allow them to germinate. Without moisture, mold spores are like an acorn sitting on a sidewalk — it will never grow into a tree in this spot. However, settled spores can be disturbed and can provoke allergic effects in people with mold sensitivities. It is important to use controlled demolition to minimize the release of spores.

As for the pieces of wood Liz saw outside Jane's house that had black marks and white scraggly lines on them, the color of mold usually is determined by the species of mold and the nutrient source it's feeding upon. You cannot determine toxicity by the color of mold. "Killer black mold" (*Stachybotrys chartarum*) is a gross misnomer, as many black molds are of the garden-variety type[6] and not dangerous. The only way to really determine what kind of mold is present and whether it is a problematic kind or not is to enlist the help of an Indoor Environment Professional (IEP) who will give a visual inspection and then take samples which will be sent to a lab for identification. The IEP will be able to evaluate the lab results and then recommend an appropriate plan of action to fix the situation and protect your health at the same time. I recommend enlisting the help of a certified microbial remediation contractor (a mold remediator) independent of the IEP to implement this plan, to avoid any conflict of interest.

Common health complaints associated with molds and mycotoxins

Not all molds are bad for your health but all molds have the potential to affect health. Molds produce allergens, irritants, and in some cases, potentially toxic substances (mycotoxins).[7] The types and severity of symptoms depend, in part, on the types of mold present, the extent of an individual's exposure, the ages of the individuals, and their existing sensitivities or allergies.[8] People who may be affected more severely and sooner than others include infants and children, the elderly, individuals with pre-existing respiratory conditions or sensitivities such as allergies and asthma, and people with weakened immune systems.

Mold exposure can come from breathing in spores or other tiny fragments, through skin contact with mold contaminants (for example, by touching moldy surfaces), and by swallowing mold. Chronic exposure can lead to hypersensitivity pneumonitis, allergic asthma, and chronic allergy symptoms.[9]

Mycotoxins may cause a variety of short-term as well as long-term adverse health effects. These range from immediate toxic response and immune-suppression to the potential long-term carcinogenic effect. Symptoms due to mycotoxins or toxin-containing airborne spores (particularly those of *Stachybotrys chartarum*) include dermatitis, recurring cold and flu-like symptoms, burning sore throat, headaches and excessive fatigue, diarrhea, impaired or altered immune symptoms, bloody nose and lung bleeding in infants.[10] The ability of the body to fight off infectious diseases may be weakened, resulting in opportunistic infections.[11]

Testing for mold

If you suspect you have a mold problem it's probably because you can already see or smell it. The first thing you need to do is determine how the mold problem got started. See the checklist below for ideas.

I recommend steering away from do-it-yourself home mold test kits. Out of curiosity I have used some of these kits; I found the results misleading. An IEP or Building Biology Environmental Inspector (BBEI) is the best way to go if you have concerns or have uncovered a problem and would like your home tested. They will know, based on a visual inspection, what tests and sampling methods would be most appropriate to help diagnose if there is a mold problem. Sample analysis should follow analytical methods recommended by the American Industrial Hygiene Association (AIHA) or the American Conference of Governmental Industrial Hygienists (ACGIH), as well as the professional judgement of the IEP. Types of samples include air samples, surface samples, bulk samples (chunks of carpet, insulation, wall board, etc.), and water samples.

Do your homework though and check the credentials of any professional you may want to consult with. It can be helpful to get a reference or two and talk with some of the people they have helped to find out more about what's involved. Unfortunately, there are some people jumping on the band wagon and calling themselves mold inspectors without any real credentials or experience. I recently spoke with a lady who had fallen very ill from mold in her home. The remediation company she hired was completely unprofessional and ended up contaminating her whole house and making the problem much worse instead of helping her. Better to be safe than sorry.

Remediation

It is impossible to eliminate all molds and mold spores in the indoor environment. However, indoor mold growth can be controlled by controlling moisture (i.e. keeping relative humidity below 50 percent) and by paying proper attention to maintenance once any existing mold problem has been addressed. To properly fix a mold problem requires specific skills, which are best left to people trained in microbial remediation, just like you would bring in a trained asbestos remediator if you discovered an asbestos problem.

When looking for a mold remediator try to choose at least two different people to take a look at the problem. They should read the IEP's findings and repair plan which will already have assessed the size of the mold and/or moisture problem and the amount of material that has been damaged. It will also have taken into account the possibility of hidden mold.

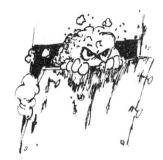

Do not agree to any work being done until you have had time to review the plan and discuss it thoroughly with the mold remediator. A good plan should include steps to fix the water or moisture problem at its source, otherwise the problem could just reoccur. The plan should cover the use of appropriate Personal Protective Equipment (PPE) and include steps to carefully contain and remove moldy building materials to avoid spreading the mold. Remediation plans may vary greatly depending on the size and complexity of the job, and may require revision if circumstances change or new facts are discovered once work has begun. The highest priority must be to protect the occupants and the remediators carrying out the work. If a large portion of your home has been contaminated, the remediation plan should include relocation of your family until the work is complete and your home is proven to be safe again.

The purpose of mold remediation is to remove the mold to prevent human exposure and damage to building materials and furnishings. It is necessary to clean up mold contamination, not just kill the mold. Dead mold is still allergenic, and some dead molds are potentially toxic. The use of a biocide, such as chlorine bleach, is not recommended as a routine practice during mold remediation. In most cases, it is not possible or desirable to sterilize an area; a background level of mold spores will still remain in the air.[12] Remember, biocides are toxic to humans as well as to mold. For a thorough and easy to read guide on mold remediation, the EPA's "Mold Remediation in Schools and Commercial Buildings" (which is very applicable to homes) is available on their website in a downloadable format at <www.epa.gov/iaq/pubs/molds.html> or can be ordered by phone at 1-800-438-4318. I recommend having your own copy to familiarize yourself with the process and to know what questions to ask remediators. The EPA's most recent document, "A Brief Guide to Mold, Moisture and Your Home," is another good resource.

Other health hazards to consider when remodeling

A lot of emphasis has been placed on mold so far but other health hazards must also be considered when remodeling, namely lead, asbestos, and fiberglass.

Lead

If your home was built before 1978 there's a strong possibility that it contains some lead paint. Even if surfaces have been repainted and covered over with lead-free paint since that time, when it comes to remodeling, surfaces will be disturbed which could release paint chips and dust that contain lead.

CHECKLIST FOR POSSIBLE SOURCES OF MOLD PROBLEMS

1. Moisture behind bath tiles resulting from cracks or caulking gaps.
2. High humidity in the basement from improper dryer vent, high water table, or clogged drain.
3. Leaking windows.
4. Wet carpets.
5. Drain pan under refrigerator.
6. AC drain pan, cooling coils, and ductwork.
7. Plant bases.
8. Roof leaks and wet insulation.
9. Water pipe leaks.
10. Dampness and poor air flow under sinks.
11. Dryer vents not connected to the outside.
12. Corners of rooms with external walls.
13. Cabinets and closets attached to external walls.
14. Faulty gutters and drain pipes that direct water onto or under the building.
15. Sprinkler systems that wet the walls or foundations.
16. Showers and shower curtain.
17. Ventilation fans.
18. HVAC ducting.

Lead is poisonous when swallowed or inhaled. Environmental exposure to high levels of lead can cause infertility in men. Pregnant women exposed to high lead can miscarry. Babies born from mothers exposed to high levels of lead may develop neurological problems, experience developmental delays, and have behavioral abnormalities.[13] Signs of lead poisoning include loss of appetite, weakness, anemia, vomiting, and convulsions. In some cases, permanent brain damage can result — even death.[14]

If you suspect you may have lead paint on the inside or outside of your home it is wise to have it tested before you embark on any remodeling. There are simple lead testing kits now available that you can use at home (see Appendix C). You can test your paint, any paint chips you find, dust, and a variety of other items in your home, such as the solder on your water pipes (used to join and seal copper pipes together) and children's toys. If you are testing paint, you will need to scratch beneath the surface to get to the layers

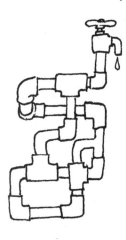

that may contain lead. Make sure you choose a discreet location so that you don't create unsightly marks in your living space. The drawback to this method is that it only gives an indication for that actual location and is not representative of the paint used in every room. You may well have lead paint somewhere else in your home.

The best way to find out if you have lead in your home is to have a professional lead inspector test it. He will use a special piece of equipment called an x-ray fluorescence (XRF) detector (see Appendix C). Even if the test shows no lead in your home, it's worth the peace of mind to know that you and your children are safe from lead poisoning.

If you yourself discover lead you should contact the National Lead Information Center which is a hotline maintained by the EPA at 1-800-424-LEAD (5323). Do not under any circumstances try to do lead abatement yourself. This is a job for a qualified professional. I have heard horror stories of people trying to remove lead from their home by themselves and ending up poisoning the whole family! Remodeling plans should be put on hold until the situation is safely resolved.

According to the EPA (2002) "In the United States, about 900,000 children ages 1 to 5 have a blood-lead level above the level of concern."

If you have already hired a lead inspector who then found that you have a lead problem in your home, you should be in good hands to get professional advice about what to do next.

Asbestos

The word "asbestos" refers to several types of fibrous minerals that are used as insulation and for their resistance to heat, acid, and fire. You can find asbestos in homes built between the 1920s and the 1970s. It can be found in hard floor materials (such as certain types of vinyl tiles), some cement and cement products (including cement/asbestos siding and roofing tiles), ceiling texturing materials, and even in some drywall compounds. It has also been used as insulation surrounding ductwork and furnaces, as well as with particular types of electrical circuitry.[15]

Health hazards associated with asbestos include asbestosis (a severe, debilitating lung disease), lung cancer, and malignant mesothelioma (a cancer of the chest and abdominal lining). These cancers can occur years after inhaling asbestos fibers: lung cancer can occur 10 to 30 years after exposure while mesothelioma generally occurs 20 to 50 years later.[16]

In my research I found much advice saying the best thing to do with asbestos in the home is to not disturb it, and that there is no danger to health unless the fibers are released and inhaled into the lungs. But this advice is not helpful when you are preparing for a remodel, which will involve disturbing structural parts of your home that may well contain asbestos.

So if you have an older home and suspect you may have asbestos, have this checked by a qualified asbestos inspector before you start remodeling. The EPA's Indoor Air Quality InfoLine can provide you with more information and a list of licensed asbestos-removal contractors to consult with (see Appendix C). This is not a job for homeowners or amateurs.

Fiberglass

Ninety percent of the homes in the United States are insulated with fiberglass insulation. The debate continues as to whether or not fiberglass is a human carcinogen.

Fiberglass is made of glass. The fibers can cut, scratch, and irritate skin. The fibers can also break off into tiny particles and the health concern is that they can get lodged in the lungs rather like asbestos, though they are not considered as dangerous. There are numerous reports linking fiberglass to pulmonary disease in production workers and installers.[17] While it is still not clear what the long-term respiratory effects of fiberglass will be, the precautionary principle would advise us to use a safer alternative when it comes to choosing insulation.

In a remodel situation, old fiberglass insulation will often be removed or at least dislodged. This very act, if done without thought and planning, can release large amounts of fiberglass particulates into the air and over surfaces including the ductwork of your heating and cooling system, where they will be re-circulated endlessly in the air for everyone to breathe. If fiberglass insulation is being removed as a result of a mold problem, it will probably contain a multitude of mold spores. As we have already mentioned, spores are easily dispersed so any spoiled insulation must be carefully placed in plastic bags and sealed before removing from its location.

The other problem with fiberglass is that it can contain formaldehyde. Some fiberglass companies are now offering encapsulated batts of insulation, which means they seal the fiberglass behind a layer of polyethylene. Formaldehyde-free insulation is now also on the market. Be sure to state your preferences in the design stage of planning your remodel. See Chapter 5 for more healthy suggestions.

Move out during remodeling

Now that you are clearer about the possible health hazards you may encounter during the process of a remodel, there is still one more thing to consider. Whether to stay and live in your home during the remodel, or leave and return after everything is completed. Many people decide to tough it out and stay living in their house through the remodel. It definitely is an additional expense and a big inconvenience to relocate the whole family. But after having read this chapter, does it really seem like a good idea when you consider everyone's health and the possible long-term consequences? I would definitely recommend moving to a safer location if at all possible.

At least plan a family vacation to coincide with your remodel and get your family away for part of the time. It will do wonders to reduce the stress levels too! For the remainder of the time you must be at home, take as many precautions as possible. Explain your health concerns to your builder and have him design a plan to completely close off any area that is being worked on. This will need to be really thought through, as there is more to this than meets the eye, as we have just been discussing.

The last word

This might seem like a lot of extra work that you were not planning on, and you're right, it is. But if you don't do it, you are leaving yourself wide open for nightmares like the situation Jane found herself in with her "remodel from hell." Taking the time to plan all this out in advance and working with the right people will actually save you time, money, your health, and your sanity. When you think about it this way, it's actually a great deal!

The Healthy New Home

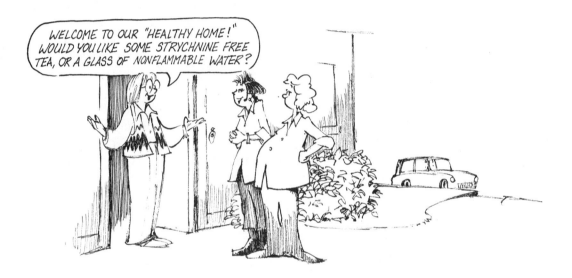

It's Sunday afternoon. Jane and Liz are driving over to see Liz's friend Steph who has just moved in to her new, healthy home. Jane and her family have spent the weekend at Liz's house due to the current impasse reached in their house remodel, which has left them without running water.

"That was a real sight we just left behind there in the living room wasn't it? Two grown men sandwiched together on either side of Tom and Jack, stuffing themselves with popcorn watching the sports channel, all of them in 'pig heaven!'" laughs Liz.

"While we are turned loose on a mission to answer the most difficult questions of this next millennium like, 'How do you stop your home from killing you?'" laughs Jane.

"Or, 'How much will your new home really cost you if you become allergic to it?'" Liz roars with laughter, "Or, 'How do you stop your home from self-composting from mold damage?'"

"Oh stop, I'm going to pee, I'm too pregnant for humor!" The laughter increases.

"Here we are, just in time, we'd better get you to a bathroom," Liz says, still chuckling.

Jane looks around Steph's cul-de-sac. "This looks nice, that's a pleasant surprise. I'm not sure what I was expecting, but I did think it would look weird somehow, but this looks very … normal."

"Yes, I'm surprised too, this whole development has been nicely done. I thought it was going to be some sort of 'hippy commune' or something. I hope I'm not going to like her new house better than mine," Liz says reluctantly.

Jane and Liz walk up the pathway to Steph's front door.

"Look how the windows and the front door are all recessed. It reminds me of the homes I saw when I was over in Italy years ago. I always liked that style of building, it makes things look timeless and as though they were built to last," Jane enthuses. "Look at that, a proper front door step. I haven't seen one of those in years."

They ring the front doorbell and a pleasant, gentle sound rings inside Steph's house.

Liz raises her eyebrows. "God, even her front doorbell has a nice ring! Mine booms out all around the house, it's enough to waken the dead!"

Steph opens the door and welcomes them with a cheery smile.

"Thanks for letting us come over Steph," Liz says giving Steph a hug.

"No problem, I'm enjoying sharing 'Mecca' with my friends," Steph answers.

"Mecca?" asks Liz.

Steph continues smiling. "That's the nickname we've given the house. We can't wait to get home at the end of the day."

A quiet thought trickles through Liz's mind. "Oh dear, I really like this place already."

"What a nice place!" Jane declares as she steps through the doorway and shakes Steph's hand.

"Liz says you're currently remodeling your house. How's it going?" Steph enquires.

"Don't ask. 'Going' is not the right word, I'm interested in the word 'gone' or 'done' and it's neither right now," Jane says, trying to inject some humor into her voice. "Maybe we could rent your basement out in the meantime?"

"You could, if we had one."

"What, you don't have a basement? What do you have?" Liz asks curiously.

"This house is built on what's called 'slab-on-grade.' It's cleaner that way," Steph answers. "Come on in and I'll give you the virtual tour with full explanations. Some things may sound unusual to you at first, but notice how you feel as we walk around. That says more than a thousand words."

As Liz and Jane enter the house, they notice a little sign on the porch by an old-fashioned bench saying, "Please remove your shoes." The girls follow the prompt and begin to take their shoes off.

"Oh thanks," says Steph. "No one wears outdoor shoes inside the house, you'd be amazed how much dirt and debris gets tracked into a home everyday on people's shoes."

"Oooo," Jane says, "your floor's warm!"

"Isn't it great! It's called radiant floor heating. It's the cleanest and healthiest way to heat your home. You heat objects, not air. It makes a huge difference if you have asthma or allergies. We used to have forced air heating at our last home. It drove my allergies nuts. It was like a merry-go-round for dust, pollen, mold spores, pet dander … you name it. And on top of that it made the air dry so we always had to use humidifiers and they kept getting moldy. It was gross. Everyone loves it in our new house, even the kids. It seems to have calmed them down, I couldn't tell you why, maybe they're just more comfortable playing on the floor now that it's warm. Oh yes, and we didn't install any carpet."

"No carpet?" Liz exclaims in disbelief.

"That's right. Carpets are like biology experiments, full of all kinds of dirt, pet dander, pollen, and who knows what. It's almost impossible to keep carpet clean, plus it usually has all kinds of chemicals in it that pollute your indoor air quality."

"Yuck!" declares Jane, "I never knew that. What else do you know about homes?"

"Well, let's see ..." Steph ponders, "it all begins with remembering what a home is really all about. I mean, think about it, don't you want your home to be a bastion of health, a place to rest and recuperate at the end of the day, a place you feel safe and protected, where everyone thrives?"

"Sign me up!" Jane interjects.

"I felt awful most of the time in our last house, I was always tired and my allergies drove me nuts. Then one evening after the kids had gone to bed I was just surfing on the Internet and I found this company that builds healthy homes and they were speaking my language, about a home nurturing you and your family and improving the quality of your life. They also talked about something called Building Biology and how your home impacts your health. Basically, if you build a home using healthy materials and don't use all the toxic chemicals that go into a conventional new house, guess what? Its good for your health. It's not rocket science, is it?"

"No!" Steph's captivated audience answers in unison.

"Anyway, I decided then and there, 'That's it, that's what I want,' and here we are. I'll never buy a home again that isn't built healthily after experiencing this one. Since we moved into this house a couple of months ago, everyone sleeps better, everyone's disposition seems happier, no grouchy kids in the morning. I have more energy and my allergies don't bother me for the first time in decades."

"That's amazing," Jane says. "I'd give anything for a good night's sleep and to have Jack, my two-year-old's, asthma go away."

Liz looks around. "Your house is so quiet, it doesn't echo like mine does."

"That's because the house is built with these big, fat insulated blocks instead of stick frame construction. You know what regular walls are like, you tap on them and they echo a bit, they sound so hollow. These walls are solid and ten inches thick. They actually absorb sound — listen." Steph slaps the wall by the window and everyone listens. Only the solid sound of silence is heard. "Right now the kids are playing outside and we can't hear anything inside. Don't you love it? And what's more these walls won't grow mold."

"Don't mention the 'M' word," Liz says quickly.

Jane sighs wistfully, lost in some sort of reverie. "It gives your house this timeless, European kind of feel, almost like you've got yourself a little castle, like this house will last forever!"

"You should see our heating bills too, much less than our last house. Thick walls keep you warm when you need it and cool when you need it. It's the old-fashioned way to work with heating and cooling, like they do in Europe, and it works just great here in America too." Steph walks off and the girls follow.

"So tell us some more about this Building Biology, it sounds fascinating," Jane says.

"One of the things that really helped me to understand what makes a home healthy is this idea that your home is your 'third skin'. You don't have to be an architect or builder to understand it. Your home is basically as important as your own skin," Steph explains.

"I bet these homes must cost a fortune," Liz interjects, looking at Jane nervously for a bit of moral support.

"It costs us about $2.50 extra a day, over the course of our mortgage, to have this healthy home. $2.50!! That's one latte a day! And for that my whole family's health is being cared for. I mean think about it … how much does it cost if you get cancer? This $2.50 a day is the best family insurance plan out there. And that's not all, half of that cost will be offset with our energy savings," Steph enthuses.

Liz and Jane exchange glances again.

Jane's eyes widen with enthusiasm. "You're kidding! I'd pay $2.50 a day if I could get rid of Jack's asthma and not have to give him those nasty inhalers."

"God, I'd have paid $2.50 extra a day to buy a healthy home if I'd known I had a choice," Liz says to herself quietly.

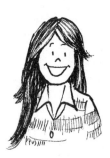

Commentary

This final chapter in the first section of the book is a discussion about what constitutes a healthy home based on a Building Biology perspective (to refresh your memory on Building Biology refer back to Chapter1). Healthy construction is a rapidly growing field. Even as I write this book new products and systems are hitting the market place to be tried and tested. The current healthy home model will possibly look different five years from now. However, this presentation encapsulates the best of what is currently available for the mainstream North American market.

Your home is your third skin

As was already mentioned in Chapter 2, seeing your home as a third skin, not only for you but also for your whole family, is such a simple concept to grasp that even children understand it. It reminds us of our fundamental need for our homes to shelter and protect us. In return we must care for our homes. To the degree that you keep your home healthy you will be caring for your whole family's health.

Let's look at the main building materials and systems used in Steph's new, healthy home.

1. Slab on grade

Steph's house is built on what's called a "slab on grade." This means that a foundation slab of concrete is poured directly onto the the building site after it has been specially prepared. This simple method of building does away with those scary crawl spaces we talked about in Chapter 3 and eliminates the possibility of animals and other nasty things living in the space under your home.

Radon mitigation

Even though the soil was tested for radon gas before Steph's home was built on this site and levels were shown to be very low, her home was still built with radon mitigation in mind. Radon levels can change over time and during different seasons, so a radon test done before construction may not be accurate a year later.

There are several options for radon mitigation. Here is the effective, inexpensive technique used for Steph's house. A perforated pipe was laid in the gravel through the center of the building envelope and runs the length of the house. A vapour barrier and insulation was laid on top, followed by a poured slab of concrete. The perforated pipe was then connected to an unperforated riser tube that vents to the outside of the building. This vent acts as a passive radon removal outlet and will probably be sufficient to keep radon from entering the house. Should radon levels rise in Steph's home any time in the future, a fan can be attached to the vent pipe to actively suction out the gas. Steph has a homeowner's manual that came with her healthy house that reminds her to check the radon levels in her home once a year and record the readings.

2. Attics you can live with

Steph's attic has cotton insulation made from blue jean manufacturing trim waste. Yes, blue jeans! This cotton insulation has become popular recently as many more people are seeking a natural and environmentally healthy alternative to fiberglass and chemically-laden insulation products. This is an important part of your home's third skin.

In assessing the environmental characteristics of insulation materials, we need to consider a broad range of issues relating to the resources going into their production, manufacturing processes, pollutants given off during their lifecycle, durability, recyclability, and impact on indoor air quality.[1]

Before laying the insulation, the attic space was thoroughly cleaned by the builders with a HEPA vacuum cleaner to ensure there was no debris or contaminants. All vent pipes are properly vented to the outside of the roof so there will be no build up of moisture or household cooking smells in Steph's attic. This space was also completely sealed from the rest of the house as a further precaution.

As the space in Steph's attic is minimal, she does not use it for storage. This is also reinforced by her homeowner's manual, which recommends not polluting attic spaces by storing cans of paint, chemicals, and other hazardous material there and taking care not to disturb the insulation.

3. Big fat walls

Besides the wonderful feel of big fat walls, the timeless look, and the fabulous sound insulation properties, it's worth discussing some of the other features of Steph's walls. Lets talk about high mass walls. High mass refers to the density of the material you are building with. Exterior walls are particularly important when it comes to high mass. Whether you want your living environment to be warm or cool, once you have reached the temperature you want, high mass walls dramatically slow down any unwanted temperature change.

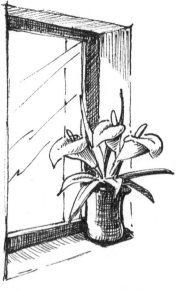

High mass walls take much less energy, mechanical equipment, and money to keep your home the way you want it.

Steph's house is built from a special wood and cement block that was developed in Europe. These blocks can be up to 12 inches thick. With a core that contains a layer of insulation called rock wool, and a hollow section for concrete to be poured into during construction. (See Appendix C.)

The end result is big fat walls that have tremendous high mass and durability. When Jane tells Steph her house feels like a castle, she's not joking. Most of us have only experienced this kind of robustness in castles, cathedrals, or old European homes. A home built this way feels like it is built to last.

The block used to build Steph's house is also known in the building industry as an Insulated Concrete Forming system, or ICF for short. But not all ICFs are created equal. I recommend avoiding ICFs made from polystyrene because of their detrimental effects on health and the environment.

A major health benefit of the wall system used in Steph's house is its ability to "breathe." Breathing in this sense means that it can take up excess indoor humidity without harming the wall and then release it as conditions change. Air can also move into and out of this medium. It's as though this wall can think for itself and it has your health and comfort in mind! Which gets back to one of the original ideas we discussed, that of our home being our third skin. Your walls are a key part in the healthy functioning of this skin.

This wall system does not require a vapor barrier either. Vapor barriers were designed to keep moisture out of buildings, but it is now clear, judging by the amount of mold found in walls constructed using vapor barriers, that they tend to trap moisture inside buildings, creating the ideal conditions for mold growth. Another feature of the block used to build Steph's walls is that it is slightly alkaline in pH, which makes it very inhospitable for mold growth or termites. In today's climate, with so many mold problems being discovered in homes, this block's mold resistant properties alone make it a superior building material.

The styrene used in polystyrene insulation is identified by the EPA as a possible carcinogen, mutagen, chronic toxin, and environmental toxin. Further, it is produced from benzene, another chemical with both environmental and health concerns.[2]

Then there is fire protection. Since the terrorist attacks of 9/11, firefighters have become extremely concerned about the extensive use of plastics such as polystyrene in construction. Plastic products can produce very toxic fumes when they burn. Steph's walls contain no plastics and therefore will not contribute to combustion or create any toxic fumes in a fire and have been given a fire rating of six hours in Europe and four hours in the U.S. (only because the U.S. does not rate materials past four hours). A fire rating means that even after a material has been exposed to fire for a certain amount of time (like six hours), it still will not burn.

Steph's house is finished with stucco on the outside and natural plaster on the inside for maximum breathability. The naturally pigmented tones of the stucco and plaster are an added aesthetic benefit to using these materials. The finished result is versatile, beautiful, and healthy.

Choosing a healthy wall system is probably one of the most important choices in building a healthy home or adding on an addition.

4. The delight of warm floors

If you have never experienced the feeling of waking on a cold winter's morning and putting your feet on a warm bedroom floor and walking warm-footed all the way to the bathroom which also has a warm floor, you have a real treat in store. There are two types of radiant floor heating. One involves heated water running through pipes usually imbedded in concrete under the floor. The other uses electrical wires that heat up from the resistance of electricity running through the wire. The first method is extremely healthy; the second method is an EMR nightmare.

Steph's house has the healthy version which uses a special form of resilient plastic pipe set in concrete. Some older versions of radiant floor heating used piping that was not very resilient and hence proved to have problems like leaks. Fortunately, new technology has created far superior products and today this kind of system is now problem-free and the best choice for health.

An added benefit of warm floors is that they are wonderful for toddlers to crawl around on or for bigger children to sit while they play and build things. Even pets love it!

Because radiant floor heating heats surfaces and not air, you are able to feel warm and comfortable and still have your windows open for fresh air — the best of both worlds. This is the benefit of designing a house right in the first place. If you have enough high mass in the walls of your house and you heat surfaces not air, an extremely comfortable indoor climate can be created that is also very energy efficient and takes very little to maintain.

As a certified reflexologist for many years, working on hundreds of pairs of feet, I have come to believe that when the feet are warm and comfortable, the whole body relaxes. Imagine a simple heating system that you don't have to think twice about, helping you to relax and reduce your stress levels! Aren't these the qualities and feelings we want our homes to provide?

Another consideration is our older family members. As people get older they often have a difficult time keeping their extremities warm. A warm floor underfoot gives them a direct experience of warmth where they need it the most, instead of having to turn a forced air heating system really high in a vain attempt to keep warm. Heated air is also very dehydrating, which can lead to severe health problems in the elderly.

You will find radiant floor heating is not only very clean but quiet too. No more listening to forced air heating switching itself on and off all night long. A radiant floor system is a closed loop contained beneath the floor so it doesn't blow dust, pollen, bacteria, and mold around the whole house. It is definitely the healthier choice for anyone who has asthma, allergies or respiratory problems. It's also good for the rest of us too!

5. Floor Coverings

When Steph discovered she had so many healthy choices for floor coverings in her new home she was eager to try as many of them out as possible. Here's what she chose:

1. For her living room she chose a specially engineered wood floor made with a maple veneer. This engineered product is much stronger and will not warp over her radiant floor heating like a regular hardwood floor might. It was also pre-finished at the factory with ultra-low VOC materials, so by the time it was installed in Steph's living room it was completely odorless, extremely durable, and gorgeous.
2. For her kitchen she chose a natural stone tile. Stone is timeless, beautiful, and durable.
3. For the master bedroom, children's bedrooms, and bathrooms she chose natural cork. Cork does not offgas or shed microfibers and is naturally moisture, mold, and rot resistant As a floor covering, cork is durable, provides acoustic and thermal insulation, cushions the foot, and is easy to clean. In addition to all of these features cork is harvested from trees in a sustainable manner.
4. For the dining room, hallways, mudroom, and other miscellaneous spaces she chose pigmented concrete in different natural tones. If you have not yet seen a naturally pigmented concrete floor you will be suitably impressed with the aesthetic look and finished result that can be achieved.
5. For her laundry she choose natural linoleum, which is made from wood and cork "flour," limestone dust, resin (from pine trees), and colorants, all mixed with linseed oil (from flax seeds) and baked onto a jute backing. An acrylic sealant is added as a topcoat. Natural linoleum is valued for its longevity and low-maintenance. Manufacturers estimate its lifespan at thirty to forty years compared with ten to twenty years for vinyl.[3]

Bamboo floors have become very popular recently. What you may not know however is that most bamboo flooring is manufactured in China and may contain nasty adhesives and finishes such as formaldehyde. Yet another example of a product you would *think* would be harmless turning out to be completely unsuitable. Formaldehyde-free bamboo is now available and definitely the best choice (see Appendix C).

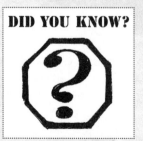

DID YOU KNOW?

Steph has no carpet in her healthy home. She has a few area and throw rugs used for decoration or some added cushion in key areas. All of them are made from natural fibers and use non-toxic dyes. The other great benefit of these rugs is how easily they can be removed and cleaned. A good shake outside is often sufficient and a little bit of sunshine helps to refresh any odors that may have sunk into them. You can also clean them with a HEPA vacuum cleaner. Some cotton throw rugs can be washed in a washing machine or the old fashioned way, in the bathtub!

6. Timeless designs and modern day functionality

When a home is designed and built to last it creates a look that is very appealing to most people. Jane commented on how Steph's home looks like one of those "timeless European" homes and feels like a castle. A lot of this is experiential. What's interesting is that when you have visited a healthy home it leaves a lasting impression. You also have something to compare other homes to. I thoroughly recommend locating and visiting a healthy home near you if you can.

The functionality of a home is another important design feature. Who is the home being built for? Who spends the most amount of time there? Do those people have any special needs? Is the home designed for a young family or a retired couple? What kind of lifestyles do the people have who live in the home? All these questions help to clarify how your home needs to function. It's time for mainstream modern designs to reflect the needs of the people again.

Recently I was working with some architects on a prototypical model of a healthy home following Building Biology principles. As I was the only female on the team it was very interesting to see the different functionality requirements we all came up with.

As a woman, a mother, a writer, and a business owner, I have many needs for my home, and I am only one member of the family. Through my eyes here are some extra functions, beyond what we have already mentioned, that I thought were important to consider when designing a healthy home:

- Mudrooms for everyone's outdoor gear, dirty shoes, and a place to wipe down a wet or muddy dog (or child), if you have one.
- A laundry room that is its own contained room with a door that can be closed and a window that can be opened. It also needs to be within easy distance from where all the laundry accumulates and away from the main "public" household spaces (see Chapter 10).
- All bathrooms and half bathrooms must have opening windows (see Chapter 8).
- There should be plenty of closet and storage space so that everything has a home.

I have found that one of the main reasons people sometimes feel overwhelmed when they first begin the journey of creating a healthy home is that they come up against how the design and functionality of where they live doesn't really work. For instance, it's quite common in modern homes today that the laundry is nothing more than a makeshift space that is fitted into a cupboard with a concertina door right off a main room like a kitchen. There is no place to sort, store, or hang clothing and if friends are coming over for the evening there is a mad dash to try and barricade the laundry door to prevent the mountain of laundry from spewing all over the kitchen floor. I'm guessing that this modern design was the

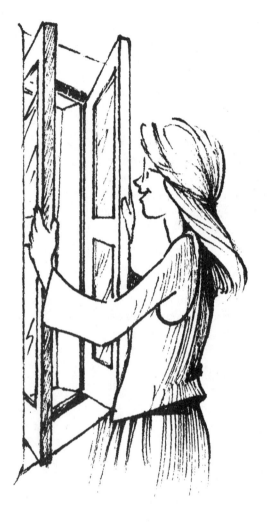

Prior to the energy crisis of the 1970s, the typical home averaged approximately one air exchange per hour. Now, in a well sealed home, the air is often exchanged only once every five hours or even less frequently, and that is not enough to ensure healthful air quality.[5]

idea of some bachelor who has his clothes dry-cleaned! No mother with a busy family can work in a situation like this without a considerable amount of stress. In the following chapters we will be addressing many challenges like this and their solutions.

7. Ventilation and natural sunlight

Many people have the misconception that air quality outside is far more polluted than indoors. Occasionally this is true, but according to the late Theron Randolph, M.D., who is considered the grandfather of environmental medicine in the U.S., "Indoor air pollution is eight to ten times more important as a source of chronic illness than ambient (outdoor) air pollution."[4] This is because exposure to indoor air pollution is constant, while outdoor air pollution comes and goes. Newborns and small children are even more susceptible to this kind of pollution. Ventilation, as in good quality fresh air, is imperative to good health.

Windows are an important feature of a healthy house. They provide light, views, ventilation, and visual character. Steph's house not only has many windows that let in lots of natural light, they are also double and triple glazed to save energy, and placed strategically for maximum natural light gain and optimum cross ventilation. Windows need to be opened on a daily basis to allow enough fresh air, oxygen, and health promoting negative ions into the home and the pollutants of daily life to be released to the outdoors. Think of your windows as part of your home's respiratory system.

Steph's house is also fitted with a special Energy recovery ventilator (ERV). In case Steph forgets to open her windows often enough or for long enough to get a healthy amount of fresh air into her home, the ERV is a simple mechanical system that does just that. It will remove polluted air and replace it with fresh, filtered outdoor air.

Here's how it works. In the winter the ERV uses warm outgoing air to heat the incoming cooler air, as well as leaving a comfortable and healthy amount of humidity inside (the incoming and outgoing air have separate compartments so that pollutants are not transferred but these compartments are close enough together that the energy can be). In the summer this process is reversed. In both seasons you get fresh air close to room temperature, combining health and comfort with energy savings. While Steph is away at work, and her windows are closed at home for security reasons, her home is being safely and efficiently ventilated. This system also filters out 95 percent of all pollens, mold spores, and dander in the incoming air while throwing all other fine particulates to the outside.

Windows are also the eyes of a home. It keeps our connection to nature and the seasons alive, which has profound effects on our sense of well- being and helps to reduce stress. Windows that look out on to some greenery are ideal. The more natural light your home lets in, the less you have to rely on artificial light and appliances. In the 1940s John Ott began studying the physical affects of light on plants and animals. This was the beginning of the modern science called photobiology. His basic idea was that light, like food and water, is vital to a healthy existence and that insufficient light, or the wrong kind, causes ill health.[6]

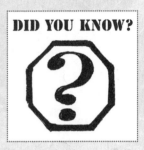

DID YOU KNOW?

A host of modern day ailments can be directly attributed to artificial l ighting-ailments such as fatigue, depression, decreased performance, diminished immunity, reduced physical fitness, and possibly impaired fertility.[7]

Exposure to artificial light, without a healthy balance of daylight, has been associated with hyperactivity, as well as changes in heart rate, blood pressure, electrical brain-wave patterns, hormonal secretions, and the body's natural cyclical rhythms.[8]

The hormone melatonin, secreted by the pineal gland in the brain during darkness or dim light, causes sleepiness; when it is overproduced through excessive exposure to dim lighting, it can indicate the clinical condition called Seasonal Affective Disorder (SAD syndrome).[9]

In Steph's house artificial lighting is used to complement natural light and so differs in each room. In her kitchen, office, workrooms, children's bedrooms, and stairways, direct lighting is used. Children's bedrooms in particular ideally need three hours of sunlight per day.[10] Their bedrooms are their workrooms and they often spend a lot of time there. In the adult bedrooms, bathrooms, and more relaxed areas of her house such as the living room, reflected and diffused lighting is used.

Visible light is made up of a spectrum of lights of different colors and wavelengths. Artificial lighting varies in its ability to provide light in the same balance of color and wavelength as natural light. Steph's house is fitted with full spectrum lighting. This contains the same balance of colors as natural sunlight, which is known to lift winter depression and improve general health. Full spectrum lighting comes in standard incandescent bulbs, reflector/flood bulbs for recessed and track lighting, and special fluorescent tubes. Steph was so impressed by the health benefits associated with full spectrum lighting that she went around her home and replaced all her older appliances, like stand up lamps and desk lamps, with the same full spectrum light bulbs. The Internet and many natural food stores carry these kinds of products now. When shopping around, do remember to choose energy-saving versions; it saves you money and the planet its resources.

8. Low EMR design

Let's start this section by recalling that electromagnetic radiation (EMR) is the more accurate term for what are often referred to as electromagnetic fields (EMF).

The basic EMR concepts were introduced and discussed in Chapter 3, from the perspective of what can go awry and where problems generally manifest. In this section we will be discussing how to do things right so that good health can prevail.

Steph's healthy home was built with what is called a low EMR design based on Building Biology guidelines. What does that mean? A low EMR design is where the electrical system for the house is designed with health in mind.

Electrical wiring for beginners

If you peel back the outer insulating plastic on typical wiring you will see three strands: one black, one white, and a third that is either green or bare copper. The black wire is called the hot wire because it draws electricity from the main panel and delivers it to light fixtures and appliances. The white wire is called the neutral wire, and it returns the electricity to the main panel after it is used. The green or bare copper wire is the ground wire and under normal circumstances it does not carry any electricity. However, if a malfunction such as a short occurs, it serves as a fail-safe protective device, carrying power back to the ground until the breaker is tripped and the power to the faulty circuit is cut off, thereby helping to prevent shock or electrocution. When the electrical system is functioning properly, the amount of electricity flowing out to appliances through the hot wire is equal to the amount flowing back through the neutral wire. This equal and opposite flow of current through the wires creates a net current of zero, which is the desired condition. When, for various reasons, unequal supply and return currents are unable to cancel each other out, a net current is present and a magnetic field is automatically created. This is where EMRs can start to affect our health.

The fundamental point is that if a house is wired properly during construction, according to the National Electric Code of the U.S., there will be no net current. This is also what I call "healthy."

The low EMR design in Steph's home began with an extensive list of specifications that were given to the electrician during construction. It then became his responsible to install the electrical system according to these specifications all the way through to having his worked tested and verified upon completion to ensure there were no errors. These specifications are too extensive to cover in their entirety here, but a few of the main features will be outlined to add to your basic understanding of what a healthy electrical system involves.

Some of the main points of a low EMR design

1. The incoming power supply for the home and the main electrical panel containing all the breakers for the different electrical circuits need to be located away from bedrooms and areas of the home where people spend good amounts of time. They can give out strong AC electric and AC magnetic fields. The best location is against an exterior wall in a garage where no one spends much time.

2. The main electric panel is laid out in a cohesive, easily accessible, easily testable format.[11] This reduces magnetic fields and makes future maintenance much easier.

3. By grouping the entry point of all utilities and providing proper bonding and grounding, any net current traveling through public utility lines will be shunted back without ever entering the home.[12]

4. All wiring in walls is shielded in metal conduit or metal flex cable and is connected to the grounding system to eliminate electric fields.

5. Because electricity will follow all available paths, metal plumbing, gas lines, cable TV lines, and telephone lines can become pathways for uninvited net current. It is therefore prudent to take simple precautions to prevent such an occurrence where site conditions allow. For example, metallic water pipes are often used as a grounding system for the electrical system in homes. If this is the case and neighbors' water pipes are also metallic and used as the grounding systems for their homes, then a neutral electrical current path will be created. This allows the electricity in neighbors' homes to affect your home and can subsequently increase your AC electric and AC magnetic field levels every time your neighbor uses an appliance. A dialectic union is a plastic joint that acts as an insulator, preventing the passage of electricity between conductive materials, such as your metal water pipes and your neighbors'. These can be easily installed where code permits, resolving the above problem. Non-metallic water pipes do not have this problem.

6. All bedrooms have "kill switches" installed. A kill switch is designed to cut off the electricity and thereby any fields in any given run of wiring. Power is not usually required during the hours of sleep. It is especially beneficial to eliminate all fields from the bedroom at night because the presence of high electric fields is most commonly associated with sleep disturbances[13] and may cause long-term health risks for sensitive individuals (see Chapter 7).

All of the above specifications were completed before Steph moved into her house. May we never know what health problems have been prevented for her and her family! All that remains to complete the low EMR design for Steph's house is for her to study her homeowner's manual to learn about the sources of AC electric and AC magnetic fields created by her own house appliances. This will be covered in more detail in part two of the book where we will focus on specific rooms.

Continual exposure to extremely low frequency (ELF) EMRs in homes can be associated with high blood pressure, nervousness, and disturbed sleep.[14]

In the UK it has been estimated that as many as one third of the population may be suffering adverse reactions to ELFs at one time or another. Research in the UK has also found that certain low frequencies act as a trigger for allergies and cause sickness, headaches, nausea, sweating, and other unpleasant reactions.[15]

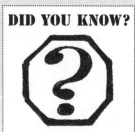

DID YOU KNOW?

Sweden has set limits for certain types of electric and magnetic field exposure; the U.S. government has not. The long-term consequences of these exposures are still being debated in this country. Millions of Americans are now unknowingly enrolled in a long-term experiment upon themselves!

Recent epidemiological studies have linked elevated risk of childhood leukemia to exposures as low and as common as 4 milligauss of AC magnetic field strength.[16]

9. Water: the elixir of life

Our health is completely dependent upon a good supply of fresh, clean water. We can survive for weeks without food but for only a few days without water. Most of us take water for granted. We expect to turn on a tap, a shower, or our washing machine and water to be right there in abundance. We also expect the water we drink and cook with to be safe for consumption. But times are changing. All of us must now think in terms of being our own EPA and assuring the quality and safety of the water in our own home. We also need to think in terms of sustainability and reducing the burden that we each place on this already overstrained resource.

In our industrialized country little or no pure water is freely available. Today's water supplies are increasingly polluted with air contaminants, agricultural and industrial chemical residues, seepage from landfills, accidental chemical spills, prescription drugs and antibiotics, and caffeine. Our water is constantly being re-used and is in limited supply —

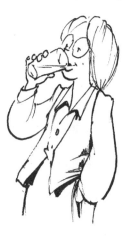

what goes down must come back up. (Chapter 3 discussed municipally treated water in more detail.)

Further contaminants can be added to your water when it is transported to your home and then through it. Common plastic pipes can leave unhealthy deposits such as zinc, cadmium, lead, styrene and also chlorine, phenol, nitrate, and other microorganisms. Copper pipes can also leach very high levels of copper into the water. Then there are problems associated with the use of water softeners using phosphates, sodium, and ion exchangers.[17]

Ultimately, we must restore the purity of our water by dealing directly with the sources of toxins in our global environment. In the meantime, we must take the matter into our own hands and protect our home environments by installing whole house and point of use water filtration systems.

What should be removed from drinking water?

1. Chlorine and chlorine by-products (trihalomethanes, chloroform).
2. Lead, aluminum, mercury, and other metals.
3. Pesticides, herbicides, organic chemicals.
4. Fluoride, viruses, parasites and chlorine-resistant protozoan cysts (*cryptosporidium* and *giardia*).
5. VOCs, SOCs, MTBE, perchlorate and solvents.

Steph's house came with a fully installed whole house carbon block water filtration system and an additional specialized unit attached to the kitchen tap for further point of use drinking and cooking water. These units were chosen based on the results of a water test done during construction. There are many kinds of filtration systems available today and only when you know what contaminants are in your water can you identify which methods will work best to provide safe and healthy water for your family's needs. The most popular methods available are carbon block, distillation, reverse osmosis, ion exchange, granular carbon systems, and KDF-55 or KDF-85 with carbon systems.

Steph's homeowner's manual also recommends that she always run the water out of her kitchen tap in the morning for a couple of minutes before using it for drinking or cooking, to run off the water that has been standing still (steeping) in the pipes during the night. The manual also recommends checking drinking water once a year for microbes and other hazardous constituents.

> The average American family uses about 220 gallons of water a day. That's about twice the average consumption for a family in Europe.[18]

Where does our water go?

As important as the quality of our water is the quantity we consume. Although the surface of the planet is mainly comprised of water, most of this is salt seawater or ice. Only about three percent is available fresh water and it is on this minute fraction that we and most other species depend. Wasting water is actually another form of pollution.

With this knowledge in mind Steph's house was built with several water-conserving devices such as low-flush toilets, water-saving shower heads, and a water-efficient dishwasher already in place.

10. Formaldehyde-free cabinets, doors and built-ins

All Steph's cabinetry, doors, and built-ins are made from wheat board that is free of synthetic formaldehyde instead of from particleboard. Wheat board is strong and tremendously versatile. With a healthy veneer on top it can be used to create beautiful doors and designer fixtures such as kitchen cabinets, bedroom closets, bathroom cabinets, door trim, skirting boards, and furniture. It's also a rapidly renewable resource. By eliminating all particleboard, which is one of the main culprits in the toxic "new house" smell, from day one Steph's new home had no noxious smells.

11. Detached garages

Steph's garage is detached from her house. It is located behind her home and connects to a quiet alleyway for entry and exit. When the garage door is opened, an exhaust fan installed in her garage is also triggered and runs for the next thirty minutes after the garage door is closed. A covered walkway connects the garage to the back door of her home, which enters into a little mudroom. As the name implies, this is where everyone leaves their muddy boots and outdoor clothes.

This design accomplishes several different things in a simple and effective way:

1. Exhaust fumes are well away from the living space.
2. The additional fan installed in the garage ensures further elimination of residual exhaust fumes after cars leave or after cars return and are cooling down.
3. The noise of garage doors and car engines starting cannot be heard inside the home.
4. Parking at the rear of homes allows the front gardens and sidewalks to be clear and safe for children playing.
5. The covered walkway provides protection from the elements between the garage and entering the home.
6. The mudroom is an excellent collection point to catch any grime and pollution from everyone's daily activities and prevent it from entering the rest of the home.

If you are designing a new home and for some reason you must have an attached garage, for example due to the size or shape of your lot, then here is another design possibility that will get better health benefits than a conventional design:

1. Still try to situate the garage to the rear of the house for the benefits mentioned above.
2. If there is a room above the garage, do not place any windows above the garage door opening; instead face them away from the garage so that car exhaust will not flow in through them.
3. Still install the extractor fan in the garage on a timer device.
4. Do not have a connecting door from the garage directly into the home. Instead have a door that connects from the garage to the outside and then a separate door that connects into the house from the outdoors. This prevents exhaust contamination from getting into the whole house.
5. Make sure mechanicals and electrical main panels are not placed on or close to a garage wall that connects to the rest of the house. These can create EMRs that can pass into your home through the connecting wall and affect people spending time in the room next to the garage. The same applies to a room above the garage.

6. It will be doubly important that the garage is maintained in the healthy ways outlined in Chapter 13, as an attached garage must be considered part of the household living space.

12. Central vacuum system

Another special feature of Steph's healthy home is that it came with a central vacuum system (CVS) already installed. Even though Steph does not have wall-to-wall carpet, floor surfaces still need to be kept clean. Damp mopping is one way to clean her floors but when used in combination with her central vacuum, cleaning is simple, very efficient, and non-toxic. Here's how a central vacuum system works. The vacuum along with its large collection bag are located outside the living space in a garage or separate mechanical room. The vacuum is connected to a piping system concealed under floors, within walls, or in the attic, ending in each room of the house at a covered outlet. To vacuum, you simply insert a long, flexible hose into the room outlet, attach the appropriate head for cleaning and vacuum as usual. All dirt and debris are sucked up and directed to the central collection bag and all exhaust air is vented to the outside of the home. Simple and clean.

13. Finishes

And finally, all finishes in Steph's house, which includes all surface materials and treatments such as paints, stains, adhesives, and sealants, are no or low-VOC and non-toxic. Finishes are the predominant source of odors in a new home and can release toxic VOCs into the air indefinitely after the home is completed unless non-toxic products are used. As an added precaution, the builders in Steph's house were instructed to keep the windows open while these last, non-toxic finishes were applied to ensure the removal of any traces of VOCs. There is so much more choice available today for no or low VOC products, which allows you to beautify your home while protecting your family's health.

Side effects from living in a healthy home

None of this is rocket science. Steph's home was designed and built with health in mind following Building Biology principles. It is beautiful, simple and undeniably *feels* very different than a conventionally built new home. I once visited a home that had originally been built from healthy materials and systems and then the owners some years later decided to do an addition to their home. For some strange reason they allowed the addition to be built from conventional building products with all the inherent toxic chemicals. Visiting this home was a profound experience. Even though the addition had been tastefully designed and furnished, no one in the family ever used the space. No one had any specific reason why, they just preferred being in the original section of the house.

At the end of the day, wouldn't you rather live in a home that you know is supporting your family's health and not harming it? As a consumer you have a lot of power to shape the future face of the building industry by demanding that homes be safe and healthy for all of us who live in them.

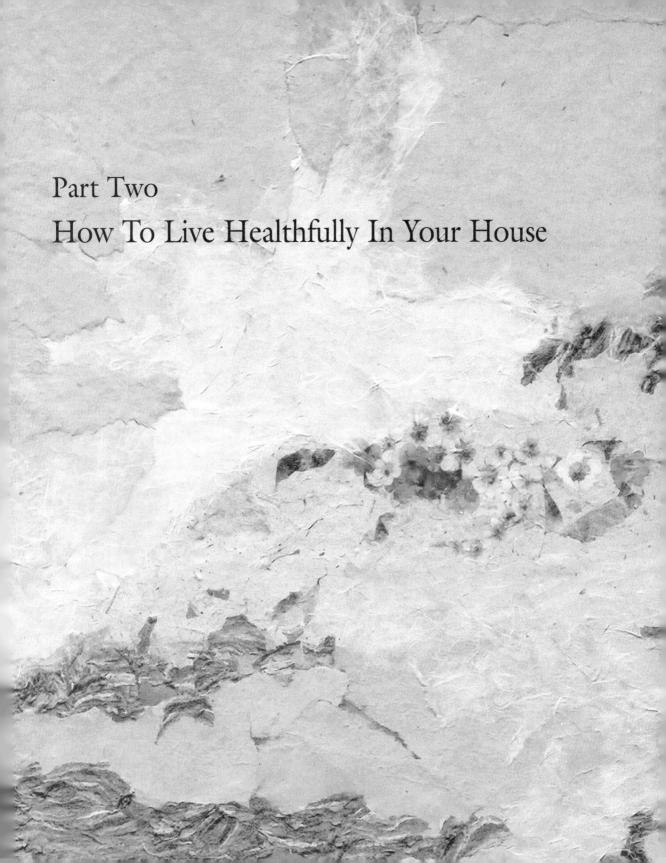

Part Two
How To Live Healthfully In Your House

CHAPTER 6

Environmental Health at Home

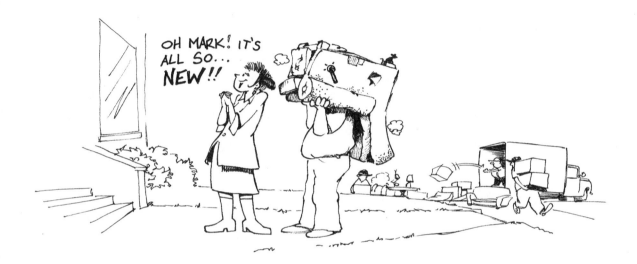

It's a bright Saturday morning as Liz and Mark drive their huge rental truck up the driveway of their brand new home. Liz has been dreaming of this day for months. She leaps out of the truck and squeals in delight as she runs to the front door. Mark dramatically sweeps Liz off her feet and carries her over the threshold.

Moments later the doorbell rings, echoing loudly around the house and startling Liz and Mark out of their celebratory embrace in the master bedroom.

"Who could that be? We haven't lived here two minutes yet!" Mark says.

"Oh, I bet it's the guys delivering the new furniture," Liz yells, already downstairs racing to the front door.

Mark looks out of the bedroom window to see for himself who it is. "That better not be all our furniture they're unloading."

Outside the scene is rather like some cartoon movie of a magical truck that has an unending stream of furniture being unloaded. In the midst of all this, two additional cars pull up in front of the house from which Liz's sister Jane, her husband Bob, their two sons Tom and Jack, and the dog promptly unload, followed in the other car by Uncle Joe.

"Right, where do you want us?" Bob asks as he rolls up his sleeves.

"I brought my tools in case we need a handyman around here," enthuses Uncle Joe, shaking a hammer above his head.

Mac the dog promptly pees on the front porch to claim his territory, Jack begins jumping up and down on the new sofa sitting on the driveway, and Tom disappears into the house without taking his muddy shoes off.

Liz looks around in slow motion recognizing the lost moment of celebration, now replaced by chaos.

As the new furniture continues to disappear inside the house, Mark opens their large rental truck ready to unload the items they brought with them.

"Blimey, is that your stuff too?" Uncle Joe declares with disbelief.

Mark throws his hands up in the air, "Liz wouldn't part with anything from the last house. I told her we didn't need all this stuff."

"Excuse me, that is not all my stuff. Who's the one with all the old vinyl Beatles albums, and all those tools for the gazillion hobbies you have?" retorts Liz appearing suddenly around the side of the truck.

"Those Beatles albums are worth a fortune and those tools have made you some pretty nice gifts over the years, I'll have you remember."

The tension is broken by Bob. "Well, let's get it inside shall we? Come on Uncle Joe, give us a hand with this table."

For the remainder of the morning and most of the afternoon, they carry a steady stream of household items inside the house. Tables, chairs, suitcases of clothes, plastic bags full of shoes, plants, a humidifier, and many boxes stuffed with miscellaneous items some of which have strange smells.

"You've got enough pesticides here to keep away any bug in a five mile radius!" Bob exclaims.

"A man's got to do what a man's got to do," says Mark in a menacing voice, as he pulls a golf club out of the bag he is carrying and takes a powerful swing at a tiny dandelion trying to grow on his new lawn. Satisfied he's made his point he continues, "Just put that stuff in the garage, would you."

Inside the house, a very pregnant Jane is unloading items from a box marked "Kitchen."

"Really Liz, I don't know why you've kept most of this stuff. I mean, look at all the new stuff you've bought."

"Well you never know when you might need it. You know me, I hate throwing things away. Anyway, this house is so big it could fit all your stuff and all my stuff combined," Liz enthuses.

"That, Liz, is a very scary thought!" The girls break into laughter.

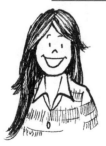

Commentary

We are now entering the second section of the book. Let's shift our focus from the structure of your home and how it has been built to how you live in your home. Regardless of whether you have a new or old home, a large or small home, a fancy or simple home, it can be shocking to realize how we all pollute our own homes on a daily basis. Sometimes our most conscientious attempts to keep our homes clean and pleasing to our senses create the most amazing health nightmares. Fortunately, help is at hand!

We are about to discuss every room in the home in a systematic way, to pinpoint possible sources of health hazards so they can be eliminated or at least reduced. That is my idea of prevention! From this point forward you are all empowered to be Ace Detectives in your own home. As we move from room to room, consider the information presented and then use your eyes, your nose, and your intuition and see what you can find in your own home. Make some changes and see if you notice any improvements. Some improvements might be seen or felt immediately, some may take up to a few months for the body to adjust itself back towards health. You have nothing to lose and possibly everything to gain. Now those are the kind of odds I like!

> "To understand the man, we have to understand his world, the environment he lives in."
> — Aristotle (c. 384-322 BC).

Living in our homes

Living in a home today is a complex dynamic. For simplicity, let's break it down into three sections:

1. Moving into your new home.
2. Setting up your world.
3. Cleaning and maintaining your home.

Be sure to read each section, as you will discover that its information actually translates into many other areas of your life at home. For example, "Moving In" refers not only to moving into a new home, but moving in to any place that you have not lived in before. Even if you are not moving anywhere, we all seem to purchase new things for our home on a regular basis. In this respect, something new is regularly moving in with you!

1. Moving in

Imagine a new home. Let's assume it's a healthy home like Steph's that is empty and ready for the new owners to move in. You have the best possible start to living in a healthy home. Surely that's the end of the story? Actually it's not. What happens next opens up many new dimensions to consider. You see, what happens next is that the owner moves in!

We have all seen or experienced a scenario similar to Liz and Bob's. The new owners arrive with truckloads of items from their last home. Beds, sofas, tables, chairs, TVs, stereos, lamps, clothes, appliances, everything from the last garage or garden shed and on and on. Unfortunately, most people don't realize that all of these items have a history and each item has the power to affect the health of your new home. Let's look at some examples from Liz and Mark's home:

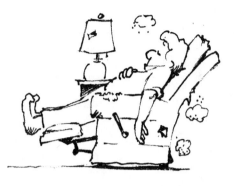

1. Mark's favorite old chair, which is stuffed with synthetic foam, is slowly disintegrating and releases fine particulates of foam and dust into the air every time he sits in it.
2. Several of Liz and Mark's framed pictures have mold on the back of them from hanging on a damp wall in their previous home. These mold spores are so tiny they cannot be seen with the naked eye. All these spores need now are the right conditions, moisture, and food, and away they will go silently multiplying and growing.
3. Liz recently acquired an antique dresser and plans to put it in her new bedroom as a feature item. However, what Liz does not know is that the dresser was previously stored in the antique shop's storage facility where pesticides are routinely sprayed to "prevent" pest problems. Her lovely dresser is invisibly impregnated with pesticide residues that may be released into the air in her bedroom and onto the skin of anyone who touches it.
4. Liz and Mark's pillows and quilt are full of dust mites.
5. Their trusty humidifier that comes out each winter contains mold from being inadequately maintained and stored while still damp.

Another scenario is where the owners go out and buy everything new for their new home, which Liz did as well. In this case a multitude of potent chemicals are introduced into the home environment all at once. The combination of all these chemicals interacting with each other creates a chemical soup that bathes and surrounds everyone.

Here are some more examples:

1. New furniture such as beds, desks, side tables, sofas, and children's furniture are often made of pressed wood such as particleboard, which contains formaldehyde. Don't be fooled by the veneer you see; many products are not made from solid wood.
2. Cushioned furniture like sofas, chairs, and beds are often made of synthetic polyurethane foam derived from petrochemicals. Fabric covers can be made from acrylic, polyester, or polyvinyl chloride fibers, which are also petrochemically derived and can have additional fire retardants, antimicrobial agents, and dyes containing heavy metals. These chemicals will continue to offgass into the air you breathe for some time as well as attach themselves to you every time you come in contact with them.
3. New stereos, computers, and electrical equipment contain plastics and glues, which can offgass for some time.

4. Curtains, tablecloths and designer fabrics often contain sizing chemicals to give them that new look, and those advertised as "permanent press" contain formaldehyde.

So what do you do? Do you go the old way or the new way? Here's what I recommend.

Something old

If you are moving old stuff in, this is an excellent opportunity to get rid of things you no longer need or use. Get everyone in the family to participate. When a whole family moves, the total volume of items can be massive. Inspect all your furniture and appliances for damp patches, moldy smells, or things that have become impregnated with smells from cooking or fragranced products. Sometimes leaving these things outdoors for a while in the sunshine will help to naturally deodorize them, but sunshine will not get rid of toxics like pesticide residues. If you do discover any questionable items, this is a good time to remove them from your household inventory. If something is spoiled or possibly contaminated, be sure to dispose of these things appropriately, which may mean calling your local recycling center or household hazardous waste facility for guidance.

I know this is hard news for those of you who are "save-a-holics" and like keeping everything, or disturbing news for those of you who are ardent recyclers and like to pass everything on. I'm an avid recycler too! I hate wasting things or adding to our burgeoning landfills and I love it when I can find a new home for something my family no longer needs or uses. But consider this: if you go to a garage sale or a second-hand store looking for a bargain, don't you assume those items are safe for you to take home and that they won't be hazardous to your health? That some other child's toy is going to be safe for your child to play with? That someone else's table or bed does not contain toxic pesticide residues from a home that has been fumigated for pests?

Americans are producing more waste with each passing year. Over the past 30 years, the waste produced in this country has more than doubled, from 88 million tons in 1960 to about 225 million tons in 2000. Today, the average American generates 4.4 pounds of trash every day. That's 1.7 pounds more trash than the average American produced in 1960.[1]

Well, this applies to you too if you are the one passing things on. Are your things safe for someone else? Anything that is questionable, err on the side of precaution and dispose of it in a way that won't pose a threat to someone else's health.

If, after reading this, you are now concerned about an item of furniture you bought at a garage sale or a second hand store yourself, you can have those items tested by an environmental inspector. If testing proves too expensive, then a precautionary measure might mean getting rid of a questionable piece of furniture or at the very least putting it in a part of the house where people don't spend a lot of time. Definitely don't put anything like this in someone's bedroom. Remember, we spend a third of our lives in our bedrooms.

If you have used pesticides yourself in your home, or employed a professional exterminator company to fumigate your home to get rid of a pest problem, then you can be quite certain your furniture and furnishings will contain some pesticide residues. If you have had a moisture problem because of a burst pipe, leaky roof, or faulty drain and did not have the problem fixed by a certified microbial remediation contractor, then your furniture or furnishings could be contaminated with mold and microscopic spores. So think twice about what's really moving in to your new home.

One advantage of older furniture is that it will at least have offgassed most of its new toxic VOCs, or if its really old, may not contain any at all. Wiping things down with either a damp cloth or warm soapy water is also a good way to remove dust and grime. Be sure to dry things properly though. If you suspect you may have a mold problem, some things are easier to deal with yourself, like soaking your humidifier in hot, soapy water and drying it thoroughly. Some things, like larger pieces of furniture that smell moldy, may need to be retired and got rid of. Vacuuming items such as sofas, beds, and throw rugs with a HEPA vacuum cleaner before you bring them into the house is another good idea.

Something new

If you are bringing in new items, be sure to choose ones that are made from natural materials and are non-toxic. Depending on your personal preference and budget there are lots of choices . Check "Appendic C: Sources and Resources" or do a little research yourself and you will be pleasantly surprised by what is now available.

If you have to bring something new into your home that smells strongly, try to let it offgass outside for a few days before bringing it in. If your sense of smell is not very strong, have someone else check it for you.

It's worth mentioning here that letting things offgass in the garage can create its own problems. It's common sense really when you think about it. Car exhaust fumes themselves contain all kinds of toxic combustion by-products, as we have already discussed in Chapters 3 and 5. These byproducts will readily deposit themselves onto anything in the garage, including any furniture you are airing out and want to bring back into the house later. Outside in the fresh air is best. Ideal places are under protected overhangs like roofs or balconies. If you don't have such a place and need to protect your furniture from the changing elements outdoors you can

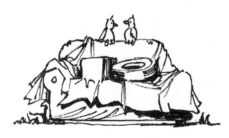

always rig a makeshift tarpaulin canopy, like when camping, over the top of everything. Just make sure there is enough open space to let air circulate.

Pay attention after you move your new things in. Notice any smells that occur or any change in your general health such as not sleeping as well, headaches, or cranky children. These could be indications of some problematic item that needs to be discovered and removed. Don't try to mask strange smells with synthetic air fresheners: you are just introducing more chemicals. The best approach is to find the source and fix it.

2. Setting up your world

Hand-in-hand with moving in goes setting up our world. Everything has to be put somewhere. Many people don't have any specific criteria for how they set their home up. It may have to be done quickly without much thought; it may be done intuitively based on what feels right; it may be done logically based on furniture that can only fit in certain places; or it may have been done following the principles of Feng Shui, the Chinese art of placement.

There is also a Building Biology way of setting up your home for the purposes of creating a truly healthy environment based on science. This is what we will be discussing room by room in the chapters to follow. Each chapter will have specific advice and tips for you to begin immediately transforming that particular space into a healthy environment.

Sometimes I get asked if Building Biology is the same as Feng Shui. No, it is not.

Feng Shui

Feng Shui is a fascinating subject with its roots in ancient China. Ancient texts indicate Feng Shui is at least 2,500 years old, with additional reports indicating it could be 3,000-4,000 years old. There are several different schools of Feng Shui; the most popular in North America are called Compass School and Tibetan Black Hat Sect school. The basic premise of the Compass School is that "direction" and building age influence a building which then affects us. The direction your home faces and where you place your furnishings will affect the flow of energy or "Qi" in your home. The Tibetan Black Hat School does not consider direction, but uses a "bagua" template that is ruled by the placement of the front door. Both schools also consider colors and shapes. These factors combine and can have positive or negative effects on the occupants.

Building Biology is a practical science that focuses on the effects which toxic chemicals, air and water quality, and EMR pollution have on our health. All of these can be measured. However, when Feng Shui was developed over 2,500 years ago people did not have microwave ovens, televisions, high tension power lines, cell phones, computers, toxic building materials, and the plethora of modern day items we now consider essential, so none of this was incorporated into the Feng Shui philosophy.

I have been in several homes that have been arranged following Feng Shui principles and found significant health problems from a Building Biology perspective. For instance, in Feng Shui you may be advised to place the head of your bed against a certain wall so it faces a particular direction to enhance the beneficial flow of "Qi" when you sleep at night. However, from a Building Biology standpoint this ignores

EMR, which affects health and is measurable. A Building biologist will always ask, what is on the other side of the wall where the head of the bed is placed and take measurements of AC electric and AC magnetic fields. There could be a refrigerator, TV, computer, or electrical main panel creating a large AC magnetic field, which easily penetrates the wall and then bathes your head in a large field all night long having a significant negative impact on your health. In Building Biology we would advise you to move your bed from this location.

I believe a blend of both approaches can be very helpful. However, if a conflict should ever arise over the placement of something significant like a bed where we spend important regenerative time, I would recommend deferring to the Building Biology recommendation first and working with the more subtle energies of Feng Shui afterwards.

3. Cleaning and maintaining your home

Once you have moved in, taking care to bring in only healthy or non-toxic furniture and furnishings, and you have set up your world following Building Biology principles, the last frontier to discuss is how you clean and maintain your home. The last two chapters focus entirely on this information. Cleaning and maintaining your home is like bathing your children and making sure they have cleaned behind the ears and are cleaning their teeth properly twice a day, every day. If these things are not monitored, problems are inevitable down the road. So too with your home. Many of the problems we are discussing in this book start with tiny seeds of neglect or a lack of understanding.

The good news is that you have a lot of control over this aspect of your home. You choose your cleaning supplies and you maintain your home. Even if you bring in other professionals to clean or fix things in your home, you still get to choose who you employ. It can be a profound experience to reconnect with caring for your home in this way. It creates a relationship that many people are too busy to experience today. Yet when you consider that your home is its own living organism and an important member of your family, this is a relationship we cannot afford to ignore.

Get your family involved

Hopefully along the way you will recruit other family members to get involved and be enthusiastic about contributing to everyone's health at home. I would like to acknowledge the efforts of all the fathers, grandparents, and extended family members who are actively involved in raising our children and caring for our homes. Every positive contribution to this effort makes a difference.

"Will you teach your children what we have taught our children? That the earth is our mother? What befalls the earth befalls all the children of the earth." Attributed to Chief Seattle.

Let's reinstate our children as our apprentices and help them learn early on in life the importance and the "how to" of living healthfully at home. Let's raise them knowing that using pesticides in and around their home can severely damage their health. Let's teach them to roll their bedding back each morning, open their bedroom window, and air their bedroom out. Let's tell them about the importance of fresh air, clean water, organic food, and the invisible polluters such as EMRs. Make it fun and acknowledge everyone's victories along the way. Think up rewards for all your efforts. Probably the biggest reward is the peace of mind you will have knowing that you are actively doing all you can to safeguard your family's health. The steady stream of little victories in your home leads to a very personal kind of inspiration, the kind that can move mountains, or a government, or a whole industry over time and get the bigger job done too!

Before our adventure begins, let's start by taking the *Healthy Home Quiz* to evaluate the current health of your family and home.

> "Illnesses do not come upon us from out of the blue. They are developed from the small daily sins against nature. When enough sins have been accumulated, illnesses will suddenly appear."
> — Hippocrates (460-377 BC).

The Healthy Home Quiz

The results of your quiz will help you identify and focus on areas that might need a little improvement. The quiz can be revisited at any time to evaluate improvements and recognize any benefits gained in your family's health. Recognizing these small, consistent improvements encourages us to keep going until we achieve the greater health gains we all hope for.

It's time to put on your detective hat and take a closer look at your home and surrounding environment! All you need is this book, a pencil, and a couple of extra sheets of blank paper. Involving your children can be a lot of fun and educational at the same time. Start by writing down the date you take this quiz. This creates a baseline of your home and family's health before you make any changes. You can take the whole quiz at one time or do it in sections.

Next, sketch a rough outline of your home's floor plan, showing interior walls, doorways, and windows, and name each room. This will serve as your map and whenever you discover something that needs further investigation or attention, mark that location with an "X." You may want to tape your map into the back of this book so you can always find it.

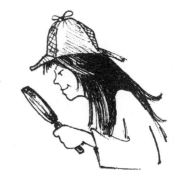

Take the quiz again at six months, after you have made some improvements, and again at twelve months, and note any further improvements. The amount of time you invest in this detective work will reap huge rewards. This quiz has been specially designed to show you the many everyday things that impact your health at home.

Pay particular attention to the health questionnaire and note everyone's health improvements along the way. It's amazing how much you can accomplish over the course of a year.

Date of first quiz_____

Date of six month quiz_____

Date of twelve month quiz_____

Your Home

When was your home built?

❏ Before 1970   ❏ Don't know

❏ After 1970   ❏ It's new

Problem: Homes built before 1970 probably contain lead paint and asbestos, both of which are serious health hazards. If your home is new you may have high levels of VOCs and toxic chemicals.

Solution: If you suspect you have lead or asbestos in your home you should have it tested by a professional. See Chapter 4. Only a trained professional should be allowed to remove these materials from your home. New homes need lots of ventilation to reduce levels of VOCs. See Chapters 3 and 5.

Remodels or Home Improvements

Have you remodeled, added any extensions or done any home improvements in the last 2 years? List any changes:

_____
_____
_____
_____
_____
_____
_____
_____
_____

Problem: New building materials and products can introduce large amounts of VOCs and toxic chemicals into your home as well as disturb older building materials that may be moldy or release fine particulate matter into the air you breathe.

Solution: If you have made changes in the last few years ventilate your home by opening windows daily and use an HEPA air filter that can trap particulates and has an added carbon filter for gases. See Chapter 17.

Water Damage

Has your home ever had any water damage such as burst water pipes, leaking roof, or faulty drains? List any occurrences and their dates:

_____

_____

Problem: Water damage can quickly result in mold growth.
Solution: Locate and fix any water damage within 24 hours to prevent mold problems.

Insulation

What kind of insulation does your home have? If you don't know then look in your attic, basement and crawl space.

_____

_____

Problem: Insulation can contain toxic chemicals like formaldehyde or fine particulates that can get into the air you breathe and cause lung and skin irritation.
Solution: If you have fiberglass insulation make sure it is covered and not bare. If your insulation contains toxic chemicals try to ventilate any fumes to the outdoors and make sure these fumes do not escape into any family living space.

Water

How old is your plumbing?

_____

_____

Problem: Older homes may have lead pipes. Lead gets in your drinking water and is a serious contaminant.
Solution: Have your water pipes replaced.

What are your water pipes made from?

_____

_____

Problem: Old copper pipes use lead solder to join seams. Lead gets in your drinking water. See Chapter 9.
Solution: Have copper pipes soldered with a non-toxic, lead-free alternative.
Where does your water come from?

❐ Municipality   ❐ Own private well   ❐ Well water

Problem: Municipal water may only be monitored for a small spectrum of contaminants and may not be checked for industrial by-products or pesticide residues. Well water needs to be monitored thoroughly too. If you have your own well, it's your responsibility to have your water checked for a thorough spectrum of contaminants. See Chapters 3 and 9.
Solution: Whole house water filtration, maintained regularly, is essential. If you have a well that has problematic organisms you will have to deal with these first before filtering your water.

Do you filter your water?

❷ Yes   ❷ No

Problem: Water today can be highly contaminated with a wide variety of substances.
Solution: Invest in a water filtration system for your whole house. See Chapter 9.

If you filter your water what method do you use?

    ❷ Whole house filtration system
    ❷ Kitchen unit attached to faucet for drinking and cooking
    ❷ Standing jug that you manually fill as needed for drinking and cooking
    ❷ Shower filters

Problem: Different systems have different filtering efficiencies. Some offer very little protection.
Solution: Have your water tested so you can decide which system will best suit your family's needs. See Chapter 9.

Have you had your drinking water tested for lead, other heavy metals, industrial chemicals, and pesticide residues?

❷ Yes   ❷ No

Problem: Never assume your municipal water is safe from all contaminants. Water can become polluted as it travels from your municipality into your home.
Solution: The only way to really know what's in the water you are drinking and bathing in at home is to take a sample from your own kitchen tap and have it thoroughly tested. See Chapter 9.

Crawl Space
Do you have a crawl space under your house?

❷ Yes   ❷ No

If yes, what does your crawl space contain? List any items you find:

_____

_____

_____

_____

Problem: Crawl spaces can contain construction debris, rodents, leftover cans of old paint, pesticides, mold, and other miscellaneous things that can damage your house and your health.

Solution: Clear out crawl spaces and dispose of hazardous materials appropriately. If you discover mold or rodents, have a qualified environmental inspector come out and design a plan to resolve the problem without introducing toxic chemicals.

Basement

What kind of basement do you have?

- ❑ Finished basement used by family members
- ❑ Unfinished basement used by family members
- ❑ Unfinished basement not used by family members
- ❑ No basement

Problem: Basements can have radon problems, moisture/ventilation problems, and be one of the most neglected parts of the house that family members use.

Solutions: Rethink your basement. Make sure it's safe for the purposes it's being used for. See Chapter 11.

Radon

Have you ever checked your home for radon?

❑ Yes   ❑ No

If yes, when was the last time?

_____

Radon levels should be checked annually. Is it time for you to test again?

_____

If no, purchase a radon kit, perform the test (see Chapter 11) and record the date and results here:

_____

_____

_____

_____

Problem: Radon is a serious health hazard in the home.
Solution: If you detect high radon levels, see Chapters 3, 5 and 11.

Pesticides

Do you use pesticides inside your home?

❑ Yes ❑ No

List any pesticide products you use in your home:

_____

_____

Problem: Pesticides are designed to kill. They are now found in many common household products from ant sprays to antibacterial soaps to antimicrobial coatings on shower curtains and rubber gloves.
Solution: Be rigorous in your detective work and read labels. Remove anything containing pesticides and find non-toxic alternatives. See Chapters 6 and 14.

Heating/Cooling System

What kind of heating and cooling systems do you have?

❑ Radiant floor heating (heated water)
❑ Radiant floor heating (heating electrical wires)
❑ Forced air heating
❑ Electric baseboard heating
❑ Space heaters
❑ Portable electric heaters
❑ Air conditioner
❑ Swamp cooler
❑ Electric fan
❑ Other

Problem: Some heating and cooling options are more hazardous to health than others.
Solution: If you are building a new house, choose the healthiest option. If you already have a system installed, regular and thorough maintenance is essential. See Chapters 3, 5 and 17.
What fuel does your heating system run on?

❑ Gas
❑ Oil
❑ Electric
❑ Other

Problem: Leaks and electrical faults may occur.
Solution: Have these systems checked at least once a year.
Does your furnace have a humidifier attached to it?

❑ Yes ❑ No

Problem: Humidifiers can become mold breeding grounds.
Solution: Check this system regularly and keep it clean.

Does your heating system have a filter?

☐ Yes   ☐ No

If yes, what kind of filter does it use and how often do you change it?

_____

_____

Problem: If filters are not maintained properly they can't clean the air flowing through them.
Solution: Upgrade to a HEPA pleated media filter and make a note to change them, whether they look dirty or not, every two to three months. See Chapter 17.

If you have forced air heating, when was the last time you had your ductwork professionally cleaned?

_____

_____

_____

Problem: Ductwork needs to be cleaned professionally on a regular basis; otherwise you can have a merry-go-round of dust, particulates, mold spores, dander, dust mites, and pollen.
Solution: If family members have asthma and allergies, you may need to have your ductwork professionally cleaned once a year. As a general rule of thumb, a thorough professional cleaning every two to three years should be enough as long as you are using HEPA filters and replacing them every two to three months.

If you have a cooling system such as an air conditioner or swamp cooler when was the last time it was maintained?

_____

_____

_____

Gas
Do you have any gas appliances such as a stove, dryer or water heater? List:

_____

_____

_____

_____

Problem: Appliances may leak gas into the indoor environment.
Solution: Have appliances checked regularly for gas leaks. See Chapter 17.

Wood Burning Stove

Do you have a wood-burning stove?

❏ Yes   ❏ No

Problem: Combustion byproducts from wood-burning stoves can be a source of indoor air pollution.

Solution: Make sure the flue is drafting correctly and that the stove is sealed correctly. Even then there can still be problems with depleting indoor oxygen levels and the escape of combustion byproducts. The best solution is to have a fireplace with a tight seal and its own fresh air intake. See Chapter 12.

Carpet

Does your home contain carpet?

❏ Yes   ❏ No

If yes, estimate how much floor space is carpeted:

_____

_____

Is any area of carpet worn, disintegrating or stained, or does it smell moldy or strange? If yes, list where:

_____

_____

_____

_____

Problem: Worn carpet will release fine particulates into the air you breathe and can be irritating. Stained or moldy smelling carpet could indicate a moisture problem and mold growth.

Solution: Replace worn carpet with a healthy alternative. Find the source of carpet stains and smells, fix them and replace the carpet with a healthy alternative. See Chapters 3, 5 and 16.

HEPA Vacuum Cleaners

Do you have a HEPA vacuum cleaner?

❏ Yes   ❏ No

Problem: Most vacuum cleaners recirculate as much as 70 percent of the debris they collect back into the air we breathe.

Solution: A true HEPA vacuum cleaner traps finer particulates and does not recirculate debris. See Chapter 16.

Ventilation

How do you ventilate your home?

- ❐ Open windows
- ❐ Use an energy recovery ventilator
- ❐ Have a whole house air filtration system that brings in fresh air from outside
- ❐ Don't ventilate the house

Problem: Without adequate ventilation, indoor pollutants can concentrate and build to dangerous levels that affect your health.

Solution: Open windows daily when you are home to allow some fresh air in. See Chapters 3, 5 and 7.

EMRs

Where is the service drop to your house? Mark with an "X" on your house map.

_____

_____

Where is the electrical main panel? Mark with an "X."

_____

_____

_____

Are there any other cables or wires that enter your home? If so list where they enter and mark with an "X" on your house map.

_____

_____

_____

Take a walk around your home and list the electrical appliances found in each room. List everything from refrigerators to electric toothbrushes. Use an additional piece of paper if you need more space.

_____

_____

_____

_____

_____

_____

Problem: EMRs are invisible sources of pollution.

Solution: Reducing the overall amount of electrical appliances or at least unplugging non-essential appliances when not in use will reduce some of the fields in your home.

Cleaning

List who cleans your home and where they clean:

_____

_____

_____

Take a walk around your home and list all the cleaning products you can find. Remember to look under sinks, in cupboards, and closets. You may discover products you didn't know you had.

_____

_____

_____

If you have a professional cleaning service come into your home, get a list from them of all the cleaning products they use in your home and write them down here:

_____

_____

_____

_____

Read the labels on all your cleaning products. Do any of these products contain toxic chemicals? (See Chapter 16.) List the products that do. You may need to phone individual manufactures to get Material Safety Data Sheets on products that do not list all their ingredients.

_____

_____

_____

_____

From the list above, circle the cleaning products that you plan to get rid of first and replace with healthier alternatives. List the healthier alternatives below, or list the kind of cleaning product you are looking for to replace each of your toxic ones.

_____

_____

_____

_____

Write the phone number here of your local Hazardous Waste facility and contact them to find out how to dispose of your old cleaning products. Do not dump these chemicals down the drain; they can damage the environment and sometimes combining certain cleaning products produces toxic gases.

_____

_____

_____

Problem: Many everyday cleaning products contain toxic chemicals that can be absorbed through your skin or inhaled while you are cleaning.
Solution: Only use non-toxic cleaning products in your home.

Hobbies

Do any family members have hobbies they do in the home?

  ❐ Yes   ❐ No

If yes, list the hobbies and materials they use:

_____

_____

_____

_____

_____

Problem: Certain hobbies require the use of toxic chemical or substances such as glues, paints, metals, and synthetic fragrances. These can have a directly negative effect on the individuals if not handled properly, as well as an indirect effect on the whole family by polluting indoor air quality.
Solution: Keep all aspects of toxic hobbies out of the home and away from children.

Smells

Do you notice, or have other people commented on, any smells in your home?

❐ Moldy	❐ Gas
❐ Damp	❐ Fragrance/perfume
❐ Stale	❐ Car exhaust fumes
❐ Smoke	❐ Electrical wires burning (sometimes smells like fish)
❐ Tobacco smoke	❐ Office smells, such as copy paper, printers etc.
❐ Chemicals	

Problem: Smells indicate something you are breathing in the air. Not all chemicals and pollutants have smells though.
Solution: Locate the source of the smell and eliminate it. Do not try to mask it with fragranced products such as air fresheners. You are just introducing more chemicals. Using an air filter is a temporary measure until you locate the source and fix it. See Chapters 16 and 17.

Pets

Do you have pets?

❒ Yes ❒ No

If yes, list all your pets that live indoors:

_____
_____
_____
_____

Do you use any pesticides on your pets such as flea collars or fur treatments?

❒ Yes ❒ No

If yes, list which products and how often you use them:

_____
_____
_____
_____

Problem: Pets can have dander and special proteins on their skin that cause allergies in some people. Many people also use pesticides on their pets which can affect the pet's health and rub off on people who touch them.

Solution: Pets can be poisoned by toxic chemicals just like we can. Use non-toxic products on your pets, for their health and for yours. See Chapter 15.

Garage

Does your garage attach to your home?

❒ Yes ❒ No

Make a list of items stored in your garage. Include old cans of paint, pesticides, gasoline, stored winter clothes, etc.

_____
_____
_____

Problem: If it does, exhaust fumes from your car will enter your home. Any toxic products stored in your garage such as pesticides or chemicals can offgas fumes into your home.

Solution: Install an independent ventilation fan to remove exhaust fumes to outside of garage. Do not store anything toxic in your garage. See Chapters 3, 5 and 13.

Yard, Garden, and Driveway

What is your driveway made from?

- ❏ Gravel
- ❏ Pavers
- ❏ Concrete
- ❏ Asphalt
- ❏ Dirt

Problem: Newly poured or refinished asphalt will offgass noxious fumes for a long time.
Solution: Use non-toxic materials, such as gravel, brick, concrete, or dirt, on your driveway. If you have asphalt that needs refinishing, choose a safer alternative. See Chapter 14.

What products do you use on your garden or lawn?

- ❏ Pesticides such as insecticides, weed killers (herbicides)
- ❏ Chemical fertilizers
- ❏ Organic, non-toxic products only
- ❏ Nothing

Problem: Pesticides are designed to kill. If they are sprayed, the pesticide product can be carried in the air and into your home. If applied directly they can still end up in your home via pets or on children's feet. Pesticides are poisons.
Solution: Follow an Integrated Pest Management program that uses non-toxic alternatives. See Chapter 14.

Do you have a sprinkler system in your yard? If you do, does your sprinkler system wet the side of your home in any location?

- ❏ Yes   ❏ No

Problem: Sprinkler systems that repeatedly wet the side of your home can create moisture problems that can contribute to rot and mold growth.
Solution: Make sure sprinkler systems do not wet the side of your home.

Do you have anything made from wood in your yard?

- ❏ Deck
- ❏ Play set
- ❏ Picnic tables
- ❏ Other wooden furniture
- ❏ Sand box

Problem: Copper Chromated Arsenic (CCA) pressure-treated wood can leach carcinogenic arsenic into surrounding soil and sand and your body if you come into contact with it.
Solution: Use non-toxic wood for outdoors. See Chapter 14.

Neighbors

Do you have any neighbors?

- ❐ Adjoining your home or immediately next door
- ❐ Several feet away but your yard shares a common fence
- ❐ You live in the country with no neighbors close by

Problem: Your neighbor's habits can directly impact your family's health. For instance, if they use pesticides on their garden they can drift into your garden and home. If they use fragranced dryer sheets and their clothes dryer vents towards your home it will pollute the air you breathe.

Solution: Keep on good terms with your neighbors. Let them know you are working on creating a healthy environment for your family. Give them a copy of this book and let me educate them on your behalf.

Location

Is your home located near any of the following?

- ❐ High-voltage power lines
- ❐ Sub stations
- ❐ Cell phone tower (sometimes disguised and on top of buildings)
- ❐ Industrial plant or factory
- ❐ Waste site
- ❐ Airport
- ❐ Non-organic farm
- ❐ Golf course
- ❐ Gas station
- ❐ High traffic main road or highway

Problem: All of the above create some kind of pollution that can impact your health.

Solution: These situations outside of your home are the hardest to remedy. You may need to reconsider where you live.

Family Health

How many people live in your home?

_____

What are their ages?

_____

_____

_____

Does any one have asthma? When did it start? How often do they have an attack? What triggers it?

_____

_____

_____

Does anyone have allergies? When and how often? What triggers them?

_____

_____

_____

Does anyone have learning challenges, poor attention span, or hyperactivity?

_____

_____

Does anyone have any sleep problems?

_____

_____

_____

Does anyone wake up tired or grouchy in the morning?

_____

_____

_____

Does anyone feel better when away from the home or outdoors?

_____

_____

_____

Does anyone smoke tobacco in the house?

_____

Is anyone sensitive to any of the following? Mark the item and put that person's name beside the substance:

- ❒ Perfume or fragranced products _____
- ❒ Laundry powder or fabric softener _____
- ❒ Soap, shampoo or hair products _____
- ❒ Cosmetics _____
- ❒ Cleaning products and cleaning product aisles in grocery stores

    _____

- ❒ Paints, stains, sealants _____
- ❒ Office smells _____
- ❒ New furniture or fixtures _____
- ❒ New clothes or clothing stores _____
- ❒ Newspaper, magazines, books _____
- ❒ Swimming pools or hot tubs _____
- ❒ Tobacco smoke _____
- ❒ Car exhaust fumes _____

❏ Diesel exhaust fumes _____

❏ Electrical equipment or appliances _____

❏ Other _____

List any other health challenges or idiosyncrasies: i.e., headaches, ear infections, frequent colds, heart palpitations, depression. Who has them and how often?

_____
_____
_____

What health improvements would you most like to see in your family?

_____
_____
_____
_____
_____

Congratulations on completing your Healthy Home Quiz!

Make a note on your calendar, right now, to remind yourself to repeat this quiz in six months and twelve months time. You could plan a special family event to celebrate the improvements you will have made.

CHAPTER 7

Bedrooms

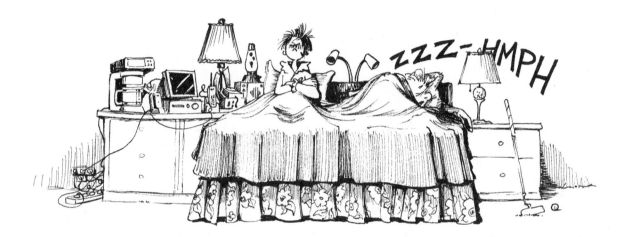

Liz makes an exasperated noise as she rolls over to see what time her bedside clock says. "3:45 a.m. ... ahhh, I'm never going to survive work tomorrow." She rolls onto her back and stares at the ceiling. It was no use, she had to admit it, she has lived in her beautiful dream home now for almost three weeks and has not had a decent night's sleep yet.

An internal conversation sparks in her mind.

"It's probably just stress. A new home. A new routine." Liz sneezes.

"I never used to sneeze during the night in our last home. I never used to lie awake night after night either. Where can all these allergies have come from? I'll stop by the drug store tomorrow on the way to work and see if

there's something else I can try. I hate not getting a good night's sleep. I hate feeling tired. I'm starting to get dark circles under my eyes. Isn't there a cream you can put under your eyes to make the dark circles go away? Is there a facelift for dark circles? Arghhh ... my neck and shoulders get so stiff at night. Stress. I wish someone would hurry up and make a pill that gets rid of stress, makes you sleep every night, stops you sneezing, and gets rid of dark circles under your eyes. I'd buy a case of that stuff."

She rolls onto her side again for another time check. "3:55 a.m. This is not OK. How come Mark's sleeping just fine?"

In the quiet of the night Liz's attention falls upon Mark's breathing while he sleeps beside her. Mark takes a load, snorey inbreath, the noise stops suddenly and nothing … for what seems like several minutes. Liz gives Mark a little nudge. Suddenly, Mark exhales loadly and makes Liz jump.

"That's so weird. I don't remember him doing this before we moved here. Maybe I just used to sleep through it. I don't know how I did though, he sounds like a faulty jet aircraft!"

Mark repeats this cycle with a variety of pauses between loud snoring breaths.

An involuntary giggle slips from her mouth. "I think I'll tape him one of these nights, he won't believe what he sounds like. Actually, I could take the tape to the doctor and see what he thinks. It just doesn't sound right."

Liz checks the clock one more time. 4:05 a.m. "I don't get it. I mean look at this bedroom. I have everything I could ever possibly need. A clock radio, a coffee maker, designer lamps that cost a fortune, a top of the line bed, a TV and DVD player, a stereo, a computer, my cell phone, my trusty humidifier, even an electric blanket to warm my bed before I get in at night. I thought a warm bed was supposed to relax you and help you sleep. Wrong. How come I have all this stuff but I just can't sleep!" Liz pulls her pillow over her head and begins to count sheep. Well it seemed to work the other night …

When Liz finally falls asleep it is 4:59 a.m. She has exactly one hour until her clock radio wakes her for the start of a new day.

Commentary

On average we spend a third of our life in bed. I know it doesn't feel that way given that so many people feel exhausted on a regular basis, but it's true. The bedroom is definitely the first place to start if you want to improve your health environmentally.

Building Biology perspective

From a Building Biology standpoint, the bedroom is the most important room in the house. People are less resistant to stress while sleeping so it makes sense to have this room be as healthy as possible. When we create a healthy sleeping environment the body's natural healing powers can work with maximum effect to help rid us of the everyday bombardment of pollution we all receive.

What is a bedroom?

According to the New Oxford American Dictionary, a bedroom is "a room for sleeping in." But have you noticed that in our modern day homes, bedrooms are often used for many other things besides sleeping? People like to watch TV in bed; chat with someone on the phone; use the computer; make a cup of coffee; listen to music. Some people like to keep pets in their bedroom; children like to play in their bedrooms … as you can see, a bedroom is not just "a room for sleeping in" anymore.

Liz has just about every possible toy, convenience, and luxury item in her designer bedroom. Could there be any correlation between these things and the fact that she can't sleep at night? Let's find out.

What does a healthy bedroom look like?

Many of today's homes have bedrooms like Liz's. But when you look at the impact all these electrical appliances, gadgets, toys, and interior design features can have on your health you may want to reconsider what you bring into your bedroom.

Don't worry! You don't have to turn your bedroom into some kind of sterile, hospital-like, austere environment (unless that's what personally helps you to relax). A healthy bedroom can look many different ways. Once you understand the basic principles, your creativity can go to town. So let's take a look at the bedroom in layers.

Nearly 40 million American men and women suffer from sleep disorders. However, sleep problems affect more women than men. In fact, according to the National Sleep Foundation poll, 53% of women aged 30-60 experience difficulty sleeping often or always: 60% of women aged 30-39, 47% aged 40-49, and 50% aged 50-60. Yet only 41% of all the women surveyed *think* they've had insomnia in the past year.[1]

The third skin layer

This layer is what you inherit when you buy or move into a new home; it is already set in stone (quite literally). The checklist below summarizes the building and system features to follow for a healthy house. Ideally, these are features to design into a new home or specify if you are planning to remodel. If neither of these options is available to you, you may still find some modified improvements you can make:

1. Exterior, high mass breathing walls.
2. Radiant floor heating (closed loop, hot water system). For health, heat objects and not air.
3. Hard floor surfaces (natural cork or linoleum, hardwood, pigmented concrete or tile).
4. Non-toxic building materials and finishes.
5. Low EMR design.
6. Windows placed strategically for natural light gain. Supplemented with full spectrum energy efficient lighting.
7. Install a whole house water filtration system.

For each of the remaining chapters, the "Third Skin" section will build on this basic list, adding specific features that promote the health of that particular room. In this case, a healthy bedroom also requiures the following:

1. Throw rugs that can be removed easily and cleaned regularly, instead of wall-to-wall carpet.
2. A "kill switch" or "cut off switch" that allows all electricity to the bedroom to be conveniently turned off at night and switched back on in the morning.

Your layer

You create the next layer. What you physically bring into your bedroom will define whether your bedroom remains healthy or starts to become polluted or compromised. Let's look closer at some of the choices Liz made for her master bedroom.

The truth about beds

After several years of making do with a rather old box spring bed Liz inherited from her sister Jane, she finally went to town and bought a brand new, top of the line, king size box spring bed. In choosing her bed she chose a popular brand name that advertises in her favorite magazines. She also knew she wanted a king size because it's big and a firm mattress because she has heard that it's better to have more support for your back at night and Mark sometimes has back ache after playing golf.

From a Building Biology standpoint, there are some other considerations when choosing a bed, like what it is made from. Because you are in direct contact with your bed for several hours every night you will be breathing in through your lungs and absorbing through your skin anything contained in your bed. You may be shocked when you read the following piece of information provided by Lifekind, a company that sells healthy beds and other household items:

When I read this information the first time it literally "stopped my mind." I had no idea that beds could contain such chemicals. How can this be allowed? Imagine receiving a low-level, cumulative exposure to harmful chemicals every night right in your own bed! And considering that babies and the elderly probably spend even more time in bed, their exposure levels are even greater.

Unfortunately this is exactly the kind of bed Liz bought. It is no longer enough to buy a big brand name bed that is marketed for its superior support or because you can electrically change its position.

Question: Are there more chemicals in your mattress or a barrel of oil?

Answer: Your mattress has more synthetic chemicals than a barrel of crude oil.

Most commercial mattresses are made entirely of petrochemical derivatives. Plus many manufactures add fire retardant chemicals and use toxic dyes to make the covers attractive. If a cotton blend was used, there can also be residues of pesticides, herbicides and fungicides.

Unfortunately, the label on your mattress (the one that says "DO NOT REMOVE UNDER PENALTY OF LAW") gives consumers no information regarding the chemicals inside their bed nor any potential health threats from short and long-term exposures to these chemicals. The usual label will just state the contents as mostly polyurethane foam and a small percentage of other synthetic fabrics such as polyester or nylon.

Most beds are actually made of such chemicals as toluene-diisocynate, formaldehyde, benzene and others that people are seldom informed of at the time of their purchase.

The label doesn't tell consumers if fire retardant chemicals have been used, and no mention is made that if the bed is involved in a fire it will produce poisonous gases such as carbon monoxide and cyanide

Mattresses and bedding can outgas over many years and introduce potentially toxic substances to your skin and lungs, which may in turn cause allergic reactions and a host of other potentially serious health problems.[2]

You need to buy a bed (which includes both mattress and frame) that meets the following healthy criteria:

1. The mattress should be made of natural materials such as certified organic cotton or pure grow wool (wool that has been sheared from clean sheep who were undipped, untreated, free ranging animals), or a combination of both.
2. For those who are also concerned about EMRs and don't want a mattress with metal springs in it (because metal conducts electricity), several other choices are available including: 100 percent natural latex, structural ash slats covered with natural latex, organic cotton and pure grow wool, and cotton futons — but make sure only certified organic cotton has been used and all the above criteria are still met. Metal supporting frames can also be replaced with wooden frames.
3. The mattress (or mattress pad placed on top of the mattress) should contain no synthetic chemicals, no glues, no synthetic foam, no fire retardants, and no moth proofing.
4. The mattress must be able to absorb and dispel moisture without supporting mold or mildew growth.
5. The frame should contain no toxic glues, no particleboard, no chemical stains or finishes.

It is also best to have your bed raised off the floor, ideally 12-16 inches so that air can circulate around and under your bed and mattress to help your bed breathe. Cleaning under your bed is much easier this way, provided you don't use it for extra storage space and fill it full of stuff. Many people with a box spring bed use a bed skirt of material to disguise the frame. Bed skirts can harbor dirt and create another place for dust mites to live in.

You can expect to pay more for a healthy bed but if you figure in the lifetime costs associated with supporting or not supporting your health every single night in a positive way, I think it's totally worth it. Creating a chemical-free environment in other areas of your life can be very difficult, but by just changing to an organic, chemical-free bed, you can remove potential chemical contaminants from one-third of your life.

Bedding

Let's not forget that beds also include sheets, blankets, pillows and pillowcases. Liz chose all new, designer bedding for her master bedroom. Because of her busy working life she chose a cotton/polyester blend of permanent press sheets and pillowcases for its "no-need-to-iron" convenience. What Liz didn't know is that this kind of bedding also contains the chemical formaldehyde, which causes immunological problems and has been linked to cancer.[3] All cotton/polyester blend fabrics have formaldehyde finishes. This finishing process combines formaldehyde resin directly with the fiber so that it cannot be washed out, ever.

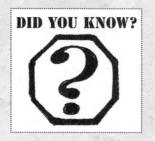

DID YOU KNOW?

Cotton products described as green, 100% natural, undyed, unbleached or colorgrown can be misleading and may actually be produced from cotton grown with polluting and toxic pesticides, herbicides, and defoliants. Only cotton labeled "certified organic" can be guaranteed to be grown and manufactured without these harmful chemicals.[5]

Growing cotton usually requires toxic soil fumigants and at least five pesticide applications. By one estimate, cotton accounts for 25% of all pesticides used in the U.S.[6]

When you consider that formaldehyde vapor inhalation can cause tiredness, insomnia, headaches, respiratory problems, coughing, watery eyes, excessive thirst, and many other common symptoms,[4] what's more important to you, permanent press bedding or your health? I have heard of one person who suffered with insomnia for many years and when she changed to certified organic cotton sheets and pillow cases her insomnia went away.

Sheets and pillowcases also come in a huge variety of colors and patterns. Liz went to a lot of trouble to match her bedding designs with her bedroom wallpaper. But those pretty colors are made from chemical dyes. Many dyes frequently include toxic heavy metals such as chrome, copper, and zinc, and sometimes contain known or suspected carcinogens. Even natural dyes, because of their poor colorfastness, are often accompanied by heavy metals in the mordant, or dyefixing, agent. On top of this many fabrics are also treated with fire retardant chemicals. When you consider the intimate contact we have with our bedding every night, it's disturbing to realize that all of these chemicals we are discussing can get onto our skin and into our bodies.

Then there are blankets. Synthetic fibers will be covered more in Chapter 10. But let's look at a trusty old favorite here: wool. Unless wool is labeled as "pure grow wool" it's highly likely to have been treated with several chemicals in its manufacture. One process is called "carbonizing," a process involving washing the wool with sulfuric acid, which dehydrates the organic matter to remove natural oils and any dirt. This chemical process can be an irritant to the skin. I have found some people who thought they were allergic to wool, only to discover they had no problems with pure grow wool that has not been chemically treated. Wool may also be treated with highly toxic mothproofing pesticides.

Pillows are of particular importance when it comes to beds. Think about it: your face rests on your pillow all night long and you inhale whatever is in it. The healthiest choices are organic cotton fill, pure grow wool fill, or a mixture of both with organic cotton covers. If you are troubled by insomnia, sinus problems, breathing problems, skin problems, headaches, and fatigue try a chemical-free pillow and see for yourself if it helps. Children usually need a pillow that has only half the filling an adult size pillow contains. Always inform the person or company you are buying your pillows from if you are buying one for a child. It's a good idea to replace your pillow with a new one every couple of years.

Liz has a "memory-foam" pillow. These pillows are marketed as being extremely comfortable because the pillow molds to the shape of your head. However, you need to ask, what is this shape-changing material made from? Any guesses?

Petroleum based chemicals.

We must start to question the long-term consequences to our health from all these nightly exposures. Synthetic foam pillows are also petrochemically derived and will break down over time releasing tiny particulates.

Wash your pillowcases at least once a week. If you wear perfume, aftershave or cosmetics, or use hair care products, change your pillowcases more often, maybe even every other day if you have allergies, asthma, or don't sleep well. Whatever is in your hair or on your skin will be deposited onto your pillowcase during the night and will steadily accumulate there creating an invisible toxic coating.

Dust Mites

Dust mites are one of the key contributors to ill health in the bedroom. These tiny creatures, only a fraction of a millimeter long, cannot be seen with the naked eye. They live off dead skin and though this sounds revolting, our homes are full of dead skin, sloughed from our bodies in everyday activities. And if this is not revolting enough, having eaten our dead skin, the dust mites then leave droppings (excrement), containing some of their stomach enzymes, everywhere. It is these stomach enzymes that people are allergic to. These allergies can lead to asthma, rare skin conditions, rhinitis (a blocked, itchy, runny or sneezy nose), sinusitis, and ear problems.[8] Besides dead skin, dust mites like warmth and humidity. The ideal room for them to grow in is an overly heated bedroom with poor ventilation and lots of fabric such as thick curtains, long pile carpet, mattresses, pillows, bedding that is infrequently washed, and cuddly toys like teddy bears.

As Liz has just moved into her new home and purchased a brand new bed and pillow for herself, dust mites have yet to establish themselves. However Mark, who will not part with the trusty pillow he has slept on every night for the past ten years, will quickly repopulate their new bed and bedding with his loyal, mature, relocated pillow dust mites.

Natural latex and wool are dust mite resistant which makes them good bed and bedding materials. Some people are allergic to latex so before buying a latex mattress, ask the manufacturer for a sample so you can test your sensitivity level (see

Fire retardants such as polybrominated diphenyl ethers (PBDEs) and other brominated fire retardants (BFRs) are similar in chemical structure to PCBs, which are still found in the bodies of people and animals more than 20 years after they were removed from commercial products in the United States. Every day, a typical American comes in contact with dozens, if not hundreds, of consumer goods that contain PBDEs, including electronics, electrical cables, carpets, furniture, and textiles. A growing body of research in laboratory animals has linked PBDE exposure to an array of adverse health effects including thyroid hormone disruption, permanent learning and memory impairment, behavioral changes, hearing deficits, delayed puberty onset, fetal malformations and possibly cancer. Research also shows that exposure to brominated flame retardants in utero or infancy leads to much more significant harm than adult exposure, and at much lower levels.[7]

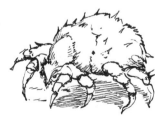

"Certified organic" means that the grower or processor has met or exceeded defined organic standards. Farms and processing facilities are inspected frequently, and detailed records must be kept. Organic cotton seeds are not genetically engineered, irradiated, or fertilized with sewer sludge. Insects and weeds are controlled with natural non-chemical methods approved by the International Federation of Organic Agriculture Movement (IFOAM).

"Natural" or "green" cotton products use conventionally grown cotton which is still subjected to pesticides, but they are free of harsh chemical bleaches, dyes, and chemicals such as formaldehyde. "100% cotton" labeling indicates that no other fibers have been used in the fabric, but does not mean that the fabric is organic or naturally processed.

how to test below). Pure grow wool mattress toppers, pillows, and comforter are great choices. You can also use "barrier cloth" mattress and pillow covers. This is a very tightly woven cloth which diminishes the dust mites' ability to move around and come into direct contact with you. Again, choose organic cotton barrier cloths.

I know this particular topic sounds awful and the picture of these tiny creatures is rather scary, but they are a major source of unidentified health problems in both adults and children.

If you want personal proof if you have a dust mite problem or not there is a simple test you can safely perform at home (see Appendix C). Basically you place a special sock over the end of the nozzle of your vacuum cleaner. Then you vacuum a portion of your carpet, your bed, and your pillow. Remove the sock along with the gathered contents and send it back to the laboratory where you purchased the sock; they will analyze the contents for duct mites and tell you if you have any and if so, how many. If you would rather have someone else do this for you, you can enlist the help of a Building Biology Environmental Inspector (see Appendix C).

A quick word about dry cleaning

The new duvet Liz bought for her bed indicates on its label that it must be "dry cleaned only." As Liz regularly has her clothes and Mark's clothes dry cleaned, this just means one extra item to take with her. No questions asked. What Liz doesn't know is that dry cleaning uses toxic chemical solvents. The term "dry cleaning" is actually a misnomer. The process is called dry only because water isn't used. Instead a liquid petrochemical-based solvent is the primary cleaning solution. Sometimes special soaps and detergents are used along with the solvent. The cleaner used by 80 percent of the industry is perchloroethylene or PERC for short, a highly neurotoxic chemical and possible carcinogen.[9]

If you do dry clean your clothes and like to recycle the hangers that accompany your clothes home, be sure to remove the paper wrapping on the hangers themselves. It will be impregnated with dry cleaning chemicals that will contaminate the rest of your closet.

Interestingly, PERC was first created to be a metal degreaser, not a garment cleaner.

The last thing you want in your bedroom is a blanket of dangerous chemicals around you all night long. Even if you air bedding out after dry cleaning before bringing it into your bedroom I am concerned that there are still chemical residues that linger and are persistent in the fibers.

Here are three options for keeping your bedding clean and healthy:

1. Only purchase bedding that can be washed. I use an organic cotton cover on our duvet and launder the cover on a regular basis along with the rest of the bedding. In the summer months when there are days of warm sunshine, I hand wash our duvet the old fashioned way, in the bathtub, and then hang it out to dry all day long. You might need someone's assistance to wring out the duvet when you have finished washing it in the tub. Then wrap it in a clean sheet to carry from your bathroom to the outside to dry; otherwise you'll leave a water trail all through your house. Can you guess how I figured out that piece of advice?

2. Sun baths. When I was a child, my mother regularly hung our bedding on the clothesline in the garden to air everything out and refresh it. Pillows, duvets, blankets, and don't forget your throw rugs too. Natural sunshine is a great deodorizer and purifier. Turn your bedding over so that as much surface area can be exposed to sunshine and fresh air as possible. If your bedding is colored you will need to keep it out of direct sunshine so it won't fade. I have all natural (neutral) colored bedding. This color can be in the sunshine and you don't have to worry about it fading. Your bedding will smell wonderful at the end of the day! If you or someone in your family has allergies, pay attention to high pollen count days and don't put your bedding outside on them.

3. If you do happen to have an item that cannot be machine or hand washed, look for "wet cleaners" instead of "dry cleaners." Wet cleaning incorporates a variety of alternative cleaning procedures, each developed especially for a specific type of item or fiber that is usually recommended to be dry-cleaned. Wet cleaners use water and water-based cleaners. They do not use the chemical PERC. They utilize machine washing, hand washing, or steam, coupled with air drying, machine drying, and/or pressing to achieve results comparable to conventional dry cleaning solvents. Look in your phone book to see if you have a wet cleaners near you. You may still need to request they use no fragranced products on your bedding.

Carpet

We have already discussed carpet in detail in Chapter 3. But here are a couple of extra considerations with regard to carpet in the bedroom.

Carpet has been associated with a growing number of health problems. In a typical carpet, toxic chemicals may be found in the fiber bonding material, dyes, backing glues, fire retardant, latex binder, and the fungicide, antimicrobial, and antistatic and stain-resistant treatments. In 1992, during a congressional hearing on the potential risk of carpets, the U.S. Environmental Protection Agency (EPA), stated that a typical carpet sample contains at least 120 chemicals, many of which are known to be neurotoxic. Outgassing from new carpeting can persist at significantly high levels for up to three years after installation. The most common carpet backing, synthetic latex, contains approximately 100 different gases, which contribute to the unpleasant and harmful "new carpet smell."[10]

Besides these chemical toxins, other characteristics are associated with carpets. They act as "sinks" and "emitters." As a sink, carpets hold onto substances such as dirt, dust, dead skin, pollen, dander, etc. They can also absorb humidity and liquid from spilled drinks and children's accidents. As emitters they can absorb and then re-emit substances such as odors and VOCs. When you consider all these factors, carpet can be quite a biologically and chemically active source of pollution in the home. Is this what you want in your bedroom, where you spend so much time?

Some people insist they want the cushioned feel of carpet in their bedroom, but think about it, do you sleep in your bed or on the floor? Where do you really want that cushy feeling most?

If your mind draws a blank when you think about what to put on your floors besides carpet, be reassured, there are many lovely alternatives available today. There are hard wood floors, bamboo, tile, pigmented concrete, natural linoleum, and cork to name the most popular ones. Throw rugs work well with all of these floor coverings and they are easy to keep clean and freshen. Just take them outside, shake them off, and let them enjoy the fresh air for a while. Once you've oriented yourself to this cleaning routine you won't ever want to go back.

Our goal in creating a healthy bedroom is to create the best quality indoor air for us to breathe during the night. We can achieve this goal by avoiding bringing anything toxic or suspicious into the bedroom or removing any items you may discover through the course of reading this book to be problematic.

Closets

Most bedrooms contain a closet of some sort to store clothes in. Some are built into the wall with doors covering them, some are recessed open spaces without doors, some are a freestanding piece of furniture called a wardrobe.

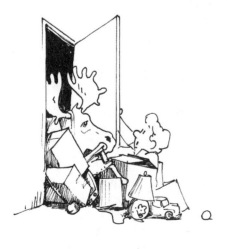

Like our modern day bedrooms, today's closets have become multi-functional sections of our bedroom that are used for hanging clothes, storing unused clothes, gathering dirty clothes, and providing a home for toys, photo albums, stamp collections, and things that won't fit in the garage any more. What does your closet look like?

Liz's bedroom has an entire wall of built-in closets. Of course they are already crammed full of a varied assortment of things besides clothes, which makes for a very precarious moment whenever anyone opens a closet door.

Ideally, your closet should contain your clothes and any other inert items needed on a daily basis. There should be no chemicals, no freshly dry-cleaned clothes, no hobby and craft items, no cleaning products, no cat litters, etc. Closets need ventilation so do keep doors open from time to time; otherwise they can start to smell strange and even grow mold. If you do notice any unusual smells remove everything and find the source. Don't put some fragranced product in there to mask the smell.

Moth balls

Just in case you have any of these in your closet, mothballs are made up of a chlorinated, toxic compound and are a suspected carcinogen.[11] Mothballs are particularly appealing to children because they look like candy. Avoid using mothballs and try a non-toxic alternative. An old-fashioned approach is to store your clothes in an airtight container and add natural pieces of cedar wood. Some people are sensitive to natural cedar smells though and may need to use some dried lavender instead.

A toxic chemical, dichlorobenzene, used widely in room deodorizers and moth repellants, has been found in the blood of over 95% of children and adults tested throughout the country.[12]

Wall coverings

Liz chose a patterned vinyl wallpaper to cover her bedroom walls. She achieved the designer look she wanted and already plans to re-do her bedroom in a different color scheme in a couple of years.

I don't recommend wallpaper, especially vinyl wallpaper, for two reasons. First, it stops your walls from breathing, and second, the glue required to fix it to your walls introduces more chemicals. If moisture gets trapped behind it, mold can grow. Vinyl also outgases noxious fumes.

When it comes to the interior surface of your walls, a natural plaster is best. It allows your walls to continue to breathe and remain healthy. Natural pigments can be added for color.

To paint your walls, use water-based, no- or low-VOC paints. There are also some beautiful lime-based paints. Be sure to ventilate the room well by opening windows both during and after painting for a few days. Do not sleep in the room until all smells have dissipated. If for some reason you must close your windows, then run a good air purifier in the room (see Appendix C) and keep the bedroom door closed so the smell doesn't spread to other parts of the house. Any forced air heating vents will need to be temporarily covered for the same reasons.

For those inclined towards more experimentation you can try milk-based paint. Good information on this is available in the book *Prescriptions for a Healthy House*. This book is one of my favorites and well worth having in your collection of healthy home resources.

Before hanging any artwork on your walls, check the backing. If it's an old piece of art, you will want to look for any signs of water damage or mold. If you find any, replace the whole frame or that part of the frame, or seek the advise of a professional mold remediator. If it's new art, again check to see what the backing is made from. You will often find cheap particleboard that contains formaldehyde. Let the frame offgas for some time until the smell has gone before you bring it into your bedroom. You could also replace the backing with something non-toxic.

Windows

Since Liz moved into her new home she has never once opened her bedroom windows. If she wants heat she turns up the thermostat, if she wants it cool, she runs the air conditioner. She has no thoughts of fresh air and actually thinks opening windows will drive her heating bills up. Does this sound familiar to you? If it does, know that you are not alone.

Since the energy crisis in the 70s people have been trained to keep windows closed to save energy. Today we are raising generations of children who don't even think to open a window to let some fresh air in. Without fresh air and adequate ventilation the everyday pollutants we generate in our homes have nowhere to escape and so accumulate to dangerously high levels indoors. Oxygen levels become depleted and carbon dioxide levels rise causing drowsiness, headaches, and poor concentration. Is it really so surprising that asthma is skyrocketing and is the number one reason for absenteeism in schools? Our children are deprived of fresh air while at the same time bombarded with pollutants. What else can we expect their little lungs to do?

If Liz were to have an air sample taken in her bedroom and analyzed at an air-quality testing laboratory, she would probably faint from shock to see the levels of toxic pollutants in her bedroom. This is another reason why she can't sleep at night and a primary contributor to the mysterious allergies she has begun to have since she moved into her new home.

The good news is, it's easy to open a few bedroom windows and let fresh air in. It won't cost you an arm and a leg either. Would you rather pay a heating bill or a medical bill? Fresh air is an integral part of healthy indoor air quality. If your home is built correctly in the first place you will be able to conserve plenty of energy and open your windows at the same time. We sleep with our windows open at night all year round: wide open in the summer, slightly open in the winter, but always open. Over the course of an eight hour night oxygen supplies diminish, especially if you have more than one person sharing a bedroom. This one simple thing — keeping windows open to some degree at night — can be a key factor that contributes to people waking up feeling refreshed and rejuvenated. Try it yourself and see.

If you live where the outside air is heavily polluted you may have to close your windows and run an air purifier instead. In this situation, sometimes you can find a period of the day or night where outdoor pollution levels drop; it just takes a little detective work. Make the most of these times by opening your windows and letting your home breathe.

Window coverings

There is so much consumer variety in our world today it's almost intoxicating! Our great-grandparents would be dumbstruck at the amount of choice we have when it comes to a simple thing like window coverings. Most window coverings are made of synthetic fabrics treated with chemicals to make them wrinkle resistant. The recommended dry cleaning process further contributes to their chemical content. Liz has great swathes of material framing her bedroom windows, with heavy curtains and a white nylon sheer curtain like you see in hotels that remains permanently drawn across her windows for privacy.

Synthetic materials are not only made from petrochemicals, they also generate static electricity, which attracts dust. Static electricity is what gives you that little electrical shock or spark when you touch something, for instance after walking around on synthetic carpeting and then touching a metal car door. Some people are very sensitive to static electricity and find it makes them feel agitated or nervous; some people have difficulty sleeping. The old natural cure for insomnia is to walk bare foot on the earth or grass for about five or ten minutes each night before bed. The earth allows any static electricity to ground itself and so leave your body. Try it and see for yourself. Either way, keeping materials that promote static electricity out of the bedroom is a really good idea.

Even natural fabrics can be problematic because ultraviolet light breaks them down over time, creating dust and the need for frequent replacements. If you must have fabric window coverings, as a general rule choose certified organic materials. Other alternatives to fabric are naturally finished wood shutters, louvers, metallic venetian blinds, or bamboo roll downs. I have even seen windows that have retractable shades sandwiched between double windowpanes.

EMRs

Whether you believe EMRs cause health problems or not, at least take a precautionary stance when it comes to the bedroom. Better safe than sorry. In my personal experience as a Building Biology when EMR is reduced in the bedroom, people sleep better (including babies and children) and feel more rested in the morning. Let me make some suggestions, then you can experiment and decide for yourself.

As we have already mentioned, the most important piece of furniture in the bedroom is the bed. Now we want to consider where to place it. Eastern traditions recommend having the head of the bed facing north. Feng Shui may recommend placing the bed in a certain location depending on the flow of subtle energy. In Building Biology one thing we look for when placing the bed is possible sources of electromagnetic radiation, which is a form of pollution (see Chapters 3 and 5).

The tricky thing about EMR is that it is invisible and the strength of some fields can fluctuate, depending on the time of day and on whether an electrical appliance's motor is running or not. We want to ensure that the head of the bed, and hence our heads, are not being bathed in electromagnetic radiation all night long when we are trying to sleep and rejuvenate.

Liz's bedroom is an EMR nightmare and is one of the main reasons why she can't sleep at night. On her nightstand alone she has an electric clock radio, an electric lamp, a cordless phone charging in its cradle, and her cell phone, which is also recharging and plugged into a power strip immediately underneath her bed. The cordless phone transformer is plugged into the wall immediately behind her head, as is the electric blanket. On the other side of the wall immediately behind Liz's head in the guest bedroom, which doubles as her home office, is an aquarium with its electrical pump running 24 hours a day … and night. This multitude of electrical appliances and gadgets right next to her head are responsible for seriously high levels of EMRs that bathe her all night long. Interestingly enough, her husband Mark has nothing on his nightstand except his watch which he removes each night before bed, no electrical sockets behind his side of the bed and only a dressing table on the other side of the wall. Could this be one of the reasons why he sleeps at night and Liz doesn't?

Detective work

Now let's do some detective work in your home. You do not need to be an electrician and there is much you can do without ever needing to lift up a screwdriver. The easiest place to begin is discovering what is on the other side of your bedroom walls. This might be an adjoining room inside the house or it might be an outside wall. On the outside walls look for anything electrical such as the service drop, which is where the electricity comes to the house, any kind of electrical wires, air conditioning units, or hot tubs. If you find anything like this, don't put the head of your bed opposite it. You also need to look outside for any high-voltage power lines or cell phone towers near your home. If you find any close to your bedroom you may have to choose another part of your house to sleep in to create the maximum distance between you and where these fields may be penetrating your home.

In Germany, where the science of Bau-biologie began, it is reported that many troubling conditions such as children wetting the bed at night; babies and children who wake frequently; adults who are insomniacs; and people who wake up tired in the morning, are relieved of these symptoms when this invisible electromagnetic radiation is removed or significantly reduced.

On the adjoining walls that are inside your house look for: the main electrical panel which is where all the circuit breakers are for the different rooms in the house, water heaters, furnaces, refrigerators, TVs, stereos, computers, aquariums. If any of these are on the wall adjoining where you want to place the head of the bed, move the appliance. If it cannot be moved, i.e. the main electrical panel, then move your bed to another wall that is free of the above. If you find yourself with absolutely no wall that is free of EMR pollution and you cannot free a wall up by moving appliances, seriously consider sleeping in another room. At least try it as an experiment and see if you sleep better. Some people notice an improvement immediately (these are usually people who are "electrically sensitive") while others need a couple of months before they notice improvement as some results will be subtle and progressive. Often the wife or mum notices her husband or child are less grouchy in the morning before they notice themselves.

When you've identified possible sources of EMR pollution on the other side of your bedroom walls, next look inside the actual bedroom. Specifically, what you bring into the bedroom yourself and how you have it set up. As a general rule, don't have anything plugged into an electrical socket immediately at the head of the bed. This may require that you rethink the use of some of your appliances. You may want to switch from an electric clock radio plugged in right next to your head to a battery operated or wind-up clock.

If you have a cordless phone next to your bed, the base usually puts out a high AC magnetic field, as does the transformer that you plug into the outlet to run the phone. Make sure this is not plugged in directly behind where someone sleeps each night. If you must have a phone in the bedroom make sure the transformer and base are several feet away from where you sleep. Electric blankets create EMRs and are best done away with completely, or at the very least unplugged every night before getting into bed. Try a hot water bottle if you like your bed warm when you get into it.

Don't run extension cables across the head of the bed or under it. Try to eliminate them or at least run them around the bed. Power strips on the floor or extenders in outlets that allow you to plug in multiple appliances should be eliminated or reduced. They indicate situations where appliances are pushing the limits, and can be strong sources of pollution. Try to reduce the amount of appliances overall in the bedroom, possibly relocating some items to other rooms in the house. If you are extremely tight on space and have to have a mini-office in your bedroom then place it as far from the bed as possible.

In Building Biology we have two ways of checking the presence of AC electric and AC magnetic fields. To check magnetic fields we use an instrument called a "Gaussmeter" (see Appendix C). It's a small device, very simple to use, about the size of a garage door remote control. Just hold it in your hand as you walk around or place it where you want to check if an AC magnetic field ispresent, i.e. around, under, and on your bed. Depending on which brand of meter you have it will either give you a digital/numerical reading or it will have a dial. Children in particular find this instrument fascinating. It's a little like magic, making the invisible visible.

When you find a source of an AC magnetic field the reading will rise. If you get a reading of 1-5 milligauss (mG) or higher, move back and forth in that location to see if you can pinpoint the highest readings. See if you can discover what is causing the field. It could be a lamp plugged in and switched on at the head of the bed, or a baby monitor plugged into the wall next to a crib. If these objects can be moved away from the bed, do so, then come back to the original place you took the reading and see if the field has decreased in strength. Ideally, work towards a reading of 0.2-0.5 mG or lower on and around the bed itself. If you cannot find the source of the field from an object in your bedroom, it may be coming from your water pipes, the wiring in your walls, an object placed against an adjoining wall in another room, or from outside.

High-voltage power lines create AC magnetic fields that can penetrate your house. This is the most difficult situation to deal with, as there is often very little you can do to remove the source. You can talk to the power company and have them come out and check everything, but getting them to move their power line away from your house is highly unlikely.

If you still have not located the source of any elevated AC magnetic fields, then you may need the help of an electrician.

For the best possible results with your electrician, rather than ask him to remove all the magnetic fields in your home, tell him you want your home to be in compliance with the electrical code and therefore free of net current. You are essentially asking the same thing only in his kind of language. It could turn out to be a simple wiring error that is easily corrected.

Some electricians are very interested in fixing electrical problems to improve health, some may not have heard of such things. If you need further help, you can contact the Institute for Bau-biologie and Ecology (see Appendix C) and ask to be referred to one of their electrical engineers or Bau-Biologie Environmental Inspectors (BBEI) who will be able to consult with your electrician over the phone. It's worth making the effort to have the health benefits of a low-EMR home.

> Electricity in the bedroom affects the circadian rhythm and the production of the neurohormone melatonin, which the pineal gland produces when one sleeps in darkness. Any disturbance in this mechanism can have a very negative health impact on the body, i.e. poor quality sleep, waking exhausted, immune problems from an overloaded body that cannot fully detox and restore itself during its natural night time cycle.[13]

The way to check for AC electric fields is a little more detailed. Results can fluctuate because humans act as electrical conductors and so will influence readings. Again, you may want to ask a certified BBEI to come to your home and take these measurements with professional equipment.

For more adventuresome souls there is a great little kit you can purchase for home use, which is very easy to use. It's called a Body Voltage Meter and it measures the AC electric field voltage on the body (see Appendix C). First you place a special grounding rod into the earth outside your bedroom window. This rod is attached to a long wire that you run through your window into the bedroom. The other end of this wire is connected to a small unit the size of a calculator called a multimeter. You lay on your bed, switch on the multimeter, and it gives you a reading showing how much electrical voltage you have on your body. If you do get a reading it means that your body is acting like an antenna for an electrical field coming from somewhere. Keep in mind, if you have fascinated children helping you with your detective work they will need to sit a few feet away from you or their little bodies will conduct some of the electricity and create an inaccurate reading. Let them have their own turn when measuring the fields on their beds.

Now it gets really exciting. Write down your first electrical reading. Then go around your bedroom, unplug appliances, and take more readings. Did the readings drop? If they did, you have some direct proof that these appliances are creating invisible fields that are affecting your body. Next try unplugging any appliances on the other side of the wall to your bed, and then take another reading. Was there any further difference? You can also switch off the electrical supply to your entire bedroom at the main electrical panel and take another reading. Be careful you are not switching the electricity off to any critical appliances and make sure to turn off any computer in your bedroom before killing all the electricity there. What is the reading now? The goal for most environmentally sensitive individuals is to lower their body voltage to ten millivolts.[14] If the reading drops significantly from switching off the electrical supply, you may want to mark this circuit on your main panel and remind yourself to switch it off each night before bed.

If the fields do not drop after turning the breaker off, see if you can find a different part of your bedroom where the fields are lower and place your bed there. If you can find no electrically quiet spot then talk to a BBEI or an electrician to find out what is happening with your house wiring. These readings may differ at different times of the day. So repeat these experiments again at another time and note any differences. Some people also take readings in their office or wherever else they spend large amounts of time. However, the bed reading is the most important.

Another solution to reducing AC electrical fields is to install a body voltage shielding cloth (see Appendix C). This is a special cloth that shields electric fields; the cloth has to be grounded to a dedicated ground rod outside, which draws the electric field to the earth instead of going on the sleeping person's body. Any static electric charge collected on the cloth runs off to the earth. The cloth looks like a simple mattress cover except that it has tiny carbon fibers woven into it. You place it on your mattress and cover it with a sheet. The fitted cover is attached to a wire that you run to the outside of your bedroom through the window to its own grounding rod. Once installed you would never know it was there. The sleep shield grounds any remaining net current, thereby reducing the AC electric field.

Here are a few EMR ideas to get you started in your bedroom:

1. Reduce the amount of electrical appliances in the bedroom. Any that you want to keep around should remain unplugged when not in use.
2. Computers and TVs don't like to be unplugged frequently; make sure no one sits close to these items for long periods of time and also check if these items are against a wall with someone's bed on the other side.
3. Large EMR producing items like refrigerators can be problematic, as they need to be left plugged in all the time. Be aware that a refrigerator's AC magnetic fields will be highest when the motor is running, so testing results will fluctuate. At least make sure no one sleeps on the other side of an adjoining wall to a refrigerator.
4. Purchase a Gaussmeter and/or a body voltage home kit and take some readings to find the optimum location for all your beds.
5. Your wiring can be another source of fields on the inside of your home. Many homes are not wired properly due to errors, omissions, and breakdown over time. New homes as well as old homes can be affected. Have an electrician check that you have no net current on your house wiring.

6. Install a kill switch (sometimes called a cut-off switch) in the bedroom. This is looks like any other electrical switch but it will cut off all the electrical power to the bedroom, which is ideal at nighttime. You may need to keep a small flashlight by your bed in case you need to visit the bathroom. Children love this!

7. If you are getting ready to build a new home be sure to request a low EMR design.

Smoke detectors and radioactivity

Smoke detectors are an important safety device in homes. Liz feels very reassured by the smoke detector installed in her bedroom. If you have one in yours or are considering installing one you should be aware that there are two different kinds.

The most common type is the ionization unit. These detectors contain a substance called *americium 241* which is a radioactive decay product of plutonium. These smoke detectors continually release ions from an internal radioactive component. If smoke is present the smoke particles will attach to these ions reducing the electric flow inside the detector, setting off the alarm. Even though the amount of radioactivity released during normal activity is considered tiny, it is still radioactive.

Another type of smoke detector is the photoelectric unit. These units work by generating a tiny light beam. If smoke is present, the beam is either blocked or distorted which causes a change in the electric flow and sets off the alarm.

As ionizing units are more common, this is the kind of unit Liz has in her bedroom. But what are the cumulative effects to Liz and Mark's health from being exposed to radioactivity every night? Which smoke detector would you rather have in your home? If you discover you have ionizing units in your home you may want to simply replace them with photoelectric units. Call your local household hazardous waste facility to find out how to handle and where to dispose of these radioactive products.

The EPA issues the following warning on their website. "Because americium emits alpha particles, americium poses a significant risk if enough is swallowed or inhaled. Once in the body, americium tends to concentrate primarily in the skeleton, liver and muscle. It generally stays in the body for decades and continues to expose the surrounding tissues to radiation. This may eventually increase a person's chance of developing cancer, but such cancer effects may not become apparent for several years.[15]

Cleaning

Use nothing toxic to clean your bedroom. Fresh air, regular vacuuming with a HEPA vacuum cleaner, laundering and sun bathing bedding, and shaking rugs outdoors are the basics. If you want to avoid any cleaning products at all there are now special micofiber cleaning cloths that will do a great job. If you do use cleaning products be economical. Most often, "a little dab'l do ya" (see Chapter 16).

Fragrance

Liz loves fragranced products in her home. Her bedroom alone contains a plug-in fragranced air freshener, a freestanding fragranced air freshener in her closet, a stack of

Approximately 95% of all ingredients used by the fragrance industry are synthetic. In a 1988 study, the National nstitute of Occupational Safety and Health found that in a partial list of 2, 983 chemicals being used by the fragrance industry, 884 toxic substances were identified. Many of these substances are capable of causing cancer, birth defects, central nervous system disorders, reproductive disorders, and skin irritation.[16]

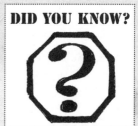

DID YOU KNOW?

By design, fragrances are composed of materials that quickly get into the air. Once in the air, these materials pose serious health concerns for many with asthma, allergies, migraines, chronic lung disease, and other health conditions. Up to 72% of asthmatics report their asthma is triggered by fragrance.[17]

The ingredients in the fragrance portion of products do not have to be revealed. Most of the materials have not been fully tested for safety and this makes it difficult to pinpoint and monitor problematic materials. There is no one agency responsible for the regulation of scented products and generally these products are a low priority among these agencies.[18]

magazines by her bed, many of which contain fragrance samples, a basket of pot-pourri on her dressing table, as well as a bottle of her favorite fragrance and three aromatherapy scented candles just for good measure. In fact Liz, like many other people today, has become addicted to fragrance. Ever though she doesn't really think about it, Liz cannot bear to do laundry unless she uses her favorite sea breeze laundry powder and adds a country fresh fabric sheet to her dryer. She has a plug in fragranced air freshener in just about every room in the house and regularly smells them to make sure they are working properly. By now you are probably asking, "How can someone become addicted to fragrance?" or "What's bad about fragrance?" To answer these questions you need to ask what fragrance is made from.

If you are not yet convinced, consider this: a single fragrance can contain as many as 600 different chemicals![19] Wearing perfume is probably one of the simplest and quickest ways to add to your body burden.

The healthiest choice for a little aroma in your bedroom is to use a small amount of pure grade, organic essential oils. Make sure chemical solvents have not been used in their extraction process. To disperse an essential oil, I prefer small electrical diffusers rather than ones you suspend from a light bulb. Light bulb diffusers tend to gather dust and can change the properties of the essential oil when heated. They can also burn or fry the oil, producing polluting byproducts. Keep in mind that even pure essential oils can be irritating to some people.

Candles in a bedroom can create a soft and relaxed mood. Choose candles made of pure beeswax or non-toxic soy without aromatherapy additives, and avoid candles with lead wicks.

Some candles on the market (mostly imported ones) contain lead in their wicks. These candles can produce lead fumes as they burn, causing a serious hazard if the fumes are inhaled. Although the Consumer Product Safety Commission voted to ban candles with lead in their wicks in 2001, you should still make sure that any candles you buy are certified to be lead-free.[20]

Breathing ozone can trigger a variety of health problems including chest pain, coughing, throat irritation, and congestion. It can worsen bronchitis, emphysema, and asthma. Ozone also can reduce lung function and inflame the linings of the lungs. Repeated exposure may permanently scar lung tissue.[22]

If the reason you got started using fragranced products in your bedroom is because it has a bad smell, find the source of the smell and fix it rather than distract yourself with chemicals. The best air freshener is fresh air.

Air filters

An air filter may be necessary if your outdoor air is more polluted than your indoor air and doesn't allow for you to open windows. There are so many different models available that this is worth researching. By the time you read this book there will be newer models and possibly better technologies available than when I wrote it (see Appendix C). Remember, air filters mostly "polish" the air. They work best dealing with minor indoor air quality issues or short term polluting problems. They are not sufficient by themselves if you are dealing with a more substantial problem like mold and mildew, VOCs from outgassing carpets and furnishings, or intolerable wall paint.

Ozone generators

Do beware of any air filter models that are ozone generators. Ozone is a pungent smelling, irritating gas. Because it is a very unstable form of oxygen, it is extremely reactive. While ozone can break down some VOCs in the air, it can also react with some existing gases, or other materials and furnishings in the home, and create new pollutants that were not there before.[21]

Several governmental agencies have filed lawsuits for unproved claims against one of the largest makers and marketers of ozone generators. The EPA has a helpful brochure entitled *Ozone and Your Health* which you can order or download at <www.epa.gov/airnow/publications.html#health>.

Ozone generators are sometimes used to remediate smoke damage in a building. In these situations high levels of ozone are used and the occupants are removed. These are specialized situations, not usually applicable to everyday use at home.

Humidifiers

Liz has had her trusty humidifier for years. She faithfully pulls it out of the garage every winter or whenever she or Mark has a cough.

Humidifiers have been used for many years to provide extra moisture in very dry environments. Forced air heating systems, such as the one Liz has in her new house, can dry out the air. A humidifier may well be a necessity. However, when a house is built with health in mind, you should not have to use a freestanding humidifier unit. The self-regulating ability of breathing walls will help to moderate the humidity levels in your home.

If you already have a humidifier and are partial to using it, remember humidifiers need to be properly maintained on a weekly basis. Liz regularly forgets to clean her humidifier, yet all it takes is a good wash with hot soapy water followed by a thorough drying of the whole unit (see Chapter 17).

Some humidifiers require you to replace a filter cartridge; be sure to do so on a regular basis and look for ones that are not treated with antimicrobial chemicals. This is not an item you want to save money on by trying to make it last longer. Humidifiers can easily become contaminated with mold and bacteria. Blowing mold spores and bacteria around your bedroom could be the start of a big problem and cause many health challenges.

Antimicrobials

It is becoming a marketing tool for manufacturers to impregnate the household products they make, such as humidifiers, with antimicrobial chemicals. These antimicrobial chemicals are pesticides. So much is still unknown about how all these chemicals affect us and interact with each other. But let's clarify one point: these chemicals are mostly designed to preserve the life of the product, not to protect your health.

I'm concerned about the popularity and mass use of antimicrobial chemical pesticides. We are already seeing more resistant strains of bacteria as a result of the over use of antibiotics. Are we heading in the same direction with the overuse of antimicrobials? If we create stronger and more resistant strains of molds and microbes because of this, will the answer be to increase the strength of the chemicals? Meanwhile, what is the impact of all this on our health? On our children's health? The truth is, no one really knows. The burden of proof that these products are safe for children should be on their manufacturers, but in reality it is on our children.

Antimicrobial chemicals can now be found in everything from shower curtains to carpets to latex gloves. Read labels carefully and avoid products with antimicrobial chemicals. All these low level chemical exposures add up. Why take the risk?

Most immediate gains

1. If you can't afford to create a healthy bed all at once, start with the pillows and work your way up through the sheets, duvet cover, and mattress cover to a new chemical-free mattress and bed frame.
2. To refresh your mattress occasionally while everything else is outside sunbathing, you can make your own spritzer very easily by putting some filtered water in a glass spray bottle and adding two to four drops of organic lavender essential oil. Shake this mixture and spray your mattress lightly. Lavender has natural antibacterial and antiviral properties plus it's very relaxing. More is not better. Just enough to refresh your mattress and allow it to evaporate fully before you remake your bed.
3. Get rid of clutter! Uncluttered bedrooms are easier to keep clean and are more relaxing to sleep in.

4. Keep electrical appliances to a minimum. Remember you are going to turn the electricity to your bedroom off at night so you may need to rethink how you like to have things set up.

5. Read all labels and see how many products contain fragrance.

6. Reduce dust mites in the bedroom. Provide good ventilation, lots of natural light, and don't overheat the bedroom. Keep humidity levels low and don't use humidifiers. Consider removing any carpet, or vacuum with a HEPA vacuum at least twice a week. Vacuum your mattress, pillows, and any curtains. Wash bedding regularly on the hot cycle to kill mites and remove their food source. Put pillows in the dryer on a hot cycle or place them outdoors in bright sunshine regularly. A pure grow wool fill pillow is the most resistant to dust mites. Cover mattresses and pillows with barrier cloth covers. Instead of making the bed each morning, roll back the covers and air the bed out each day. Replacing cuddly toys with ones stuffed with pure grow wool is best, and regular laundering on hot wash and high dry cycles is necessary. There are some products available that claim to control or reduce dust mites. These usually involve coating your carpet with a substance or solution. I personally have not tried any, but if you are interested make sure any product you try is proven to be non-toxic before using it.

7. If you are unsure about how you will tolerate a product once it is applied or installed in your home, give it this little home test before you buy it. Place a sample of the product in question in a large glass jar with the top screwed on tightly to allow fumes to accumulate. The following day, open the jar and take a sniff. How does it smell? OK or awful? Also watch for any other signs besides odor. Watch for any dizziness, headache, sneezing, coughing, or mood changes. This method of testing has its obvious limitations. While the test gives information about the product in question, it does not give any indication about cumulative or synergistic effects when it's combined over time with other chemicals.

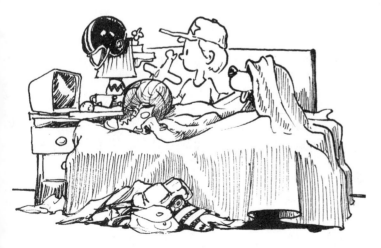

Children's bedrooms

All of the previous information about healthy bedrooms also applies to children. However, there are a few additional things to consider. Children generally spend more time than adults in their bedrooms because they sleep more and often play there too. Their bedrooms can be filled with just as much clutter as their parents', it's just different kinds of clutter. Toys, art and hobby supplies, electrical gadgetry, books, and snacks are just some of the most common items.

The repercussions of sleep apnea and poor sleep for children are vast. When children do not get the sleep they need, they are at risk for health, performance, and safety problems; difficulties in school are often the result. However, sleep deprivation in children is often overlooked or attributed to attention-deficit or behavior disorders.[23]

SLEEP APNEA SYMPTOMS IN CHILDREN

Nighttime:
- Snoring
- Breathing pauses during sleep
- Restless sleep
- Mouth breathing
- Difficulty getting up in the morning, even after getting the proper amount of sleep

Daytime:
- Hyperactivity
- Inattention
- Behavior problems
- Sleepiness

The healthy bed

Depending on your budget, there are improvements you can make immediately in your child's bedroom. The biggest and most important investment is a completely healthy bed. You can follow the guidelines mentioned previously for which bed items to purchase first. Upgrading to a healthy mattress and frame is a good investment as soon as it's possible.

Get rid of any polyester bedding and even if you cannot replace it with organic cotton to begin with, at least get 100 percent cotton. Before putting new bedding on the bed you will need to wash it. Here's what I recommend: add one half to one cup baking soda to the wash, rinse, then follow with another wash this time adding one to two cups of white vinegar. You may need to repeat this sequence a few times to take out some of the finishing chemicals and odor from the fabric. Check to see if you have any old cotton bedding that you can reinstate with a good wash. Older cottons will have had more chemicals washed out and if they are really old may not have been subjected to the same toxic fabric treatments used today. Sometimes you can find green, natural, or organic cotton bedding on sale in some of the environmental catalogues (see Appendix C), or call and ask if they run seasonal sales that you can plan for.

Lift the mattress up and look at your child's bedframe. Is it made of solid wood or does it contain particleboard? Many children's beds have a particleboard base that the mattress sits on. Or if the bed has built-in drawers underneath you may find they are made of particleboard too. Sometimes you can remove these and replace them with a few solid wood slats or drawers. If you can't remove them, then it's a good idea to paint on a special product to seal and reduce the offgassing process and protect your child from breathing in chemicals such as formaldehyde all night long (see Appendix C).

Train your children to pull back the covers on their bed each morning and air it out. This lets the moisture generated while sleeping, evaporate. It's a simple task that even the youngest child can accomplish and it will help to reduce moisture buildup, mold growth, and dust mite problems that can occur in mattresses.

Furniture

As parents we have a lot of control over the furniture we bring into our children's bedrooms. The main thing to look out for is furniture made of particleboard and plywood. Particleboard is used so extensively because it's cheap to buy. New furniture made of particleboard is the worst offender for offgassing large amounts of formaldehyde. With existing furniture, check the bed, the back of bedside tables and drawers, desks, and worktables. If you discover particleboard you can either seal it as mentioned above or get rid of it. Older pieces of particleboard furniture will have offgassed some of their formaldehyde, but I am still concerned about low level amounts affecting our children while they sleep. Remember, the only truly safe level of a toxic chemical is zero and the only way to be sure of that is to not have any particleboard in the bedroom at all.

There are now several healthier choices for solid wood children's furniture depending on your personal taste and budget (see Appendix C).

> Some less expensive box springs are constructed of plywood or particleboard, both of which commonly contain formaldehyde, according to the U.S. Environmental Protection Agency. Some plywood manufacturers also use pentachlorophenol, a probable human carcinogen, to preserve plywood.[24]

Toys

What else does your child have on their bed? Some children like to have cuddly toys, dolls, action figures, and other unique and interesting things close by while they sleep.

The question to ask is, what are these toys made from? There have been many concerns raised in the last few years about PVC (better known as vinyl) toys and the chemicals they contain. Take an inventory and see how many PVC toys you can find. Replace as many as you can with toys made from traditional materials such as wood, cloth, and natural rubber. These alternative materials were often used for toys before the rapid increase in plastics and are among the best alternatives.

There is a helpful fact sheet from Greenpeace called *Toxic Toy Story*[25] which explains what to look for and what to avoid. In general try to keep plastics to an absolute minimum. This includes toys, storage boxes, shelf units, and dress up clothes. This may require some rethinking but is definitely worth it when you consider toys made of PVC contain toxic additives that can leach out and be ingested by your children and affect their health.

Pets

Try to keep pets off the bed, particularly if your child has asthma and allergies. Pets are usually not very good at wiping their feet after they have been outside roaming around

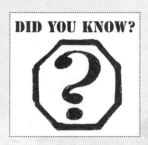

PVC (polyvinyl chloride or vinyl) is widely used in toys and other children's products. For soft applications, such as toys designed for chewing ("teethers"), softeners or plasticizers are added to give the desired flexibility. Although a range of chemicals are used as softeners, phthalate esters (phthalates) are by far the most commonly used.

Phthalates do not bind to the PVC, remaining present as a freely mobile and leachable phase in the plastic. As a consequence, phthalates are continuously lost from soft PVC over time. Contact and pressure, such as that applied during teething or play, can increase the rates at which these chemicals leach from the plastic.

Children in contact with soft PVC toys may, therefore, ingest substantial quantities of phthalates during normal play, especially from toys specifically designed to be chewed. This is of concern as phthalates are known to present a number of hazards. Although acute toxicity appears to be low, phthalates have been shown to cause a range of adverse effects in laboratory animals following longer exposure, including damage to the liver and kidney and, in some cases, effects on the reproductive tract.[26]

and so bring an unknown variable into your child's bedroom (see Chapter 15). If pets are allowed in the bedroom, I think it is well worth the expense of a small air purifier to help with hair and dander. Regular thorough vacuuming will also be necessary.

EMRs

Electromagnetic radiation in children's bedrooms has been associated with all kinds of nighttime disruptions: everything from crying babies to bedwetting. Take a look around your child's bedroom to see how many electronic appliances and gadgets you can find. Unplug or remove as many items as possible. Our goal is a low EMR bedroom. What is on the opposite side of the wall to where the head of the bed is? How close are any major electrical appliances to the head of the bed, i.e. computer or TV. Pay attention to bed frames that are constructed like a bunk bed only instead of a lower bed there is a desk. If a child has a computer, TV, or stereo on the desk they can be sleeping right on top of a large source of EMRs. Also look for any remote control toys that put out radio waves. Don't keep these near or under the bed either.

Many young children today also have wireless phones and cell phones in their bedrooms. A more in depth discussion of cell phones is beyond the scope of this book, but if you are a parent who allows your child to have a cell phone, I highly recommend reading the book *Cell Phones: Invisible Hazards in the Wireless Age* by George Carlo and Martin Schram. There are some amazing photographs of computer-imaging showing how radiation from cell phones penetrates younger skulls far more deeply than those of adults.[27] Be sure your child is not sleeping with a cell phone under their pillow or right next to their head. Better still, keep them out of the bedroom altogether.

Finally, if you can get your children to participate, turn the electricity off to the bedroom at night. For children who are scared of the dark, you can have a nightlight in their bedroom that is on an extension cord to an electrical outlet outside their bedroom. Older children think it's a great adventure if you give them their very own battery operated flashlight for nighttime trips to the bathroom. After a while your children will be sleeping so deeply at night they won't need a light in their bedroom.

Light

Young children spend a lot more time in their bedrooms than adults. In some ways you could call them their daytime offices. Natural light is essential for their health and well being. John Ott, in his now famous book *Health and Light* told us back in 1973 that light is a nutrient rather like food, and, like food, the wrong kind can make us ill and the right kind can keep us healthy.

Make sure your children open their curtains or blinds in the daytime and don't have any large pieces of furniture blocking light from their windows. Installing full spectrum light bulbs is a simple way to create more natural light. Many natural food stores now carry these light bulbs or you can find them through the Internet.

Food

Enforce a "No food in the bedroom" rule. Keep cookie and pizza crumbs confined to the kitchen or dining room where they are easily vacuumed up. Food debris, no matter how small an amount, will attract all kinds of pests and can trigger allergies.

Healthy Air Quality

Creating a healthy bedroom for our children is a top priority. Maintaining it will require some effort. Children's bedrooms are high traffic areas so a certain degree of monitoring will be needed. I am constantly amazed at the things I discover in my son's bedroom. As children get older and desire more privacy, monitoring can become difficult. At the very least teach your children to open their windows and let fresh air in each day.

If your child likes to do art and hobbies in their bedroom, make sure they use non-toxic and "non-smelly" products (see Chapter 11). Watch out for miscellaneous things that may not seem obvious polluters at first like fragranced scratch and sniff books for younger children.

Regular cleaning of children's bedrooms using non-toxic cleaners is essential (see Chapter 16). Get your children involved. My son has been helping to clean his own bedroom since he was four years old and now at eight does a great job all by himself. Even if they protest, get them involved and reward them afterwards. It's the old fashioned way of apprenticeship. They need to learn from us by working alongside us. If they know it's important to you, whether they acknowledge it or not, it will become important to them. This way a healthy home will become second nature.

Of all the people I have worked with over the years, I find the greatest successes often happen with children. So don't be concerned that your child is going to have a terrible time changing over to a healthy bedroom. Children are much more adaptable at making these changes and they are very quick to catch on, maybe because they don't have all the preconceived ideas we adults accumulate with time. Just make change fun for them (and you too!). Help them help you remember to keep things healthy around the house. Encourage them to do school projects on healthy living practices you do at home. Call them science projects and let them educate their friends at school. However we can, let's get the word out.

Protecting over a third of your child's life by creating a healthy bedroom may be the single best thing you can possibly do as a parent. Even if your child doesn't have any apparent health problems, they are still being bombarded every day with environmental toxins. So let's not wait until something is broken and then try to fix it. The truth is we are all being affected.

Most immediate gains

1. Go through your child's toys and pick out ones made from PVC to begin with and get rid of them. Unfortunately, I don't recommend recycling them at a garage sale. These are items we don't want to pass on to some other less informed parent or child. You may need to call your local recycling center or household hazardous waste facility to find the best way to dispose of them.

2. As an incentive for children to part with some of their toys, allow them to choose something new that is healthy and proven to be safe. Call it an upgrade.

3. Place your child's bed in a low EMR zone. If you can't find one, you may need to change their bedroom to another room.

4. Create a reward system to encourage your child to participate in keeping their bedroom healthy.

5. Make it a habit to air out the bed and open a window each day. just like remembering to clean their teeth.

6. Look for miscellaneous polluters like fragranced products, solvent markers, and nail varnish, and remove them from the bedroom.

7. Replace particleboard furniture with solid wood, or at least seal particleboard with a product designed for that purpose (see Appendix C).

8. Start creating a healthy bed by getting rid of polyester or poly/cotton blend bedding and replacing them with organic cotton, or reinstate old, well-washed 100 percent cotton bedding. Replace your child's pillow with a slender organic cotton or a pure grow wool one.

9. Check the label on your child's nightclothes. Get rid of polyester or anything treated with fire retardant chemicals (see Chapter 10). Organic cotton nightclothes are best (see Appendix C).

New baby's bedroom

This chapter on bedrooms would not be complete unless we spent a little time focused on the smallest and newest member of the family. Your baby.

In anticipation of the new arrival, parents often go to great lengths to prepare the baby's bedroom with extra-special care. Usually the baby's room undergoes a major improvement if not a full-blown remodel as in Jane's house (see Chapter 4). Ideas are gleaned from baby magazines or frequent trips to the local home improvement store. Today there is an abundance of things to choose from. Babies never had it so good!

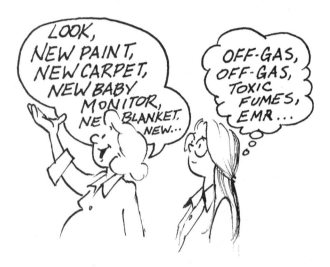

Unfortunately, one vital piece of information is usually missing from these well thought out plans — a piece of information that could have a dramatic impact on your baby's immediate health and well being. What could this be? The chemical impact from all these decorating materials and new furniture. You would think that stores selling these items would inform you of possible health hazards to your baby, but they don't. If they did, new parents and other family members would be appalled.

As babies enter this world they face more chemicals in their very own bedroom than their ancestors of a hundred years ago were exposed to in a lifetime.

After reading this far into *Homes that Heal,* you will be much more familiar with where these chemicals are to be found. However, let's recap a few of the main culprits. Paint, new carpet, carpet backing, carpet adhesive, wallpaper and adhesives, crib frame, crib mattress, bedding, drapes, and even those cute little toys that hang over the crib! Some parents even spray pesticides to prevent any "bugs" from living in baby's room, oblivious to the fact that these are toxic chemicals designed to kill. The list continues with air fresheners, antibacterial soaps, a host of baby toiletry products, and disposable diapers.

The good news is that with the right information, you can do something about it. Here are some simple guidelines to follow.

Decorating and remodeling

Plan to do any decorating or remodeling as much in as advance as possible, hopefully at least a few months. This will give any materials used or new furnishings bought, time to offgas some of their VOC content. Common VOCs you may have heard of are toluene, benzene, formaldehyde, acetone, and solvents, all of which are hazardous to health. These VOCs result in a slow release of chemicals into the air and can be very harmful to a new baby's delicate lungs, skin, and nervous system.

Next, look to any surfaces you wish to change. This includes painting walls and ceilings, wallpapering, and covering floors. Lead paint has been banned for some time now so a new healthy home won't have a problem like this. If you do have a home built in the 1970s or before, you should check for lead (see Chapter 4). When choosing paint, buy low or no VOC paint. Water-based latex paint has fewer toxic VOCs than oil-based paint. Keep in mind though, that even the least toxic paints will release some VOCs into the room for days or weeks after painting. You don't want a pregnant mum or a new baby inhaling unnecessary indoor pollutants. If you are pregnant, have someone else do the painting for you.

Be sure to ventilate the room while painting and for several days after. Opening windows works fine. You will need to close the door to the room being painted and cover any vents on forced air heating systems so that VOCs will not get into the rest of the house. Absolutely avoid paints that contain mercury compounds as fungicides as these can be emitted while the paint dries. Mercury is a toxic metal that can damage a person's nervous system and brain.[28]

I personally don't recommend wallpaper, especially wallpaper made with PVC, as it diminishes the wall's ability to breathe, as well as outgassing. Wallpaper also requires glue to attach it to the wall. Pigmented natural plaster is a lovely alternative. This is the healthiest wall and ceiling covering. For more information on floor coverings see Chapters 3 and 5.

Furniture

Pay particular attention to furniture, as we mentioned above. Much of what is available is not healthy. Choose solid wood furniture finished with something non-toxic like beeswax.

If you are looking for a baby-changing table avoid ones with PVC mats on top. There's nothing wrong with doing things the old fashioned way when it comes to changing diapers. Fold a thick towel in two, put it on your bed, and change your baby there.

On the subject of plasticizing chemicals, think twice before you give your baby a pacifier or teething toy made of PVC. Silicone pacifiers are currently considered safer; for teething toys, consider non-toxic wooden ones (see Appendix C).

Cribs and Bassinettes

What your baby's crib or bassinette is made from and what it is painted or coated with is of vital importance because your baby will be spending lots of time there. As a baby does not have a protective blood-brain barrier until it is six months old, chemicals can travel unchecked throughout its body with tremendous effects even on the delicate brain and nervous system. Cribs can contain toxic stains, paint, or polyurethane finishes. Have you ever seen a teething child chewing on some part of its crib? I have. Are these chemicals edible? I don't think so. Choose instead a solid wood, non-toxic finished crib. Look for ones that can convert from a crib into a toddler's bed later. It helps make your investment last longer (see Appendix C).

Most baby mattresses are full of the same chemicals we mentioned earlier in this chapter, with added fire retardants, and are often covered with PVC plastic in case your baby wets the bed. The best choice would be an organic cotton or pure grow wool futon. They are available in crib and bassinette sizes (see Appendix C). Wool is naturally flame retardant and dust mite resistant. You can purchase a natural wool moisture pad to put on top of the futon to protect your baby's mattress without chemicals or PVC.

SIDS

There have been some interesting studies done by Dr. Jim Sprott in New Zealand on Sudden Infant Death Syndrome (SIDS). This tragic occurrence is a very real concern for many parents of new babies. Dr. Sprott believes that SIDS is caused by a mold buildup in crib mattresses which then generates a toxic gas in the presence of certain chemicals. To protect babies from this kind of exposure, he recommends wrapping baby mattresses in a special non-toxic plastic sheet (see Appendix C) following a specified protocol, and ensuring that bedding used on top of a wrapped mattress does not contain any phosophorous, arsenic, or antimony chemicals. He also points out that the risk of cot death increases as a mattress is re-used from one baby to the next. To find out more about this topic read *The Cot Death Cover Up* by Jim Sprott.

Bedding, clothing and other miscellaneous fabrics

Any fabric that comes into contact with your baby should be free of chemicals. Be aware of synthetic crib bumpers, as babies invariably nuzzle up next to them and so will breathe in large amounts of anything in or on the fabric. Organic cotton crib bumpers are available.

Add diapers and clothes to this. They are your baby's second layer of skin and need to be free of toxins such as pesticides and fire retardants. Many people don't understand the health impact of these mass-marketed products. Once again, organic is best. The skin is the largest eliminative organ of the body. In babies it is of particular importance because while their other eliminative organs are still maturing, babies rely on the their skin to keep them healthy and feeling well.

Diapers

Current information on the health and environmental effects of disposable diapers is staggering-everything from how plastics disrupt hormones to the intense amount of heat generated in disposable diapers. For more information on this subject read *Natural Family Living* by Peggy O'Mara and/or subscribe to *Mothering Magazine*, which has excellent articles on all aspects of raising healthy children, including diapering options, and is full of great resources for purchasing a lot of the items we have been discussing.

Toys

Don't be tempted to fill your baby's crib full of stuffed animals and toys made of synthetic fibers. You'll be introducing another layer of petrochemicals into your baby's world

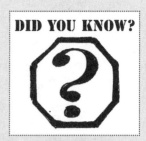

DID YOU KNOW?

A study published in the October, 1999 issue of the *Archives of Environmental Health* found that laboratory mice exposed to various brands of disposable diapers suffered increased eye, nose, and throat irritation, including bronchoconstriction similar to that of an asthma attack. Dr. Rosalind C. Anderson, lead author of the report, "Acute Respiratory Effects of Diaper Emissions," explains that the diapers were tested right out of the package, one at a time. Even in a mid-sized room, the emissions from one diaper were high enough to produce asthma-like symptoms. Solvents and other substances are typically added to these products during the manufacturing process in order to affect malleability and other properties. "Even if you don't want these chemicals in the final product, it's hard to take them out. We are finding chemical off-gasses in all sorts of baby products besides diapers, including baby mattresses and mattress covers," Dr. Anderson says.

What chemicals were released from the diapers? Tolune, xylene, ethylbenzene, styrene, and isopropylbenzene, among others.[29]

- Your baby will go through an average of 5,000 diaper changes before she is toilet trained.
- Disposable diapers constitute the third-largest source of solid waste in landfills.
- 18 billion diapers a year are put into our landfills.[30]

and inviting dust mites to move in. There are some beautiful soft organic cotton and pure grow wool toys now available that may well become a family heirloom! Some people believe it is best to put nothing in the crib with your baby to prevent other hazards like choking or suffocating.

Lead is another contaminant in toys. It could be in the paint of an old wooden toy. Babies like to put everything in their mouth and when they are teething watch out — they can quite easily eat the paint off an object. More recently, lead has shown up in some crayons too, particularly crayons made in China. You may think that your baby is too young to be playing with crayons but if you have older children, sometimes items such as crayons can mysteriously end up in your baby's crib.

Personal Care Products

Other sources of chemicals that could come into contact with your baby's delicate skin are personal care products. Baby soaps, lotions, diaper rash creams, talc, shampoo and bubble-bath can all contain synthetic chemicals. Read labels thoroughly and make sure you know what's in a product before you buy it. Don't just trust the marketing efforts on the front of the package that may call a product "natural." This term really does not mean anything in today's commercial climate (see Chapter 8). Your own personal care products also come into contact with your baby: your lotion, soap, perfume, and hair care products. A good

The National Institute of Occupational Safety and Health has found that one third of the substances — both natural and synthetic — used in the fragrance industry are toxic.[31]

rule of thumb is to find the purest personal care products for your baby then use them too (see Appendix C). It's best to avoid any fragranced products.

EMRs

Check your baby's crib and any other places where your baby sleeps or takes naps with a Gaussmeter for AC magnetic fields. There should be no more than 0.2-0.5 mG. Sleeping in high EMRs may make baby restless and agitated. Remove as many electrical appliances and gadgets as possible from your baby's bedroom. This includes baby monitors and nightlights. Before baby monitors, parents used to keep their baby's bedroom door ajar and stay close by so they could hear them. It still works wonderfully today! Make sure appliances that need to remain are at least six feet away from where your baby sleeps. Be sure to check the other side of any wall you place your baby's crib against for refrigerators, computers, TVs, washer and dryer machines, and any other electrical appliance or fixture.

AC electric fields are different from AC magnetic fields and should also be avoided. A body voltage test is the best way to measure electric fields in the crib (see earlier in this chapter). Shutting off the electrical circuit to the baby's room at the main panel or breaker box will ensure wires in the walls are free from voltage (unless there is a wiring problem). Lamps with two pin plugs should be unplugged when not in use as they can create strong AC electric fields. Because scientists continue to find links between EMR and childhood cancers, prudent avoidance is the best strategy.

One final piece of advice. It may be wise to let family and friends know your non-toxic and healthy preferences so that they can be sure to shower you with the right gifts when the time comes!

Children are routinely exposed to mixtures of carcinogens, neurotoxins, and respiratory irritants. Diesel exhaust, for example, contains dozens of chemicals listed as *hazardous air pollutants* by the EPA, including known and probable human carcinogens. Producing conclusive evidence that children are endangered is extraordinarily difficult even for single chemicals, and especially for the mixtures experienced daily by children and others. Testing necessary to understand the health effects of being exposed to the mixtures we all experience in daily life has never been attempted. The mixtures themselves are so complex and varied over time that it is usually not possible to identify a consistent pattern of exposure, or to assing blame for illness to a single chemical. Given these conditions, no one can conclude that children are sufficiently protected.[32]

CHAPTER 8

Bathrooms

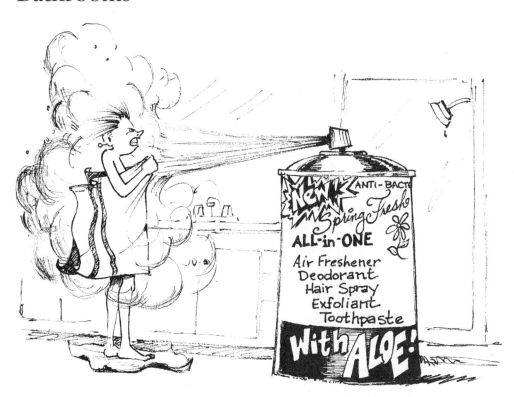

The alarm clock rings to herald a new day. "It can't be morning already," Liz groans as she thumps the snooze button for just a few more minutes of precious sleep. Another sleepless night transforms into another desperately tired morning.

After several rounds with the snooze button, Liz commands her body to rise from the bed. She drags herself towards the bathroom.

As Liz's mind begins to power up for the day her thoughts jump around like an overweight frog. There are several things she must remember to do before she leaves for work. Liz glances at herself in the mirror and notices her eyes are slightly puffy. "Oh great," she moans. Somewhere in the back of her mind she is pondering how these new allergies began just after she moved into the new house. It couldn't be the house though … right … it's new. But how come she wasn't bothered at all last weekend when they stayed at the beach …?

Liz turns on the shower and lets the water run a minute to warm up. The bathroom fills with steam. As the hot water starts to wake her up she wonders why it seems to take her forever these days to get going in the morning. She reaches for her favorite bright colored soap with antibacterial properties and a "sea breeze" fragrance. Next, she reaches for her expensive shampoo, recommended by her hairdresser, that's "all natural" and contains aloe. Then, the matching conditioner. Liz shaves her legs with a disposable razor that has a special "moisturizing" strip that contains more aloe. As she steps out of the shower she feels dizzy for a brief moment and a little short of breath; she resolves to exercise more frequently. Maybe she should ask her doctor about these new allergies and shortness of breath, or maybe she should ask her friend Steph at work. She used to have allergies.

Liz dries herself with a thick, brightly colored towel that matches her new bathroom ensemble. She grabs a piece of color-coordinated toilet paper as she sneezes. Liz notices the plug in scented air freshener by the mirror

and wonders if she needs to replace it yet. She takes a deep sniff; it still smells pretty strongly. "Hmm, maybe that wasn't a good idea," a faint voice says in the back of her mind. She marvels at how convenient it is to have all these lovely fragranced products for her home and how she no longer has to smell those strange smells she used to notice in certain parts of the house. Liz feels the first stabs of a headache begin. "Oh no! Not a headache again. Better get some coffee quick."

Liz quickly finishes off in the bathroom with "morning fresh" antiperspirant/deodorant; all natural body lotion with vitamin E; super-mint toothpaste and mouthwash; cosmetics (super-mat foundation, extra-long lash mascara, all day lipstick); a quick touch up with nail varnish on her chipped acrylic nail and finally a little hair spray to keep everything in place.

By the time she makes it to the kitchen she really needs that coffee. Liz is now feeling tired again and her headache is starting to really bother her. She knows there were some things she was supposed to do before she left, but she can't for the life of her remember what they were. Liz is irritated and its still only 7:00 a.m. "Why do my days start out like this?" she wonders. No time to think about that right now; grab the coffee and go!

Commentary

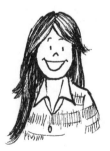

Where would we be without bathrooms? Modern homes can have anything one, two, three or more bathrooms plus half bathrooms too. With so many of them in our homes they must be a very important part of daily life. Yet it wasn't that long ago when a bathroom simply meant an outside building containing a toilet. It was considered unsanitary to have these facilities inside a home. My parent's home in England still has an ancient but functioning out-house kept as a relic, though occasionally it still gets used in an emergency when the whole family gathers and an extra toilet is very handy.

Building Biology perspective

Designing bathrooms into homes has become standard architectural practice. But this shift from outdoors to indoors has brought with it new challenges to the health of buildings. With multiple bathrooms comes increased plumbing. Increasing plumbing increases the possibility of faulty parts or workmanship. Undetected slow leaks, like we saw in Jane's kitchen, can harm the building and the inhabitants' health. Burst pipes can wreak havoc within minutes. Dislodged seals around drains in showers can create more undetected leaks. Hair and debris in drains can lead to blockages, overflows, and sewer gases. The volume of humidity and condensation produced by multiple showers and baths each day creates moisture challenges which if unchecked can lead to mold problems.

Let's take a closer look at the bathroom in layers.

The third skin layer

First, follow the basic checklist in Chapter 7. The ideal building features for a healthy bathroom also include:

1. Never use carpet in a bathroom; it will inevitably become damp, inviting mold and bacteria infestation.
2. Good ventilation is critical. Install an exhaust fan that moves enough CFM (cubic feet per minute) of air to effectively remove moisture.
3. Half bathrooms, which may only contain a toilet and small washbasin, should have a window that opens. Fresh air is the best air freshener. Mechanical ventilation is also essential in a bathroom.
4. Showers have glass panels to contain water.

Your Layer

OK, time to confess, how many people have mornings that start out like Liz's? Alarm. Shower. Coffee. Work. If you have young children you can probably skip the shower and the coffee and go straight to the work of raising your children. By 7:00 a.m. Liz is already irritated and can't think straight. Whatever happened to waking up rested and revitalized? Or starting your day with mental clarity and feeling enthusiastic about life? How do you feel first thing in the morning? How would you like to feel?

Everything you bring into your bathroom, from the towels to the toilet paper to the personal care products can affect your health. If we were to add up the amount of products and their chemical contents commonly found in bathrooms we could probably qualify even the most conservative bathroom as a mini hazardous waste site.

Everyone knows the importance of a good night's sleep. Ask any parent with young children. Sleep deprivation, whether short-term or long-term, affects your health, your mood and the quality of your life

Liz's question, "Why do my days start out like this?" is an important one. Let's see if we can find some answers for her.

Allergies

Liz's lack of sleep weakens her immune system and places additional burdens of stress on her body. Not surprisingly, some health problems are starting to show up. Since moving into her new home Liz has developed allergies and a few other troubling symptoms. She has puffy eyes in the morning, gets short of breath when she's not even exercising, has frequent headaches, and experiences mood swings ranging from irritation to depression.

For those of you with access to the Internet, I would highly recommend visiting the website of the Environmental Working Group, and reading their interactive article called *Body Burden: Pollution in People.* There are nine case studies and if you click on any individual it will show the specific chemicals and pollutants they found in their bodies. One of the participants is journalist Bill Moyers. It's a real eye-opener. <www.ewg.org/reports/bodyburden/dynam-contams.php>.

Recognizing that you are allergic or reacting to something in your home can be challenging. Most people are familiar with common allergens such as cat and dog dander, pollen, and dust. But in our homes we are exposed to so many other environmental substances in our air, water, food, and personal care products that pinpointing all the triggers has become a highly complex problem. We are rarely exposed to one single chemical or substance in isolation but rather an interacting mixture of many that can fluctuate throughout the course of a day. Usually the process of elimination is where the most answers are found.

Even our trusted family physician may not be able to help us find the cause of our problems unless they have had some specialized training in environmental medicine. Doctors no longer make house calls and so do not see us interacting with our home, school, or work environment where we experience our symptoms and where the best clues often lie.

For years Liz has been exposed daily to low-level amounts of chemicals just from her personal care products. Her body responds with tiredness, occasional headaches, sneezing, and dry coughs — all of which are mild allergic reactions. She has become so accustomed to feeling this way that she thinks it's normal, or attributes it to stress. However, when she moved into her new home, the additional burden from toxic building materials, new furniture, and furnishings filled her barrel to the point where it began to overflow. She now recognizes she has allergies and other symptoms but does not know what's causing them. How many people do you know, maybe yourself included, that can relate to this story? It's a very important point to understand.

> Millions of people are undergoing needless drugging, hospitalization, or even surgery because the environmental cause of their problem is not understood.[1]

For some people this turning point — when the barrel overflows — marks the beginning of health problems that may trouble them the rest of their life. Others may recover their health but remain sensitized to certain chemicals. I am one of those people who can still lead a normal life, but I remain sensitized. Whenever I am exposed to diesel exhaust fumes I instantly get a bad headache. Fragranced products also give me headaches and sometimes make me nauseous. It can be hugely inconvenient to feel fine one minute and awful the next.

The fact that Liz's symptoms subside when she is away from home gives her a clue to where the main source of the problem could be. The most immediate gain for Liz would be to start opening her windows at home, all of them, and ventilate the whole place.

If you or a child of yours are currently experiencing allergies or other symptoms I would recommend reading the book *An Alternative Approach to Allergies* by Theron G. Randolph, M.D. and Ralph W. Moss, Ph.D.

Showers

Now for Liz's shower. Many municipalities treat their water with chlorine to kill bacteria (see Chapters 3 and 5). When chlorine reacts with organic matter in water, such as dirt, leaves, and sewage, it forms substances called disinfection byproducts (DBPs). One group of DBPs are known as trihalomethanes (THMs). Chloroform is one of the most toxic THMs and is considered carcinogenic.[2] One under-reported fact is that THMs are primarily formed by chlorine reacting with our own bodies. Reaction with sweat is the main source, followed by skin, hair, and urine.

Chlorinated water, its byproducts, and other chemicals are easily absorbed through the skin when bathing and showering; these chemicals also enter our body through inhalation. Most VOCs will vaporize at temperatures lower than 90 degrees. The average shower is 105 degrees. The result is a shower full of toxic gases that can lead to eye, nasal, and respiratory irritation, and possible other effects we don't yet know to look for. At the very least chlorine has a drying effect on your hair and skin. This is why Liz is short of breath when she gets out of the shower and her skin feels so dry she has to coat herself with body lotion.

Shower filters

Our water now contains numerous toxic chemicals and residues including pesticide residues, heavy metals, arsenic, lead, radon, and industrial chemicals, some of which were banned years ago. All of these chemicals can react with each other creating their own new toxic substances. During a seven to ten minute shower in warm water, you will inhale and absorb through your skin more chemical contaminants than you would ingest from drinking a gallon of the same water. Is it any wonder some people don't feel well after taking a shower? The same goes for a bath too. How often do we bathe our children and have them play for 20 minutes or so in the water? They are much more vulnerable because of their smaller bodies and immature immune systems.

Water filtration in homes has become essential. Depending on your budget, at least install shower filters in bathrooms. Different filters have different capacities. Some companies may claim their shower filters remove 90-100 percent of the chlorine present, but the size constraints of the shower pipe, combined with the fact that water is heated and running through the system at an average rate of ten liters per minute, prevents any more than 75 percent removal by even the best system. Most average less than 50 percent, and less than that during summer months when chlorine levels are highest.[3]

Here are some of the current choices available:

1. Most showerheads contain a natural copper/zinc mineral media called KDF-55 filtering medium. It removes free chlorine by reversing the electrochemical process that originally separated the chlorine from sodium in a brine solution. The chlorine is able to recombine with a metal ion, normally zinc, to form a soluble zinc chloride that washes out of the filter and is considered harmless to humans. KDF is also bacteriostatic and tends to reduce or eliminate fungus and mildew build up in the shower enclosure. These filters need a certain amount of water pressure to filter efficiently and filter replacement will vary depending on the quality of water passing through them.

2. Another model incorporates a two-stage filtering system. Stage one uses KDF-55 to remove chlorine and enhance pH balance. Stage two uses a carbonized coconut shell media to remove synthetic chemicals and VOCs. I have found this system to be the most effective (see Appendix C).

3. There are also little filter "balls" you can dangle from your bath faucet to fill your bath with. These use either KDF or a crystal medium to filter. These are the least effective of all. Independent testing has shown these often only filter out about ten percent of the chlorine.[4]

Another option is to fill the tub with filtered water from the showerhead.

Whichever model you choose, regular filter replacement is the key to their efficiency. If your budget will allow, the best way to go is a whole house filtration unit. These use larger filters with denser mediums and are more efficient. This method provides filtered water throughout your house for showering, cleaning teeth, cooking, laundry, and washing dishes (see Chapter 9).

The National Breast Cancer Fund has published many recent reports on the "Chlorine Connection," and documented that the one common factor among women with breast cancer is that they all have 50-60 percent higher levels of chlorine byproducts in their fat tissue. Today in America, a woman dies of breast cancer every 13 minutes.[5]

Over the years, several women have consulted with me because of skin problems. They were helped tremendously by simply installing shower filters and removing chlorine from the water. They had all spent lots of money on expensive skin care to soothe and moisturize their skin, some had consulted dermatologists, but simply purifying the water their skin came into contact with did the trick.

Shower curtains

All showers require some means of protecting the rest of the bathroom from water damage. The most popular choices are glass panels or shower curtains. In Liz's master bathroom she has glass panels in her free-standing shower and in her downstairs bathroom she has a decorative shower curtain for her shower in the bathtub.

Glass panels are attractive, inert, and permanent and therefore are the healthiest choice. Shower curtains, on the other hand, are often made from or contain an inner layer of waterproof vinyl. Vinyl is also known as polyvinyl chloride or PVC. It is the worst plastic both from a health and environmental standpoint. New vinyl shower curtains can offgass chemical odors such as vinyl chloride, which can cause cancer, birth defects, genetic changes, indigestion, chronic bronchitis, ulcers, skin diseases, deafness, vision failure, and liver dysfunction.[6]

As vinyl curtains age they become brittle and crack and so need replacing regularly. Both incinerating old vinyl and producing new vinyl creates dioxins, some of the most dangerous chemicals on the planet. My advice is to choose safer alternatives.

Watch out for shower curtains that are impregnated with antimicrobial or antibacterial treatments. These contain pesticides designed to protect the product, not your health.

Healthier shower curtain choices are organic cotton canvas, 100 percent cotton-duck and all-hemp. Hemp is probably superior to cotton in this application because it is naturally mildew resistant. Regular laundering will keep your shower curtain clean, though to remain mildew-free these natural fibers need to dry out thoroughly and quickly between uses and that can only happen in a well ventilated bathroom.

The production of plastic accounts for the single largest use of chlorine and PVC is the most common of all chlorinated plastics. Vinyl chloride, the chemical used to make PVC, is a known human carcinogen, according to the World Health Organization's International Agency for Research on Cancer (IARC). Workers in PVC manufacturing facilities and residents of surrounding communities can be affected by exposure to these chemicals. Some studies have found higher rates of testicular cancers and a rare form of liver cancer among workers in PVC plants. These cancer-causing chemicals and lead, the nerve-damaging metal often added to PVC, have contaminated water, soil and air around these facilities, which are often located in poor communities. According to Greenpeace, low-income, African-American communities in particular are disproportionately impacted by PVC manufacturing facilities.[7]

Ventilation

Remember to open windows and run ventilation (exhaust) fans while taking a shower or bath. Windows need only be opened a little even in cooler weather as this will help replace the amount of air the exhaust fan is extracting without creating negative pressure inside the bathroom. Negative pressure is created whenever an amount of air is removed from a space, rather like a vacuum. This vacuum will try to fill and balance itself by sucking air from other sources, choosing the path of least

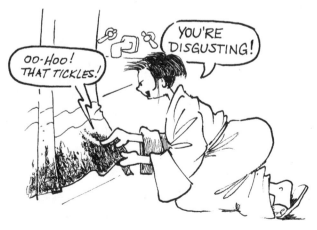

It is estimated that an average family of four in an average house puts two to three gallons of water into the air every day from all sources.[8]

resistance. If there are cracks in walls and floors or gaps around ductwork and pipes air can enter through these sometimes minute openings, bringing with it air that may be contaminated.

Make sure the exhaust fan in your bathroom has enough CFM (cubic feet per minute) of air movement to effectively remove moisture. If you are building a new home ask your builder about this. Do not assume the right size fan will be installed. If you already have exhaust fans installed, call the manufacturer, give them the name/model of your fan and check with them. If it is not sufficient, upgrade to a more effective model. If your fan has an on/off switch consider having it rewired by an electrician so that it always operates when the light is on. Run your fan for several minutes after taking a shower to allow all the moisture to escape

Personal Care Products

Bathrooms are home to a veritable "chemi-copia" of personal care products. In Liz's shower alone she has two kinds of soap, her recent favorite which matches her bathroom colors and has a fragrance she likes and one that is antibacterial that Mark likes, a fragranced shower gel which doesn't get used very often, two kinds of shampoo (his and hers), conditioner, shaving cream, razors with moisturizing strips, and a fragranced nylon body scrubber.

In the bathroom cabinet and arranged around the wash basin you will find toothpaste, mouthwash, a tube of teeth whitening cream, hair dye, aftershave, perfume, antiperspirant deodorant, body lotion ... I'm sure you get the picture. All these products contain a wide variety of chemical compounds and synthetic substances, many of questionable safety. This is an important point. Don't you think we are entitled to know what's in the products we liberally apply all over our bodies and our children's bodies each day? Federal government regulations continue to allow incomplete ingredient disclosure on the labels of many personal care products.

Let's look at some specific products Liz likes to use. Antibacterial soaps have become popular by catering to our cultural fear of germs. Our overuse of antibiotics and products like these has contributed to the creation of "super bugs" that can now resist many of the products we created to kill them. It is hard to get one up on nature; in the long run, she usually wins! An antibacterial product is designed to kill bacteria; it is essentially a pesticide. Do you want to start your day with a head to foot dose of pesticides? Washing thoroughly with good old-fashioned soap and water works great and is a much healthier choice. Children need to be taught to how to wash their hands properly; otherwise they will only wet them and not accomplish much.

Always read all the ingredients in a product and as a general rule of thumb, if you can't pronounce it, it's probably synthetic and petrochemically based, and not natural at all.

Also, pay attention to *where* the marketed ingredients are in the list of ingredients. For example, with Liz's shampoo, if aloe is listed at the top of the ingredient list, aloe should be the main ingredient in that product. If however, aloe is listed low down or even at the bottom of the list it means that aloe is the smallest percentage of ingredient in the whole product. So a product containing only a tiny amount of aloe may be marketed as if that were the main ingredient, misleading you into thinking it's a healthy product. The same goes for the conditioner and even the razor. I was amazed recently when I went to buy some shaving razors; I had to scour the complete aisle to find one that didn't have a moisturizing chemical strip. If you want a natural way to lubricate and moisturize your skin before you shave, use a liquid plant-based Castile soap. It works just great without exposing you to yet more chemicals.

While studying dermatology many years ago, I was taught that you should never put anything on your skin that you wouldn't be willing to put in your mouth. What a scary concept in today's "better living through chemistry" world of personal care products! What you put on your skin does go into your body. Rather than getting your vitamin E from your body lotion, which is probably also chock-a-block with synthetic lubricating chemicals, sister chemicals to things you usually put in your car engine, I suggest you get it from your food or a high quality supplement with guaranteed purity.

What are the effects of all these products on our children? Why do most commercial brands of toothpaste carry warnings telling us not to swallow them? If you make toothpaste a "kid friendly" bubble-gum flavor, don't you think some children might just swallow it occasionally? But how would you as a parent know that? And how would a child's allergic reaction, which could present in a variety of different ways from a sudden change in behavior to a complete loss of concentration, ever be connected to the regular use or consumption of an "innocent" thing like toothpaste? If you are interested in seeing some proof of these kinds of exposures on children, Dr. Doris Rapp's video *Environmentally Sick Schools* is very revealing.

Cosmetics

Cosmetics are part of the broader category of personal care products. We are interested in specifically looking at those that have the ability to impact our health and our home. Cosmetics are the least regulated products under the Federal Food, Drug and Cosmetic Act (FFDCA). The FFDCA does not require premarket safety testing, review, or approval for cosmetics.[12] Yet every day we apply cosmetics to our skin.

Synthetic: A substance that is formulated or manufactured by a chemical process or by a process that chemically changes a substance extracted from naturally occurring plant, animal, or mineral sources, except that such term shall not apply to substances created by naturally occurring biological processes.[9]

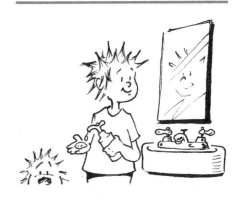

A recent study published in the *Journal of Applied Toxicology* drew attention to a possible connection between chemicals in deodorants and breast cancer tissue. The British researchers found a group of chemicals known as parabens, used as a preservative in thousands of cosmetic, pharmaceutical, and food products, in 18 of 20 breast tumors tested. Numerous studies have shown parabens can mimic the effect of estrogen, which can drive breast cancer tumor growth.[10]

It is estimated that we all carry about 400-500 chemicals in our bodies that did not exist just 60 years ago.[11]

Let's look at a couple of cosmetic products to give you the basic idea and you can take it from there with whatever products you may personally use.

Nail products are very odorous and contain solvents such as toluene, amyl, butyl, and ethyl acetate, which are all neurotoxins.[13] Solvents dry by evaporation, which means that a percentage of these chemicals will end up in the air you breathe as well as directly on your skin. Many parents apply nail varnish to their children's finger and toenails without realizing the toxicity they are inflicting. Nail varnish is not designed to be eaten, but children do eat it when it's on their nails. Furthermore, nail polish remover contains acetonitrile, a chemical that breaks down into lethal cyanide when swallowed.

Then there are aerosol hair sprays. Do read labels and find out what ingredients they contain and consider the following: the product is supposed to go on your hair, dry, stiffen it, and stay there, but I have yet to see an aerosol product that sprays in one direction only. Much of the product ends up in the air around you, which you then breathe in. Is it a good idea to end up with all those fixative chemicals in those delicate lungs of yours that need to stay flexible and moist? Consider also how much hair spray that ends up rubbing off onto your pillow as you sleep at night then gets breathed in. I have had clients with troubling acne and allergies get great results from stopping their use of hair spray and using a clean pillowcase every night. Fortunately today there are some companies providing non-toxic — even organic — products that allow us to create the look we want without sending us to an early grave.

And finally, a word on home-use hair dyes. Read labels and find the least toxic product. Be sure to ventilate the space while you use these products as again they will affect the quality of the air everyone breathes. Some parents allow their children to dye their hair different colors. Let's not expose them to more chemicals than we need to.

The skin is extremely permeable. Cosmetic ingredients most certainly are absorbed through the skin. Some chemicals may penetrate the skin in significant amounts, especially when left on the skin for long periods, as in the case of facial make-up. One study showed that 13 percent of the cosmetic butylate hydroxytoluene (BHT) and 49 percent of the carcinogenic pesticide DDT (which is found in some cosmetics containing lanolin) are absorbed through the skin.[14]

In 1990, some twenty-nine hundred children up to age four were admitted to hospital emergency rooms because of nail preparation-related poisonings.[15]

Neither diethanolamine (DEA) nor triethanolamine (TEA) is carcinogenic. However, if products contain nitrites, which are used as preservatives, the presence of DEA or TEA can cause a chemical reaction during formulation or even as the products sit on the shelves. This reaction leads to the formation of nitrosamines. Most nitrosamines, including those formed from DEA and TEA, are carcinogenic.[16]

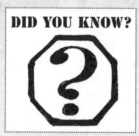

DID YOU KNOW?

The full extent of the effects that toiletries, cosmetics and personal care products have on our health cannot be covered adequately here. The sheer amount of products on the market is massive. Many people suffer from allergies, irritation, and photosensitization as a result of using these everyday products, all the while filling their barrels and accepting these uncomfortable complications as the normal cost of grooming. The examples discussed here are meant to highlight some of the problems and to encourage a better way of choosing personal care products for your family. To help you decipher labels and steer you towards healthier products I suggest reading *The Safe Shoppers Bible* by David Steinman and Samuel S. Epstein, M.D. The Internet also has some very helpful websites for evaluating the safety of common personal care products such as *The Green Guide* by the Green Guide Institute (see Appendix C).

Maybe the most important stance we can take, given the current lack of help and protection from the government, is to always read labels and only buy products that fully disclose their contents and that use proven, non-toxic ingredients.

A study published in the February 15, 2001 issue of the International Journal of Cancer found that women who use permanent hair dyes once a month are twice as likely to get bladder cancer as women who don't dye their hair. Especially dark dyes have been linked to cancers like multiple myeloma and non-Hodgkin's lymphoma. While dye is not a carcinogen on the level of cigarettes, there's reason enough to be wary. That the FDA has no power to pull unsafe dyes off the market shouldn't reassure you.[17]

Colored towels and toilet paper

As Liz steps out of the shower she is now covered head to foot in a cocktail of chemicals. It's no wonder she's a little dizzy, breathless, and starting to get tired again. Even the bright, fluffy towel she dries herself with contains chemical dyes to give it that bright color, as does her matching toilet paper. A dye is a colorant. Natural dyes usually come from plant material. Synthetic dyes mostly come from aniline (a compound derived from benzene) and coal tar. Since World War 1 these synthetic dyes have become very popular because they are cheap and easy to use. The synthetic dye industry has boomed, and today it's been estimated that 2,000 specific synthesized chemical compounds are available.[18] Dyes can be very unstable. Look at towels or clothing that have been washed several times. Don't they fade? So where does the dye go? If the dye is released it can be absorbed by the skin. To help fix dyes into fabrics, additional chemical compounds are used called mordents. And formaldehyde resin is often added to fibers. Even white towels and toilet paper have been bleached with chlorine to give them that bright, white color we all love so well.

Liz has 100 percent cotton towels — a better choice than a cotton/polyester blend — which incorporates synthetic fibers. However, as they are not certified organic cotton, her towels may contain pesticide residues. Cotton is the most contaminated of all natural fibers: seeds are treated with

If every household in the U.S. replaced just one 12-pack of 400 sheet virgin fiber bathroom tissues with 100% recycled ones, we could save:

- 4.4 million trees
- 11.6 million cubic feet of landfill space, equal to over 17,000 full garbage trucks
- 1.6 billion gallons of water, a year's supply for over 12,700 families of four
- and avoid 275,000 pounds of pollution.[21]

The wastes that paper mills discharge into the environment after paper is bleached with chlorine contain dioxins. And dioxins don't readily break down, which means that over the years they've been accumulating in our air, water, and soil. Once they're out there, they enter the food chain and we're exposed to them through the food we eat. Dioxins are now so widespread in the environment that virtually every man, woman, and child in America has them in their bodies. In fact, each day we ingest 300-600 times more than the EPA's so-called "safe" dose. As they accumulate to critical levels inside us, their effects begin to show.

Dioxins are deadly. In fact, dioxins are believed to be the most carcinogenic chemicals known to science, and the U.S. EPA's Dioxin Reassessment has found dioxins 300,000 times more potent as a carcinogen than DDT (the use of which was banned in the U.S. in 1972). There's no way to sugar-coat the effects dioxins have on people and the environment. Recent research has conclusively linked dioxins to cancer, reproductive disorders among adults, deformities and developmental problems in children, and immune system breakdowns. And dioxins can cause these effects at exposure levels hundreds of thousands of times lower than most hazardous chemicals.[19]

fungicides, and herbicides and pesticides are used repeatedly and heavily worldwide.[20]

The problem with so much of this is that these chemicals are invisible, and we don't equate color with chemicals. Many of us have just trusted that these products we come into such close personal contact with must be safe, never thinking in terms of "How did they make that bright color?" It's time to ask those questions, be informed, and shop with health in mind.

The healthiest choices are certified organic cotton towels and bathmats. Toilet paper should be bleached without chlorine, be unscented, and use no dyes (see Appendix C). Having recycled content is a kind choice for the planet.

Air fresheners

As we discussed in the previous chapter on bedrooms, air fresheners contain chemical fragrances (also see Chapter 10). Many fragrance chemicals affect the brain and nervous system. Some effects are immediate and transitory while others are chronic.

For example, let's look at headaches. Some people experience headaches even from fragrances they really like. A headache could come on immediately or start up 20 minutes later, it's different for different people. This is the case with Liz. When she checked to see if her plug-in air freshener was still working, she gave herself a massive fragrance hit. This hit often creates an excitatory effect in the nervous system and gives people a little high which they then associate with liking that fragrance. However, what goes up must come down. By the time Liz's headache kicks in she's in the kitchen and doesn't have time to stop and make the connection to what caused it. This delayed response confuses many people. Children are particularly vulnerable to fragrance products as their nervous systems are still developing.

If this rings a bell for you, the next time you get a headache or notice a mood change, stop and think about where you've been, what you've done or who you have been around in the previous 30 minutes. This detective mentality will pay off once you start uncovering chemicals in your environment that are affecting your health and well being.

Also, a brief word here on the extensive use of fragranced products in the home. If you are trying to disguise a particular smell or odor that you find unpleasant or bothersome it would be wiser to find out what's causing it. Bathrooms can start to smell musty very quickly if ventilation is not adequate.

Other problematic smells can be the "new" smell associated with a new home or a particular new product you just introduced into your home. Simple solutions are opening windows for natural ventilation and running good air purifiers when you have to close the windows. If one particular product

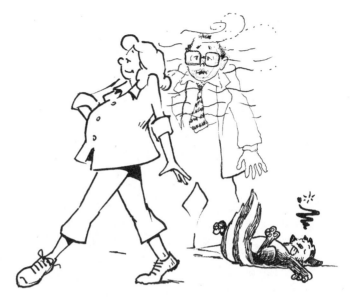

is offensive, such as Liz's vinyl shower curtain, remove it from the home completely and replace it with one of the healthy alternatives that have been suggested.

EMR

Beside wiring problems and outside sources, electrical appliances are the main source of EMRs in the bathroom. Hairdryers and electric toothbrushes are probably the most common ones. Hairdryers can generate huge AC magnetic fields. Take a reading with your Gaussmeter while your hairdryer is plugged in and working and see what reading you get. It's not uncommon to have AC magnetic fields of 50-100

In homes where aerosol sprays and air fresheners were used frequently, mothers suffered from 25% more headaches and 19% more depression, and infants under six months of age had 30% more ear infections and 22% higher incidence of diarrhea, according to a study at Bristol University in England that was published in *New Scientist* in 1999.[22]

milligauss! Fortunately, we are not exposed to these fields for very long (unless you are a hair dresser by profession). To reduce EMRs in your bathroom, unplug appliances when they're not in use.

Carpet

Bathrooms by their nature tend to have wet floors or wet patches on a regular basis. Carpet will absorb this moisture and can easily become moldy. Sometimes mold will be visible, sometimes it will not. Liz has carpet in her bathrooms and already the downstairs bathroom in her brand new home has a leak. Mold is already quietly growing in the carpet underlay. Even if she were to pull up a corner of her carpet to inspect it, mold spores are so tiny she would not necessarily be able to notice anything. Many carpet underlays are multicolored which can make it very hard to distinguish signs of spoilage.

Hard surfaces are much easier to keep dry and some floor coverings such as natural linoleum are supposed to be more resistant to mold. Use organic cotton bathmats next to the bath or in front of the shower to absorb wetness. The key is to remember to lift mats up off the floor to allow them to dry thoroughly between uses and to launder them weekly.

Full spectrum light

People look and feel best when surrounded by natural sunlight (see Chapters 3 and 5). Unfortunately, most of us spend over 90 percent of our time indoors where ordinary light bulbs do a poor job of reproducing the full spectrum of light created by the sun. The imbalanced light produced by ordinary bulbs causes eyestrain and fatigue, distorts the color of objects, and reduces contrast. Though you might not spend a lot of time in your bathroom, some of the activities we perform there, such as tweezing eyebrows and shaving, greatly benefit from more natural light. In particular, applying cosmetics in full spectrum light will produce much better results. You may find some of your color choices are not as attractive as you thought once viewed with natural light. It's good to know what everyone sees when you step outside! Full spectrum light bulbs provide a more balanced light by filtering out the excess yellow and green light emitted by ordinary light bulbs. And they last four times longer than ordinary bulbs.

A flawed system

If you are hearing this kind of information for the first time, by now you may be experiencing everything from being overwhelmed to disbelief to anger. How can these products that we so trustingly use each day be allowed on the market?

For the past quarter of a century, government and the private sector have relied heavily on a system called *risk assessment* for making decisions. This model focuses on how much of a hazardous activity, product, or substance is safe. This translates into: how much damage can the environment or our health tolerate? This model rarely takes children's special health vulnerabilities into consideration with any accuracy.

Risk assessment is generally used to judge the potential effects of a single chemical substance or compound as emitted or released from one source. In reality, people are exposed to complex mixtures from multiple sources on a daily basis. Risk assessment does not take this into account. Mounting evidence shows that chemicals act differently in children, especially in their brains, than in adults. During critical windows of fetal and early childhood development even tiny amounts of toxic chemicals can cause catastrophic damage. We need to embrace a

Alternatives assessment is a simple, common-sense alternative to risk assessment. It is based on the premise that it is not acceptable to damage human and nonhuman health or the environment if there are reasonable alternatives. The approach calls for taking precautionary measures even if some cause-and-effect relationships have not been fully established scientifically. The process must involve examination of the full range of alternatives, including no action at all. Equally important, it must be democratic, and it must include potentially affected parties.[23]

better decision-making technique called *alternatives assessment* that incorporates the guidance of the precautionary principle.

The bottom line is that you don't have time to wait until the government and the various agencies figure out what's safe and what's not. Tomorrow you will find yourself in the grocery or department store faced with decisions to make about what products to buy for your family and home. How will you make those decisions?

The information contained in this book will help. Take it with you when you shop, even after you have understood and integrated all its important information. We all need reminders and ongoing support. I forget things all the time because life is busy. So do keep this book around and consult it regularly. Keep it in the laundry room on top of the washing machine and each time you go in there to do some laundry pick the book up and flick through it again and remind yourself of some of the basics. Or keep it by the stove so that while you are waiting for something to cook you can pick it up to jog your memory. I really believe that the purpose of education is action, not knowledge. Unless we get active and start changing things in our homes, health problems will still befall us. Will education alone help you to prevent cancer or will getting all those chemical cleaning products out of your home help more? Only you can decide in the end and all you need is a little common sense.

Most immediate gains

1. Don't use fragranced products in the home. Even your personal fragrance or hair product could affect your child when you are around them or give them a hug.
2. Install a whole house water filtration system or, at the very least, shower filters in your bathroom. Remember to replace them regularly. Washing your face in unfiltered water can aggravate your skin.
3. Unplug all appliances after use to reduce EMRs.
4. Bathtime toys. If you leave them in the bathtub and don't empty them out or wring them out they become the perfect breeding ground for mold. A few years ago I was horrified to see a black slimey substance shoot out of the air hole of my son's rubber duck one bath time when he squeezed it to make it quack.
5. Switch out light bulbs and replace with full spectrum energy efficient bulbs. Full spectrum lamps and desk lamps are also available.
6. Give yourself a "chemical-free holiday." Whenever you are staying home for the day or even half a day, rest from using all your usual personal care products including cosmetics.
7. Develop the habit of always reading labels and teach your children too. Being an informed consumer can't start too early.
8. Take an inventory of all your personal care products. Get rid of anything toxic or questionable and replace with healthy alternatives. You may need to call your

local household hazardous waste facility for guidance on disposal, don't just pour them down the drain. Look on the Internet for products you can't find in your local stores.

9. Switch over to organic cotton towels and save the old ones for cleaning or mopping up spills.

10. Make sure the exhaust fan in your bathroom has enough CFM (cubic feet per minute) of air movement to effectively remove moisture.

CHAPTER 9

Kitchens

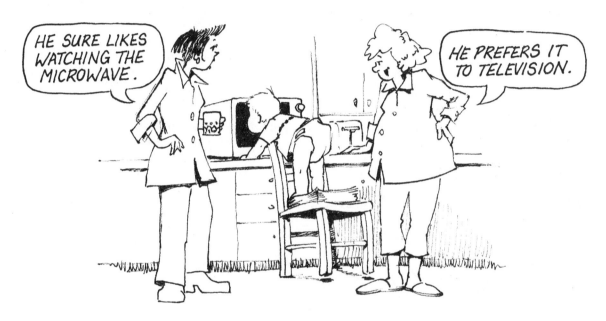

It's a quiet Sunday morning. Liz and Mark have been enjoying the novelty of cleaning their new house, which doesn't take very long since they only spend time in about a third of it.

While Mark disappears into the garage to tinker with a few projects he has in progress, Liz sits down to a cup of freshly microwaved coffee and a copy of her favorite women's magazine which contains a sample of the latest new fragrance. She sniffs the magazine and smiles. "Not bad!" she declares out loud to her empty kitchen.

The kitchen door suddenly bursts open.

Liz just about leaps out of her skin in surprise.

"Aunty Liz, Aunty Liz!" yells her nephew Jack as he runs towards her with the force of a bullet.

Liz's pregnant sister Jane appears through the door some seconds later smiling and out of breath. "Thought we'd pop in and keep you company for a while. How are you doing in this beautiful new home of yours?"

"Well Jack just about gave me a heart attack, but apart from that, I have to tell you this place is a dream come true. Do you fancy a coffee, I just made myself one."

"Oh, tea for me please," Jane says.

Liz puts another cup of water in the microwave to heat.

"Jack see!" declares Jack as he drags a chair across the kitchen and positions it right in front of the microwave. He promptly climbs up and pushes his face against the glass door of the microwave to watch the cup go around on the turntable.

"Do you think its OK for him to do that?" Jane asks, in a concerned tone of voice.

"Of course it is. They're no different than any other electrical appliance," Liz says.

"Jack loves coming over here and watching your microwave. I think he prefers it to TV. Ours broke and I've been wondering whether to get a new one or not," Jane says, still sounding hesitant.

"I'd be lost without my microwave, I do everything in it. It's so quick and easy and I don't have to mess up the rest of the kitchen," Liz enthuses.

The microwave pings to show its cycle is complete. Jack's face is only momentarily disappointed before his next idea. "Popcorn Aunty Liz!" Jack says, clapping his hands together.

Liz places a packet of microwave popcorn in the microwave and lets Jack press the start button. Again Jack places his face against the glass door and waits with rapt attention for the exploding to begin.

As the two women sit with their drinks, Liz sighs and looks around her new kitchen with a big smile. "This is the life! Don't you just love that new home smell!"

"Yes, it's great Liz, I wish I could afford a smell like that," Jane says wistfully.

The moment is punctured by the sound of popcorn exploding. "Yeeehaa!" yells Jack.

Commentary

Kitchens are the heart of our homes. Deep within all of us is an ancestral memory of gathering around the hearth for warmth, food, friendship, and to experience a feeling of connection to the place we call home.

Building Biology perspective

Bau-biologie is sometimes translated as "building with nature" or "building for life." These particular translations seem most appropriate when discussing kitchens. Our connection with nature reminds us of our own interconnectedness. Our kitchen needs to be vitally connected to the rest of our home. Like the heart that pumps the life force and blood throughout our body and the emotional center that when nourished sustains us in our busy and often unpredictable lives, kitchens help keep us alive.

In the old days kitchens were called common rooms. They were a kind of kitchen/living room where a multitude of activities took place. Women cooked, sewed, and weaved. Children played and the baby in its cradle was always next to the hearth. Men gathered in the evenings around the kitchen table to discuss local matters. The central focus was the large hearth because it was the only source of heat.

But kitchens have dramatically changed over the years, particularly since World War II when the family structure began to change. Women began working outside the home and the around-the-clock job cycle resulted in the disintegration of family dinners as a gathering point of the day.[1] In addition, post-war food production introduced new ways of cooking and serving food so that the kitchen lost much of its focus and for many families became nothing more than a place for heating and dispensing commercially prepared foods.

Design

The design of modern kitchens often reflects these changes. Some kitchens are too small, some too large, and many have no comfortable place to sit and enjoy a meal or keep the cook company. The hearth is gone, replaced by a stove or microwave oven. A kitchen may still function, but where has the connection gone that once drew everyone to the kitchen? Where has that sense of home gone?

I believe that if we put our attention back on the kitchen, if we orient ourselves towards health and remember our home is a living organism, then family and friends will return to the kitchen and we will rekindle the nourishment needed to strengthen and protect our bodies in these environmentally harsh times.

The third skin layer

Follow the basic checklist, and then ass the following ideal building features for a healthy kitchen:

1. Never use carpet in the kitchen, it will inevitably become damp from spills and accidents inviting mold, and if kitchen carpet is not kept meticulously clean the daily deposit of food debris will invite pests. Area rugs can be used for decoration or a little extra cushioning underfoot in spots like in front of the kitchen sink.
2. Windows need to open to allow the moisture generated from cooking and cleaning to escape and let fresh air in. Also, a sturdy ventilation hood should be installed over the stove. This needs to be vented to the outside of the house.
3. Any built-in items such as kitchen cabinetry are free of synthetic formaldehyde.
4. Large EMR-generating appliances such as refrigerators are placed away from places where people spend large amounts of time and preferably are placed against an outside wall.
5. A point-of-use water filtration system is installed and attached to the kitchen water tap.
6. Water pipes are made from non-toxic materials.

Your layer

Let's take a look at Liz's kitchen and discuss the best and worse case scenarios.

Water

Water is one of the main features of any kitchen. Water to cook with, to clean with, and to drink. Good quality water is essential for health. Unfortunately, as we have already discussed in Chapters 3, 5 and 8, you can longer assume that the water brought to your home is safe for consumption. Filtering your water at home now needs to be considered as important as having a roof on your house.

Liz's new house came without any water filtration installed. Her water is delivered from her local municipality in concrete pipes and her home distributes water through PVC pipes. Today, this is considered normal purely because it is the modus operandi, not because it's a great set up proven to protect people's health from all known harm.

In order to decide which system of filtration is best for your home, you need to find out what's in your water. Your public water company is required to regularly test the water they deliver to your tap for eight contaminants (fecal bacteria, fertilizer, mercury, lead, zinc and cadmium, some pesticides, and some industrial chemicals — dioxin, PCBs, styrene, benzene, tetrachlorethylene) and report their findings to the EPA and the state. Water utilities are supposed to tell customers at least once a year, in their waste water bill, what pollutants have been detected in their drinking water and whether water quality standards have been violated. For more facts, or to see if your public water provider has posted their report on the web, visit: <http://www.epa.gov/safewater/dwinfo.htm> You can also phone your local company and ask them to send you a copy of their most recent report.

> Either we filter out the contaminants in water before we consume it or we force our body to be the filter.

If you are among the 40 million Americans who get their water from a private well, then only you can provide your family the protection necessary from potential pollutants in your water. Have the water from your tap tested each year. Contact the Environmental Drinking Water Hotline at 1-800-426-4791. This is a private company contracted by the EPA to supply names of state certification officials. They will have a list of certified labs that meet EPA standards. If your water is contaminated, the hotline can provide you with important information to help you protect your family.

In general, installing a whole house water filtration system will provide better quality water to your whole house. However, in the kitchen I believe it is necessary to install an additional point-of-use filtration unit, attached to the main tap you use, for additional filtration. At first this may seem like overkill but consider this: if you have old copper pipes with lead solder, lead pipes, or pipes made from PVC, these pipes can leach their own pollutants into the water carried between your whole house water filtration unit's point of filtration and your tap. As a precautionary measure always run your kitchen tap for a couple of minutes each morning before running your filter to flush out any contaminated water stored in the pipes overnight. Then your water is ready for drinking or cooking.

Fluoridation

Water fluoridation has been very controversial over the years. Those for it say it reduces dental cavities, those against it say it causes other health problems. If the source of the fluoride added to drinking water is contaminated, then additional toxins may be added to water such as lead, arsenic, radium, and alumina.[2] Find out if your water is fluoridated and where the fluoride comes from. If you decide you want to remove fluoride you will need a special filter.

Once you have discovered what's in your water, you are ready to select the best filtering system for your home (see Appendix C). Don't be fooled by salespeople who make claims they can't substantiate. Ask for written documentation of exactly what a system will filter and then compare two or three different models before you decide. Once installed, mark on your calendar when the filters will need to be replaced (see Chapter 17). This is really important. It's false economy to try to make filters last longer by not replacing them in a timely fashion. Filters become inefficient when not replaced promptly.

Bottled water is not the answer either. According to *Bottled Water: Pure Drink or Pure Hype?* a study by the Natural Resource Defense Council, "While much tap water is indeed risky, having compared available data, we conclude that there is no assurance that bottled water is any safer than tap water. We have no way of knowing the actual quality of bottled water."[4]

Bottled water is expensive ($1 to $4 a gallon). We think it's higher quality, when in fact the quality of bottled water is at best unknown. For as little as ten cents a gallon, filtering your own water at home with a well-chosen system is by far more economical, more convenient, and is the most reliable way of producing the highest quality healthy water. If you need bottled water for travel or to take to work, fill your own glass quart jar at home with filtered water and take it with you. For children at school, I suggest a stainless steel thermos that does not break or leak easily, and is easy to clean.

One final source of water in the kitchen to consider is refrigerators with cool drinking water functions and ice makers. Make sure this water is filtered or do not use it. Even if you have a whole house water filtration system I am still concerned about the water pipes within the refrigerator. What are they made from? How do you clean them? If they are

In December, 2003 Representative Glenn Donnelson (R. Utah) was interviewed about community water fluoridation. He made the following comments:

"Most people do not realize that the fluoride chemicals placed in water are not the same fluoride chemicals placed in toothpastes, mouth rinses, and topical gels. More than 90 percent of the chemicals used to fluoridate water in the U.S. are not pharmaceutical grade. Instead, they come from the wet scrubbing systems of the superphosphate fertilizer industry. These chemicals, known as silicofluorides, are sodium fluorosilicate and fluorosilic acid and are classified by the EPA as hazardous waste. But when they are sold for as little as a penny, they are classified as a product. Silicofluorides are contaminated with toxic metals and trace amounts of radioactive isotopes such as lead, mercury, arsenic, uranium, radium, and cadmium. In fact, recent testing by the National Sanitation Foundation suggests that the level of arsenic in these chemicals are high and of significant concern. .

"A major concern is that the Food and Drug Administration (FDA) has never approved fluoride for safety or effectiveness. Chemicals added to water to make it safe or potable are within the jurisdiction of the EPA. When a product, substance, or chemical are added to the public water supply for the purpose of treating or preventing a disease, that chemical must have an approval health claim by the FDA. To say that 'fluoridated water will decrease tooth decay' is an illegal health claim."[3]

Used by industry to degrease metal parts, trichloroethylene (TCE) is now estimated to be in 34 % of the nation's drinking water. The EPA classifies TCE as a probable human carcinogen.[5]

Of the over 2,000 contaminants found in potable water, as of June 2003 the EPA has established standards for only 87.[6]

Municipal water treatment is primarily set up for disinfection rather than water purification.

A new study reveals that even exposure to "safe" amounts of lead damages children's intelligence. In fact, lead's effect on intelligence is proportionately greater at low blood levels, meaning most of the damage is caused before the maximum level is reached.[7]

Chloroform is a colorless liquid which evaporates very quickly but breaks down slowly once in the air. It is one of the most hazardous urban air toxic pollutants, according to EPA's National Air Toxic Assessment (NATA). Most people ingest chloroform in their water and inhale it as it evaporates from water uses. The typical home indoor air concentration obtained from monitoring studies is two micrograms per cubic meter ($\mu g/m3$) for indoor air. The carcinogenic health benchmark that provides a protective level for chloroform is 0.043 $\mu g/m3$. Chloroform is classified by the EPA as a probable human carcinogen. Chronic human exposure to chloroform through inhalation can cause adverse health effects in the liver, such as hepatitis and jaundice, and central nervous system effects, such as depression and irritability.[8]

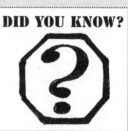

DID YOU KNOW?

plastic they can leach chemicals into the water, and if not flushed out and cleaned regularly they may become moldy and contaminate your drinking water. To be sure your ice is safe to use, only use water that has already been filtered. This may require going back to using little ice trays and filling them regularly with your own filtered water.

The only way to really rest assured that your family is drinking good water is to take care of it yourself. Have your water checked annually. Things change. New pollutants are constantly finding their way into our water supply. The effort required to protect your family's water supply is a great investment when it comes to something as important as the water you drink, cook, and bathe in.

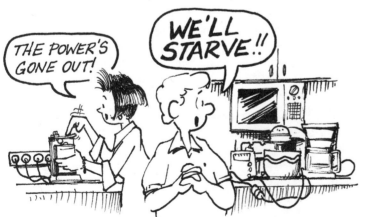

Appliances

Every kitchen comes equipped with a variety of appliances. But how many appliances do you really need and how many do you use on a regular basis?

Let's discuss some of the main ones first.

Refrigerators

Refrigerators store and preserve our food. They are also the biggest energy users in the kitchen. In a healthy kitchen there are a few considerations.

First, because of the high AC magnetic field refrigerators generate when their motors are running, they should be placed away from places where people spend large amounts of time sitting or sleeping, including whatever is on the other side of any adjoining wall. In Liz's home, the refrigerator is placed against a wall on the other side of which Mark sits all day in his home office. He receives a significant EMR exposure just from the refrigerator.

> Some 20-40 percent of household energy is consumed in the kitchen.[9]

Also, place your refrigerator away from the stove, dishwasher, or water heater. In fact they all should be as far apart as workably possible. It requires tremendous amounts of energy to keep a refrigerator cool, so placing it next to heat-generating appliances adds further energy burdens to your refrigerator's efficiency.

Secondly, the style of refrigerator you choose (or already have) is important. Self-defrosting models have a drip pan located somewhere under the unit. These drip pans are notorious for bad odors and microorganism growth. They should be cleaned monthly. When choosing your refrigerator make sure the drip pan is easily accessible from the front and has adequate clearance underneath for ease of cleaning. Liz has not read her owner's manual for her new refrigerator and so doesn't know that the drip pan needs to be cleaned regularly. It's a good idea to keep the cooling coils clean too — they're located behind or underneath the refrigerator — otherwise they can become coated with dust, which affects your indoor air quality. When kept clean your refrigerator will work much more efficiently and save energy costs.

Thirdly, keeping the inside of your refrigerator clean is essential. Some people like to keep their refrigerators jammed full of food and forget to clean it out weekly. Food spoils, mold grows, and all your food risks being contaminated. An pleasant thought, but uncommonly true (see Chapter 16). Keeping your refrigerator less cluttered makes it easier to clean and is more energy efficient as you won't need to keep the refrigerator door open as long while you try to find what you are looking for.

Stoves

There are many different options when it comes to stoves, but basically they can be defined as electric or gas.

Gas

Natural gas and propane ranges have been popular for a long time. Some chefs will cook only on gas stoves because they allow for better timing and temperature control. The down side is that they release polluting combustion byproducts including carbon dioxide,

In a study of 47,000 chemically sensitive patients, the most important sources of indoor air pollution responsible for generating illness were the gas stove, hot water heater, and furnace. Exposure to gas fumes primarily affects the cardiovascular and nervous system, but can affect any organ of the body. Some of the earliest symptoms include depression, fatigue, irritability, and inability to concentrate.[10]

carbon monoxide, nitrogen dioxide, nitrous oxides, and small amounts of formaldehyde. Older models that have a continuously burning pilot light are the most problematic as they produce combustion byproducts continuously. There can also be problems with leaking gas pipes. A large leak can cause an explosion, but smaller undetected leaks can have quite insidious health effects. One Environmental Inspector colleague told me he finds leaking gas in 60 percent of the homes he inspects.

If you already have a gas stove or are anticipating buying one, the newer models now have electronic ignitions which removes the problem of pilot lights continually creating combustion by-products. Another idea is to have a gas fired range-top with an electric oven.

Pay attention to the color of the flame your gas stove produces. If your stove is functioning correctly, the flame will burn bright blue. If you have a yellow flame this indicates incomplete combustion. Deadly carbon monoxide fumes are produced in great quantities as a result of incomplete combustion. If you discover yellow flames, have a qualified service person come out immediately and check your stove. As a precautionary measure there are now little home kits for monitoring carbon monoxide levels in your kitchen (see Appendix C).

Electric

Liz has an electric stove and oven, though she doesn't use them much as she prefers her microwave oven. Electric stoves are considered cleaner than gas stoves and are definitely the kind of stove recommended for people who have environmental sensitivities. However, all electric cook tops, ovens, and ranges produce elevated AC magnetic fields. Obviously, when cooking, some exposure to EMRs is inescapable with an electric stove so you may want to check the strength of the fields with a Gaussmeter (see Chapter 5).

Different electric stoves may vary in their field strength. See if you can establish a comfortable balance between creating distance from the stove while at the same time being close enough to cook. It would be prudent not to lean against your electric stove while waiting for something to cook.

British researchers reported in the medical journal *Lancet* that in a study of 1,159 people, women who cooked with gas stoves were more likely to have asthma than those who cooked on electric.[11]

Electric stovetops now come in several styles. Traditional stovetops have spiral elements to cook on. These must be kept clean otherwise grease and cooking debris will combust on the elements creating indoor pollution. Only use non-toxic cleaners on the elements otherwise you will be introducing more chemicals into your kitchen air every time you switch on your stove and the elements heat up. There are also models that have plate-style elements and models that have a radiant glass surfaces. Both of these are much easier to keep clean because of their flat surfaces. Beware of free or recommended cleaning products that can accompany a new stove. They can be horrendously toxic.

Ovens

Ovens are prone to cooking spills and debris. They need to be cleaned regularly to prevent food incineration smells and pollution. Continuous-cleaning ovens have coatings on their walls that release noxious fumes. Self-cleaning ovens produce other substances that create air pollution and many commercial brand oven cleaners are toxic. The best way to clean your oven is to use baking soda on fresh spills and then rub (see Chapter 16).

Microwave ovens

It is estimated that over 90 percent of American homes now use microwave ovens for meal preparation.[12] Liz does most of her cooking with her microwave oven because it is quick and does not create as much mess in her kitchen.

Microwave ovens function quite differently from conventional ovens. A microwave oven uses a device called a magnetron which produces microwaves that penetrate through food containers and into food where they excite the water molecules creating friction which produces heat. This is what cooks the food. Microwave ovens also emit high AC magnetic fields.

The health and safety of microwave ovens in the U.S. is still controversial. Russia has done the most research on microwave radiation and it is interesting to note that in 1976 the Soviet Union banned the use of microwave ovens.[13]

The main concerns are:

1. Microwave ovens can leak microwave radiation. The debate is over how much leakage is safe?
2. What happens to the food cooked in microwave ovens?
3. What happens to us when we eat it?

I would advise a precautionary approach when it comes to using microwave ovens. Better safe than sorry. Here are some ideas:

1. If you can do without a microwave oven, do without it. If you can't, then try to reduce your use. Go back to heating water on the stove when making a cup of tea.
2. When using your microwave, press the start button and move away at least four feet. Twelve feet would be better. This is especially true for children who may like to watch the food while it is cooking. The oven door is the most dangerous place for microwave leakage.
3. Have your microwave professionally checked for any leakages at least once a year or purchase your own microwave detector so you can check more often (see Appendix C). Any detected leakage is unacceptable.

4. Keep the seal around the microwave door free from food debris and make sure nothing is trapped in the door such as a paper towel before using.
5. If your microwave behaves unusually, i.e. it starts making funny noises or you see a few sparks fly, stop using it and have it checked by a professional.
6. Do not microwave food in plastic containers. Only use ceramic or ovenproof glass (such as pyrex) with oven-proof glass lids or plates.
7. Place microwaves at a distance from main food preparation areas. Should they be leaking microwave radiation, you will be at a safer distance.

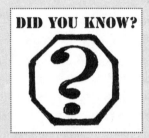

DID YOU KNOW?

These modern ovens for rapid cooking and grilling can lead to neurological reactions, hormone alterations, cell damage, difficulties with gall bladder and bladder, digestive disturbances, and can lead to cataracts.[14]

Researchers at Stanford University School of Medicine in Stanford, California have noted that a mother's breast milk, when reheated in a microwave oven, loses some of its infection-fighting properties. Microwaving breast milk was found to break down antibodies and proteins that normally inhibit bacterial growth and help a newborn fight infection. Microwaving breast milk appears to compromise its immune-fighting abilities. (The practice of collecting and freezing breast milk, then reheating it in microwave ovens, has become standard in most neonatal care units today).[15]

A "microwave-safe" or "microwavable" label on plastic containers only means that they shouldn't melt, crack, or fall apart when used in the microwave. These labels do not guarantee that containers don't leach chemicals into foods when heated; the U.S. Food and Drug Administration does not regulate these labels and has not developed any standards for them. As a precaution, *Green Guide* science advisor Lisa Lefferts always avoids using plastic in her microwave. "You don't want hot, fatty food touching plastic in the microwave," she cautions. "Plastic plus hot plus fat is the worst combination. That's because most chemicals that leach from plastic are lipophilic (they love fat) and temperature speeds up the leaching process into the fat."[16]

Dishwashers

Eighty percent of the cost of running a dishwasher is in heating the water.[17] Water needs to be heated to high levels to really clean well. Liz's home is not equipped with a whole house water filtration unit and so her water contains a whole host of chemicals including chlorine and other substances. Running the dishwasher is essentially like taking an enclosed shower. The heated water will volatilize these substances into the air creating considerable indoor air pollution (see Chapter 8). Combined with this you have the chemicals and substances found in commercial dishwashing detergent such as chlorine and fragrance. Further chemicals are added if you use solutions to prevent water marks on glassware. This chemical cocktail can leak fumes into the kitchen when the dishwasher is operating and in the steamy mist when the door is opened after washing.

I am also concerned that chemical residues remain on the washed dishes and utensils. Do some detective work and next time you run the dishwasher, see if you notice any smells and then inspect your dishes and utensils. See if you can smell, feel, see, or even taste any residues. If you can, then you and your family are ingesting dishwashing detergent in small amounts every time you eat or drink. No one knows the long-term health effects of these exposures.

Dishwashers also vary greatly in their ability to clean and the amount of noise they produce. If you are in the market to buy a new dishwasher, choose one with energy-efficiency settings, that cleans thoroughly, and is quiet. Noise pollution at home is another important health concern.

Try the following tips for your dishwasher:

Many people report such symptoms as headache, fatigue, burning eyes, and difficulty breathing when exposed to even the small amount of chlorine released during normal dishwashing. [18]

"One day people will have to fight noise as we must fight cholera and pestilence now."
— Robert Koch, M.D., Bacteriologist, 1905 Nobel Prize Winner.

1. Be sure to open a window when you use your dishwasher.
2. If you have a range hood that vents to the outside of your home run this as well.
3. Use a non-toxic, fragrance-free, biodegradable dishwashing detergent.
4. Instead of using chemicals to prevent watermarks on glassware, use vinegar.
5. Only run your dishwasher when you have a full load and try to run it at the end of the day or when people are not around. If you have a kitchen door close it.

Smaller appliances

Liz's kitchen contains a vast array of smaller appliances that are all plugged in and ready to go. But given that neither Liz nor Mark are gourmet chefs and neither of them spend much time cooking in their kitchen, you have to wonder why they have so many appliances. Liz would tell you that they are really just decorative and they are there in case she needs them. The main health concern here is the amount of EMRs being generated unnecessarily. Even if an appliance is not in use, it will still create an AC electric field while plugged in.

Take stock of your own kitchen and see how many smaller appliances you have which are plugged in. Can any of these be unplugged while not in use? Can any of these be stored and put away until needed? It is much simpler and quicker to clean your healthy kitchen when you have fewer appliances to navigate around.

I have been able to get our smaller kitchen appliances down to only two: a toaster and a CD player. Everything else is stored until needed. One final tip. Do let the rest of the family know that you will now be unplugging smaller kitchen appliances when not in use. This will prevent family members from panicking and thinking appliances are not working or broken, and it will also encourage them to join your efforts and remember to unplug appliances after they have used them too.

Ventilation

A healthy kitchen needs great ventilation. Everyday cooking and cleaning generate significant amounts of indoor pollution. Liz does not open her kitchen windows and though her stove's range hood looks nice and new it is pathetically weak. This combination has the potential to generate lots of humidity and condensation, which over time can create ideal conditions for mold growth. It also allows an accumulation of VOCs and other pollutants to build to very high levels.

Opening windows while cooking or running the dishwasher will help, but for best results, install a good quality range hood above the stove and properly vent it to the outside of the home. Some range hoods merely filter the air through a carbon filter and then recirculate it. These do not remove kitchen pollution sufficiently.

It is wise to invest in the largest available range hood with variable speed controls. Some models have remote fans that are quieter when operating. When using your range hood always open a window to supply the make-up air that will be needed to replace the vented air. Otherwise negative pressure will be created and the air needed to replace the vented air will be pulled through the path of least resistance. This means air could be pulled from a fireplace chimney creating a dangerous backdraft of air that can be much more polluted than the air you are trying to vent.

PVC

Liz's kitchen has a new vinyl covered floor. Although it is easy for her to keep clean and gives her the look she wants, what Liz doesn't know is that it is also silently offgassing toxic chemicals such as vinyl chloride from the vinyl and an array of solvents from the adhesive used to fix it in place.

But Liz's floor is not the only source of PVC in her kitchen. She has PVC water pipes, and in her cupboards and drawers she has more PVC in the form of food packaging such as the plastic trays in her boxed cookies, cling wrap which she likes to wrap everything in, especially when she microwaves food, and PVC bottles. Unfortunately, this means that Liz and Mark are exposed to plasticizing chemicals (which can disrupt hormones) through food every day. What will the long-term health effects be?

Of the ten billion pounds of polyvinyl chloride (PVC) resin produced annually in the U.S., 60 percent is used in construction. The most prevalent use of PVC in construction is for piping of water, gas and sewer drainage. Vinyl is used in 66 percent of all American kitchens as flooring. Other construction uses include: window frames, doors, wire sheathing, imitation leather, furniture and vinyl wallpaper.[19]

Floor coverings

Kitchen floors are subjected to much wear and tear, dampness, and large amounts of food debris. At least Liz has a hard floor covering which will be easier to keep clean than a carpet. I have lived in a home with a carpeted kitchen, and I will never do so again. We are enthusiastic cooks in my family and some food inevitably ends up on the floor requiring constant cleaning, scrubbing, and maintenance not only for cleanliness but also to prevent pests.

Hard surfaces are the best for kitchen floors. If a little extra cushioning is required in key areas of the kitchen where you stand for large amounts of time, such as in front of the sink or stove, a thick throw rug or mat will usually do the trick. These will need to be vacuumed or shaken outside on a regular basis.

Cabinets

Many kitchen cabinets contain formaldehyde and other toxic chemicals. When cabinets are new, as in Liz's kitchen, the VOC levels are very high. With time these levels will drop but what will happen to someone's health in the meantime from breathing in these fumes on a daily basis? I am also concerned about storing food in new cabinets with high formaldehyde levels. I have found no studies done on the possible contamination of food stored in high formaldehyde cabinets, but it seems plausible that as chemicals volatize in confined areas like cupboards, these chemicals could contaminate the food stored there. I posed this question to Jack D. Thrasher, Ph.D. who is a toxicologist/immunotoxicologist and author of the book, *The Poisoning of Our Homes and Workplaces: The Truth About the Indoor Formaldehyde Crisis.* He replied, "Since formaldehyde easily forms covalent bonds it could bind to food. After all, this is the mechanism by which formaldehyde antibodies are determined." Anyone fancy formaldehyde-flavored cereal for breakfast?

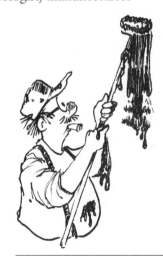

Liz's best solution is to open her kitchen windows and ventilate the space. She could also paint a special sealant on her cabinets to try to stop the chemicals from escaping. If you are planning to build a new house or remodel your current kitchen, be sure to choose formaldehyde-free cabinetry.

Paint

Liz's kitchen has been painted with oil-based latex paint that contains benzene, formaldehyde, toluene, and xylene, which are all known carcinogens or neurotoxins. These chemicals can offgass into the air for an indefinite amount of time and vapors can be circulated to the rest of the house through her forced air heating system.

There are now many healthier choices available for paint. Look for no-VOC or low-VOC paint with limits set by California's South Coast Air Quality Management District (SCAQMD). Natural milk paints are another no-VOC option, but they must be used quickly once mixed and are prone to mildew, making them unfit for bathrooms or kitchens. Even paints made from certified organic plants might give off natural VOCs from citrus or pine-based solvents, which can cause

Oil-based paints rely on VOC-emitting solvents such as mineral spirits to control their drying time, but conventional water-based latex paints aren't necessarily milder. They can contain such VOCs as formaldehyde and the suspected carcinogen acrylonitrile, as well as ethylene glycol ethers associated with lowered sperm count, and fungicides and preservatives to combat mold and mildew.[20]

allergic reactions in some people. It's a good idea to test any paint before covering a whole wall. Pregnant women should never paint or even enter a freshly painted room until it has dried and been ventilated for at least 72 hours.

Pests

Kitchens are a source of food and water to more than just your family. Pests will happily try to move in if they have easy access to these resources. Unfortunately, many people are quick to grab a pesticide product to kill the intruder without realizing that these products can cause significant harm to the rest of the family (see Chapter 14).

> Of the pesticides legally allowed to be used on food crops, the EPA considers 60 percent of the registered herbicides, 90 percent of the fungicides, and 30 percent of the insecticides to be potentially carcinogenic.[21]

Toxic pesticides do not solve pest problems. Only when you find the source of the problem and fix that will you truly get rid of any pests in your kitchen. Here's a mini crash-course of non-toxic ways to get rid of indoor pests:

1. First identify what pests you have and roughly how many there are.
2. Next, do some detective work and see if you can find where they are getting into your kitchen. Repair, caulk, or seal any points of entry such as cracks, crevices, and holes around pipes. Be sure to use non-toxic caulking.
3. Look around your kitchen to find what is attracting them. Remove any sources of water and food. Empty any standing containers of water and check around the bases of plants. Don't leave dirty dishes overnight in sinks. Look for crumbs and debris in carpets or rugs. Clean work surfaces immediately after cooking and remove food left out in the open such as fruit or bread. Take garbage out daily and if you have pets, don't leave their food out all day. Good housekeeping will easily remove these pest attractions.
4. If you are still attracting pests after doing all of the above, contact one of the organizations that specialize in helping homeowners with non-toxic ways to solve pest problems, or look for resources specifically addressing Integrated Pest Management (IPM) strategies.

Food

Although this is a book about how your home impacts your family's health, we can't talk about the kitchen without briefly mentioning food. Kitchens are the heart of the home and likewise the food we prepare in them gives us vital nourishment. From the perspective of body burden and chemical load we must figure into the picture how much of our commercial food is heavily laden with chemicals. We are dealing with pesticides, herbicides, fungicides, chemical fertilizers, heavy metals such as mercury, dioxins, genetically modified organisms (GMOs), colors and preservatives, to name but a few.

Children eat more per pound of weight than adults do. Their exposure to toxic chemicals in food is therefore considerably higher. Combine this with a rapidly growing and still maturing body and its easy to see why many children are experiencing health problems. The best way to avoid all of these chemicals is to simply buy organic food.

We must consider the quality of food we eat as part of the overall picture of achieving and maintaining good health. It really can tip the balance for or against us. The more we support organic farmers the lower their prices will become. I have found that when you eat organic produce that is in season it is often the same price, if not lower, than non-organic food. It tastes better too.

Cookware and food storage

Over the years, concerns about cookware continue to surface. In the 1970s aluminum cookware was linked with Alzheimer's disease because of the elevated levels of aluminum found in the brains of some Alzheimer's patients. Many people have since phased out using aluminum pots, pans, and cooking foil as a preventative measure.

Recently a new concern has surfaced. The safety of non-stick coatings such as Teflon have been called into question because of a group of chemicals called "perfluorochemicals" (PFCs). Originally these indestructible chemicals were considered biologically inert. However recent scientific findings now show them to be "highly toxic, extraordinarily persistent chemicals that pervasively contaminate human blood and wildlife the world over."[23] PFCs can be found in non-stick pans, furniture, cosmetics, household cleaners, clothing, packaged food containers, products designed to repel soil, grease, and water, including carpet and furniture treatments, food wraps, sprays for leather, shoes and other clothing, paints, cleaning products, shampoo, and floor wax.

> The U.S. Environmental Protection Agency estimates a 1 in 1000 chance of contracting cancer from dioxin exposure through a typical American diet.[22]

Faced with such a long list of household products where do you begin removing these chemicals from your life? As a first step, I would recommend getting rid of any non-stick pans and replacing them with glass, stainless steel, or cast iron; all of them are tried and true for safety. Then look for any old products you may already have like scotchguard water repellant for shoes, and get rid of those. Let each product you remove and replace with a healthier choice be a little personal victory: one less toxic chemical for your family to have to deal with.

Another important consideration, besides the type of cookware you use, is how you store your food. As we have already discussed, some plastics can leach chemicals like hormone-disrupting phthalates into whatever they come in contact with. If you currently use plastic containers to store food in, switching to glass would be a better choice. Instead of the plastic sandwich bags we send our children to school with, use cellulose sandwich bags (see Appendix C). These switches are easy and simple. Nowhere in the house are small improvements felt as much as in the kitchen.

> In studies the 3M Company submitted to the government in 2001, scientists reported finding PFOA (one of the PFC chemicals) in the blood of 96 percent of 598 children tested in 23 states and the District of Columbia.[24]

Reduce, reuse, recycle

Every kitchen generates waste. What we do with it is the interesting question. Throwaway packaging is the worst offender and yet we have become so accustomed to it we hardly even notice it. Fortunately, as a global community people are becoming more aware of

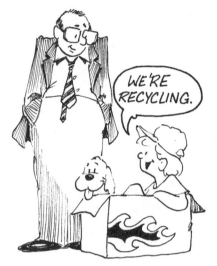

the need to recycle. We cannot continue to generate massive amounts of waste. The first step you can take is to reduce the amount of waste your family generates. Next time you are at the store, choose products with less packaging. Interestingly enough, many of the companies that make healthier products also use less resources and less packaging. Our physical health and the health of the planet are interconnected.

Next, pay attention to products that can be reused. I prefer to buy food like organic peanut butter in glass jars instead of plastic. These jars are great to reuse for raisins, left over food, or for children to put water in when painting. Much of the waste that ends up in everyday kitchen trash is recyclable. Contact your local recycling facility to find out what can be recycled in your community and where you need to take your recycling to. Some communities provide curbside collection.

Compost

Composting your kitchen vegetable and organic waste scraps is a wonderful way to reduce waste and generate something very worthwhile: truly organic compost. This kind of compost is full of nutrients and makes excellent soil fertilizer for your garden, trees, or plants. A healthy replacement for chemical laden fertilizers (see Chapter 14). If you don't use it yourself, ask a neighbor who likes to garden if they would like it, or ask a local farmer.

All you need to get started is a small container with a lid to put your compost items in. It's a good idea to keep it out of the sun so the heat won't make it smell bad. You need to be careful not to keep food waste in your kitchen for very long because mold grows very quickly on it and people with mold allergies might react to it. Take your compost out every day or two and add to a composting bin or designated composting area in your garden. Do not put animal products in compost. There are several good books on composting and organic gardening (see Appendix C).

Returning to the hearth

You are now suitably armed with a huge amount of information to transform your kitchen into a place that can nurture and restore your family's health on a daily basis. Welcome your family and friends back into your kitchen and stoke the hearth fires again, even if that can only be done metaphorically. For your home's longevity, keep its heart healthy!

Most immediate gains

1. Just say no to PVC. The only way to avoid PVC is to identify it first! On packaging, look for the "3" or the letters "PVC," often found next to the three-arrow recycling symbol. For other PVC products, you'll have to ask the manufacturers what materials were used. Lots of alternatives to PVC are available.
2. Be rigorous in your detective work and find all products containing pesticides, such as antibacterial soap, antimicrobial coatings, etc. and replace them with safe alternatives.
3. Create a welcoming family space in your kitchen.
4. Run your tap water first thing each morning to flush out the water that has been standing in water pipes overnight.
5. Buy organic food.
6. Switch from plastic sandwich and storage bags to cellulose bags.
7. Store food in glass jars.
8. Get rid of non-stick coated cookware such as Teflon.
9. Replace your old refrigerator with a newer energy efficient model that has an easily accessible drip pan. Clean the drip pan regularly.
10. Install a point-of-source water filter on your main kitchen tap.
11. Open up new cabinets and let them completely air out.
12. Replace antibacterial impregnated sponges with natural cellulose sponges and organic cotton cloths that can be regularly laundered (see Appendix C).
13. Granite counter tops can contain radioactivity. If you have a lot of granite in your kitchen or are planning to install it, have it inspected by an environmental inspector to ensure that radiation levels are safe.
14. Sometimes a mobile air purifier is helpful to dissipate strong cooking smells in the kitchen.
15. Watch where you put the baby's high chair and make sure it's not close to any source of high EMRs or a microwave oven. Babies can spend a lot of time in their high chairs while mothers cook or clean the kitchen.
16. Get rid of your microwave oven.

CHAPTER 10

Laundry

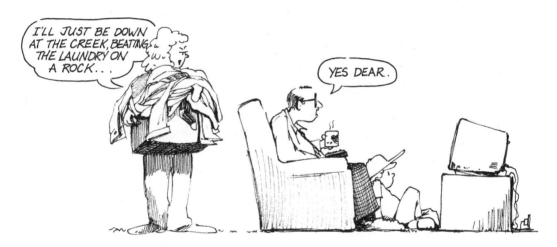

As Jane looks at the piles of laundry on the floor she wonders how her family ever came to have so many clothes. "Unreal," she mutters under her breath as she empties the last pile from her arms onto the floor. A sudden contraction takes her by surprise, forcing her to steady herself against the washing machine. "I'm not giving birth till I've got all this laundry done," she declares in a determined voice.

Jane's laundry is a little recessed alcove off her kitchen. It has just enough space to fit a washer and dryer and has one shelf to store all her laundry products. It has a concertina door that can be closed to separate it from the rest of the kitchen. Mostly the door is left open as there is always some laundry to be done. With no room for storage, laundry in process often takes up part of the kitchen. On any given day you will find piles of dirty clothes scattered near the washing machine waiting to be washed, and freshly laundered clothes drying over the backs of dining chairs or hanging from doors.

As Jane sifts through the next pile of clothing to be washed she pulls out two pairs of Tom's trousers which have grass stains, and three shirts of Jack's, two with a miscellaneous assortment of juice and food and one with marker pen stains on it. "Oh great, where did he get that from?"

Jane scans her laundry shelf looking for help. What an arsenal of cleaning products she has collected. First she tries a special spot

165

remover stick that says it removes grass stains on Tom's trousers. Then she finds another spot remover that says it works on food and stubborn juice stains. This is a new product she just bought at the store because she had a 50 percent discount coupon. "This should be good and it's 'odor-free' which must mean its more healthy." She sprays the bottle and a cloud of mist covers not only Jack's shirts but half of her other laundry. Jane sneezes. "That's powerful stuff!"

The final cleaning challenge is the shirt stained by the marker pen. "Let me see, I'm going to need something really strong for this one." Her eyes fall on a large container of chlorine bleach. "That should do it." Jane retrieves a bucket from the kitchen, fills it with water, and adds a good dash of bleach. The familiar smell of bleach wafts through the kitchen. Jane suddenly becomes light-headed and quickly sits down at the adjacent kitchen table.

After several minutes Jane revives and returns to her laundry project, although she now has a vague headache. "I've just got to get this laundry done or there will be nowhere to sit for dinner." She removes one load from the washing machine and transfers it to the dryer adding a couple of fragranced dryer sheets. Another load is added to the washing machine, including Tom's trousers, Jack's shirts, a cup full of "morning fresh" laundry detergent and a cup of "country bouquet" fabric softener. She hits the start button. "Voila ... a job well done," she declares as she heads for the sofa to take a much needed nap.

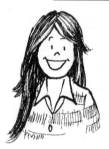

Commentary

Modern laundries are so well equipped with household cleaning products that they could be considered amateur chemical warfare laboratories. With our emphasis on speed and convenience we have become blinded to the important and far reaching effects our laundry can have on our home and our family's health.

Building Biology perspective

The laundry room is an extension of the bathroom. Our bathrooms clean our physical skin (the first layer) and our laundry rooms clean our clothes, bedding (our second skin), and other household items. Sadly the laundry is often one of the most neglected spaces in the home. Taking a bath or shower is pleasurable and can be relaxing or revitalizing. Doing the laundry however does not usually give us that same self-satisfaction-but what if it did? What if you could derive satisfaction from doing your laundry? I'm sure I've got you smiling by now, even if it's just because you find this idea ludicrous, but at least entertain the idea and let's see how you are feeling by the end of this chapter.

> The simple truth is that the way we allow chemicals to be used in society today means we are performing a vast experiment, not in the lab, but in the real world, not just on wildlife but on people.[1]

Let's take a look at the laundry room in layers

The Third Skin Layer

Follow the basic checklist and then add the following ideal building features for a healthy laundry room:

1. Radiant floor heating can be "zoned" so that different parts of the home can be maintained at different temperatures. As the laundry room is a less used room in the home and tends to become warm during use, it can be set at a lower temperature. This saves energy and makes this room more comfortable.
2. Never use carpet in a laundry. Laundries are prone to dampness from high humidity levels or can become wet from mechanical errors such as leaking pipes and faulty valves, inviting mold growth.
3. Even a small laundry space should have a window that can be opened to allow the moisture and any smells generated from washing and drying to escape. Mechanical ventilation is also very helpful provided it is vented to the outside of the house and away from other windows.
4. A small sink makes hand washing delicates and overnight soaking much more convenient.
5. Situate the washer and dryer against an exterior wall. These appliances generate high AC magnetic fields when in use and should be kept away from where people sleep or spend long periods of time.
6. Laundry rooms should be separate from main living spaces and have a door that can be closed. They should be large enough to comfortably contain: a washer and dryer, a small sink with a work surface next to it, adequate built-in shelving and/or cupboards (formaldehyde-free), space to hang items to dry, space to sort laundry, and preferably a built-in fold-away ironing board (with a non-toxic cover).

Your Layer

What do we bring to our laundry rooms? Washers, dryers, washable items such as clothes and bedding, and of course cleaning products. Let's look closer.

Washing machines

Washing machines can be divided into top-loaders and front-loaders. Top loaders, as the name implies, load the washing from the top. They have a vertical drum with an agitator that cleans by moving items back and forth. Front loaders load from the front like dryers, have a horizontal drum, and clean by continually tumbling items. Tumbling creates a better scrubbing and rubbing action than the back and forth action of top loaders. Because of this, front loaders require less water and less detergent.

Until recently, washers and dryers had porcelain-on-steel or stainless steel interiors. Now more machines are using plastic. As we have already discussed, plastics can emit

Recent studies have implicated widely used synthetic compounds such as phthalates, an ingredient in plastics, and alkylphenol polyeth oxylates, which are found in plastics, detergents, and many other products, in hormone disruption.[2]

noxious fumes as well as leach plasticizing chemicals such as phthalates into whatever they come in contact with. Who knows the health consequences to our children's developing bodies if tiny amounts of hormone disrupting chemicals are imbedded in their clothes several times a week.

Jane's washing machine is a rather old top loader. The good news is, it has a porcelain-on-steel interior. The bad news is, it has rather cheap rubber hoses that connect her water lines to the washer. As these cheap rubber hoses quietly deteriorate under the force of continuous water pressure, they can leak slowly, until one day they announce their expiration with a mini-flood. Jane has had one such flood; fortunately she caught it in time and was able to mop up the water promptly with thick towels. If these slow leaks go undetected, massive mold problems can result.

If this has ever happened to you and you have never checked under the floor covering in your laundry, you might want to carefully peel back a corner of your flooring and see if the floor is damp or has any visible signs of mold growth. I emphasize the word "carefully" as mold spores can be very easily dislodged and dispersed. If you do discover a damp floor or mold, find a qualified Indoor Environmental Professional to come out and do a thorough evaluation (see Chapter 4 for guidance).

For those of you shopping for a new washing machine, choose one that uses less water, such as a front loader, and has a stainless steel or porcelain-on-steel interior. Try to find one that allows you to adjust the water usage to match the size of the load, has an economy cycle, and can wash more delicate items. If you need to make do with what you already have and that includes rubber hoses, consider replacing these with the more sturdy version that uses a braided stainless steel mesh on the outside. Visit your local hardware or home improvement store to find them.

Dryers

There are two basic types of dryers: those that dry using heated electric elements and those that dry by burning natural gas. Although gas dryers are more energy efficient than electric dryers, they cause the same pollution problems as gas stoves:

1. Combustion by-products may not be completely vented to the outdoors.
2. There can be seepage from small gas-line leaks.
3. Sometimes a slight odor of natural gas or combustion by-products is left in the items dried.

For all of these reasons, electric dryers are considered a healthier choice.

All dryers should be vented directly to the outdoors. Do a little detective work next time your dryer is running and see if you can locate your dryer vent. There will be moist air coming out of it. What you think is your dryer vent could turn out to be something else. If you discover your dryer vent does not run all the way outside your home, consider adding a well-sealed extension pipe and venting it all the way to the outdoors.

Another consideration is the location of your dryer vent outdoors. If a vent is located directly under a window to one of the main rooms in the house, and if windows are open (as I'm always recommending) when the dryer is in use lint, moisture, and odors will end up right back in your home. This could lead to allergic reactions, asthmatic attacks or other respiratory and neurological problems. If this is the case, keep any windows near the vent closed while the dryer is in operation.

Jane has an electric dryer that vents into her attached garage. This does not qualify as "outside" and in fact is quite problematic for a variety of reasons. First, large amounts of lint accumulate and cover a portion of her garage, creating more debris to be tracked back into the house. Secondly, the high amounts of humidity generated from the dryer put additional moisture into her garage and items close to the vent are prone to mold and mildew growth. Thirdly, whenever anyone enters the house through the garage when the dryer is running, the strong fragrance from the dryer sheets she uses comes back into the house, significantly increasing indoor pollution levels. And finally, when her dryer is not in use, exhaust fumes from the garage have an open pathway directly back into her home.

Another thing to be aware of is the use of heat recovery ventilators (HRVs). Some heat recovery devices are available that recirculate the hot air from the dryer back into the house. Unfortunately most of these do not filter fine particulates sufficiently and if a gas dryer is being used, combustion gases can be released into the indoor air instead of being vented outside. While the principle of these devices is to save energy they need to be installed wisely to protect health and well being.

Both washers and dryers generate strong electromagentic radiation. These appliances are usually placed against an outside wall because dryers require venting to the outdoors. If they are placed against an inside wall, check that there is no bed or favorite sitting place on the other side of the wall. Try to keep your distance from these appliances when in use (AC magnetic field strength quickly falls off with distance), or leave the room and come back later when they have stopped. Don't let young children park themselves in front of glass-doored washing machines to watch it work. Preventing EMR exposures whenever possible is a good idea.

Drying clothes naturally

You can't beat the smell of laundry that has been dried outside in fresh air and sunshine! Whenever weather permits, don't forget this natural resource we have. Drying synthetic fiber clothing in mechanical dryers often produces static electricity in clothing that can feel uncomfortable (natural fibers don't usually do this unless they are laundered along with synthetic fibers). When clothes are dried outdoors, no static electricity is generated and clothing always feels great. Why not choose the "feel good" method whenever you get the chance.

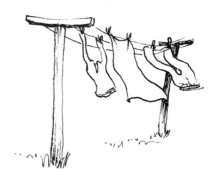

Installing a retractable dryer rack in your laundry is another good idea. This will allow you to dry items naturally all year round.

Laundromats

If you do not have your own washer and dryer and have to use a public laundromat here are some considerations. Residues from other people's laundry can accumulate in public washers and dryers. You have no idea who just used the machines you are about to use. As a precautionary measure I would advise spending a little extra money to run the washing machine adding a large cup or two of vinegar before you use it for your own washing. The vinegar will help to clean residues out of the washer. See if you can also find a dryer that does not smell of fragranced dryer sheets, and leave the door open to ventilate while you wash your laundry.

Another option is to ask a friend or neighbor who has their own washer and dryer if you can use theirs to do your laundry. Turn it into a regular social event! You could also offer to pay them what you would normally pay at the laundromat to offset their increased energy costs. Be creative.

Clothing and fibers

The first step in successfully laundering a piece of clothing is to find out what it is made from. Natural fibers include cotton, wool, silk, linen, ramie, and hemp. Synthetic fibers include polyester, nylon, and acrylic. Rayon and acetate are considered manufactured fibers regenerated or derived from cellulose fibers. Annie Berthold-Bond's book *Better Basics for the Home* has an excellent section on how to launder items made of different fibers. I keep a copy handy in my laundry. With a little guidance and practice most things can be machine or hand washed at home using healthy laundry products (see below).

Untreated, natural-fiber fabrics offer many health advantages over petroleum-derived synthetic alternatives:

1. Natural fibers breathe, allowing heat to disperse and perspiration to evaporate from our bodies. Some synthetic fabrics have been engineered to breathe, but most have not.
2. Natural fibers are made from renewable sources and biodegrade.
3. Organic natural fibers don't put a layer of toxic chemicals next to your skin for it to absorb all day long.
4. It can be easier to remove odors such as tobacco smoke and fragrance from natural fibers than from synthetic fibers.

It is getting particularly hard to find children's clothing made from 100 percent natural fibers. In addition some children's sleepwear is treated with toxic flame retarding chemicals or is made from polyester that is inherently flame resistant. You might think twice when you read the following information.

Polyester is the most commonly used synthetic fiber. It has become popular because it is as versatile as cotton. Do remember though, cotton is natural, polyester is chemical. Which would you rather have against your children's skin?

Take a quick inventory of your family's clothes. How many garments contain synthetic fibers? Don't forget to include underwear. I do wonder if somewhere in the future a connection will be made between the lifetime use of synthetic fibers in bras and the incidence of breast cancer. But who would ever fund such a study? And if someone did, would the information ever make it into the general public's hands?

You may be pleasantly surprised that your family already has many natural fiber garments. Be sure to wear these the majority of the time. If you find polyester, nylon, and acrylic set them aside to be phased out and replaced with natural fibers. Fortunately children grow so fast it won't be long until they are ready for something new. I definitely recommend organic cotton when it comes to underwear, which covers our most delicate and vulnerable skin (see Appendix C).

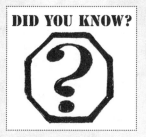

DID YOU KNOW?

Understanding Textiles by Phyllis G. Tortora says "Polyester shrinks from flame and will melt, leaving a hard, black residue. The fabric will burn with a strong, pungent odor. Some polyesters are self extinguishing. Melted polyester fiber can produce severe burns."[3]

Three of the chemicals used in manufacturing synthetic fabrics have known side effects. Benzene is known to depress the central nervous system, causing headaches, dizziness, nausea, and convulsions. Ammonia causes burning sensations in the eyes, nose and throat, pain in the lungs, nausea, tearing, coughing, and an increased breathing rate. Ethylene glycol is that same poison we find in our windscreen washer fluid.[4]

Ethylene glycol, which is used to make polyester, evaporates slowly at room temperature and readily when heated. The chemical from which ethylene glycol is made, ethylene oxide, has been linked to leukemia, stomach cancer, brain tumors, and possibly breast cancer, genetic damage, and birth defects in laboratory animals.[5]

Irons and ironing boards

I hope you are now convinced that wearing natural fiber clothing is a good idea. As you move away from synthetics and their no-need-to-iron convenience towards natural fibers such as cotton, you will need to reinstate your iron and ironing board.

If you have not used your iron in a long time, check the cable and plug to make sure they are still in good working order and check the flat ironing surface (the sole plate) for any coating or discoloration that may have been burned on. If it's time for a new iron, invest in a good quality one. Look for irons with stainless-steel sole plates. Stainless steel is inherently

Nowadays, most irons and ironing-board covers are coated with tetrafluoroethylene plastic, better known as Teflon. Given that heating plastic makes it outgas its toxic fumes, irons and ironing-board covers seem odd places to put it, particularly since a nonstick finish is not even necessary. Tetrafluoroethylene fumes can be irritating to eyes, nose, and throat, and can cause breathing difficulties.[6]

non-sticking and so does not require the application of synthetic chemical compounds to its surface.

Also check your ironing board to see what the cover and padding is made from. It is quite common for these to contain Teflon-coating and flame retarding chemicals (see Chapters 7 and 9 for more on toxicity). Do you really want your clothing coming in direct contact with toxic chemicals like these? It is probably safe to assume that the heat from the iron will volatilize any chemicals from the ironing board cover or padding into the air you are breathing while ironing and may even deposit chemical residues directly into your clothing. The safest choice is an undyed, untreated, 100 percent cotton cover and pad (see Appendix C). Try the following experiment. Wash some laundry without using any fragranced products. Then iron a garment that is made from 100 percent cotton and notice and smell. Then iron a garment with polyester in it and notice that smell. Do you find any difference?

Choosing an iron with a steam function is another good idea. Steam helps eliminate wrinkles fast. Only use filtered or distilled water in your iron though. Hard water buildup can clog the steam vent openings, and remember what happens in the shower with unfiltered water? Any chemicals and substances become volatilized into the steam that you then breathe in. This can happen with the steam from your iron if you don't use filtered water. Another little exposure: another drop in the barrel!

Laundry products

Modern commercial cleaning products are a manifestation of the popular saying from several years ago, "Better living through chemistry." Are we all chemists? No. Do we all know what these chemicals really do? No. Do we know if these products are really safe for our family's health? No. But they have to be safe if you can by them at the store, right? Wrong.

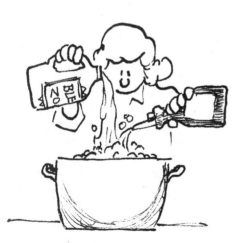

Because our clothes are continuously in direct contact with our skin, it is essential to choose laundry products that will not only clean clothes properly but are proven to be safe for human health.

Now that you know to look at clothing labels to find out what fibers your clothes are made from, you need to learn the how to decode the symbols found on labels that tell you how to launder each item. See the following chart: "Fabric Care Language Made Easy." Out of necessity, I designed an at-a-glance laundry chart to help me remember all this information. I keep it on the wall above my washing machine. The idea was popular with friends and now these charts are available to help anyone who wants reminding of the basic guidelines to follow for successful, healthy laundry (see Appendix C).

Your Guide to Fabric Care Symbols

MACHINE WASH	BLEACH	TUMBLE DRY	DRY	IRON	DRY CLEAN

MACHINE WASH

TEMPERATURE

Cold/Cold

Warm

Hot

CYCLE

Normal

Permanent Press

Delicate/Gentle

OTHER

Do Not Wash

Hand Wash

BLEACH

Any Bleach (when needed)

Only Non-chlorine Bleach (when needed)

Do Not Bleach

TUMBLE DRY

HEAT SETTING

No Heat

Low

Medium

High

Any Heat

CYCLE

Normal

Permanent Press

Delicate/Gentle

OTHER

Do Not Tumble Dry

DRY

Line Dry/ Hang to Dry

Drip Dry

Dry Flat

Dry in the Shade

Do Not Dry

Do Not Wring

IRON

TEMPERATURE

(Dry or Steam)

Low

Medium

High

OTHER

No Steam

Do Not Iron

DRY CLEAN

Dry Clean

Do Not Dry Clean

Courtesy of:
The Soap and Detergent Association

Fabric Care Language Made Easy

Here are some general guidelines to follow:

1. It's very helpful to pre-sort your laundry, not only darks and lights, but also by fiber, cotton, silk, synthetic, etc. Laundry sorters are available that make this process super simple. They consist of a metal or wood frame with two or more removable 100 percent cotton canvas laundry bags (see Appendix C).
2. Use the least amount of soap or detergent necessary to do a good job. This might require a little trial and error but it will make rinsing more effective and save you money.
3. When a larger amount of soap or detergent is required for a tough cleaning job, double up on rinsing; otherwise product residues can be left in fibers that can cause allergies and skin irritation.
4. Try to wash each load on the shortest and gentlest cycle. This creates less wear and tear on fabrics.
5. Some washing machines allow you to select the amount of water per load or have an economy setting. Use the least amount of water and the coolest temperatures that still allow effective cleaning. These functions help minimize fading and shrinkage and help save water. Hot water is required to kill dust mites though.

Selecting cleaning products

When it comes to selecting cleaning products you have several choices. You can buy ready-mixed commercial brands; you can use simple, single ingredients like Castile soap and vinegar; or you can make your own recipes. There are now solutions to fit everyone's budget and busy schedules.

Detergents and soaps

Detergents were originally developed specifically to clean synthetic fibers. Not surprisingly, many detergents, like synthetic fibers, are made from petrochemicals and can contain chlorine bleaches, optical brighteners, quaternary ammonia, artificial fragrances, metasilicates, free silica, cationic fabric softeners, borine, petrochemical surfactants, toxic algaecides and sanitizers, coloring, and fillers. Fortunately, there are now natural and healthy alternatives available that are also kinder on the environment (see Appendix C).

Some people prefer liquid laundry detergents rather than powders. Liquids dissolve completely where powders may not. Again, read labels and choose the gentlest ingredients. Also look for products labelled "fragrance-free."

Natural fibers can be cleaned effectively with plant-based soaps. These are what our grandmothers used for years and they still work well today. One example is Castile soap, originally made from olive oil and today made from other vegetable oils as well. You can find it in most health food stores as a liquid or bar. If you choose the bar variety you will need to shave it into really thin flakes and use hot water in the wash to melt the soap. Use cold water in the rinse to stop the soap from sudsing and if any residue or scum is left behind you can rinse your wash adding one half cup of white vinegar.

Fabric softeners and dryer sheets

Fabric softeners never existed before synthetic fabrics. One of the reasons they were invented was to disguise the offensive smell that synthetic fibers give off when heated during laundering or on our warm bodies. Often the chemicals themselves used in fabric softener, such as quaternary ammonia, smell so strongly that according to Jim Rimer, founder of Bi-O-Kleen products, "they require up to 50 times more fragrance to try to mask their own noxious odors."[7] Hence fabric softeners are usually highly fragranced products. Fabric softeners also leave an invisible residue on fabrics to reduce static cling (another of their functions). This does not wash out and can be a skin irritant.

Healthier alternatives are:

1. Add a quarter cup of baking soda to wash cycle to soften fabric.
2. Add a quarter cup of white vinegar to soften fabric as well as eliminate cling.

Speciality cleaning products

All of us run into situations where a special product is needed to remove a stain or brighten our whites. By now you have probably figured out that these products can be toxic too. Jane likes to use liberal amounts of chlorine bleach and stain removers on her children's clothes. What she does not realize is that she is exposing herself to strong concentrations of these chemicals while doing the laundry. This is what caused her light-headedness and required her to go and take a nap afterwards.

Have you ever felt light-headed, dizzy, or tired, or experienced a mood change such as becoming irritable while doing the laundry? If you have, it could well be due to a chemical exposure or chemical cocktail in your laundry. I wonder how many people hate doing laundry because it genuinely makes them feel unwell. If this rings any bells for you try the following experiment. Replace your laundry products with healthy, fragrance-free ones and do a load of wash that only contains natural fibers. Open a window or ventilate the space and leave the room while the

The chemicals found in commercial fabric softeners and dryer sheets are often carcinogens such as benzyl acetate, limonene and camphor. Many cause central nervous system disorders, headaches, nausea, vomiting, dizziness, and a drop in blood pressure. Benzyl alcohol, ethyl acetate, linalool, alha-ter-pineol, and many of these chemicals irritate the skin.[8]

Generally, chlorine is a dangerous chemical to keep in your house. In 1993, 40,000 household exposures to chlorine were reported to poison control centers, more than any other chemical. Particularly dangerous are fragranced chlorine bleaches and products made with chlorine bleach plus surfactants. Disguising the odor—actually making the experience of inhaling chlorine bleach pleasant — can lead to over-exposure, as we inhale the fumes unchecked. Another danger lies in mixing household products containing chlorine, either intentionally or unintentionally. These mixtures can create chlorine gas and chloramines, both of which are toxic gases that can injure the deep tissues of the lungs. Although the number of reported incidents is relatively small, the percentage of accidents with moderate to serious outcomes is high.[9]

In 2000, cleaning products were responsible for nearly 10% of all toxic exposures reported to U.S. Poison Control Centers, accounting for over 206,000 calls, over half of which were about children under the age of six. According to Philip Dickey of the Washington Toxics Coalition, the most acutely, or immediately hazardous, dangerous cleaning products are corrosive drain cleaners, oven cleaners and acidic toilet bowl cleaners, and anything containing chlorine or ammonia.[10]

The neighborhood dry cleaners may look innocuous enough. But by some estimates, dry cleaners rank only second to diesel exhaust in terms of cancer risk from air pollution. Traditional dry cleaning methods use a toxic solvent known as perchloroethylene (PERC). Like all solvents, PERC dissolves readily and of gasses into surrounding air space, whether it's the neighborhood next to a drycleaners, or the clothes closet in your house. At high exposures, PERC causes cancer in lab animals, and is also linked to kidney, liver and reproductive problems.[11]

washer or dryer is operating. Did you notice any difference in how you felt? Even if you didn't notice anything profound this is definitely the best way to reduce any possible exposures while doing this household job.

There are several healthy versions of speciality cleaning products now available such as chlorine and fragrance-free bleaches and solvent and fragrance-free stain removers (see Appendix C). You can also make your own cleaning products (see Chapter 16). Read labels and educate yourself about which companies create the best products; fortunately there are still some companies out there who are committed to making healthier products that are gentle on the environment!

Finally, store all your laundry products up on shelves or in cupboards where children cannot get to them. Put "Mr. Yuk" stickers on all of them and teach your children to leave these products alone (see Chapter 16). Better safe than sorry.

Dry cleaning

As we have already discussed dry cleaning in Chapter 3, we will only add a couple of reminders here. The best strategy is to stop buying things that need to be dry cleaned, especially children's clothes. With existing items, avoid dry cleaning whenever possible and instead try to find a wet cleaners. Some fabrics that carry a "dry clean only" label can be washed by hand successfully with a little extra care.

If dry cleaning is unavoidable, do air any items out thoroughly before bringing them into your home or wearing them. Remember the garage is not a suitable place to air items out if you park your car there. They will just become further contaminated with car exhaust fumes. Outside in a protected place is best.

Remove plastic wrapping from dry cleaning as soon as possible and dispose of it responsibly. It will be impregnated with toxic chemicals. Definitely don't keep it in the house or try to recycle it. The same goes for any paper wrapping on the clothes hangers that comes home with your dry cleaning. Some people like to keep these, so be sure to remove the paper, wipe the hanger down, and then air them outside for a while.

New clothes

New clothes often have a "new" odor and feel. This is due to the presence of chemicals such as formaldehyde, used for its wrinkle-resistant properties, and sizing chemicals used as a temporary stiffening glaze to make new clothes look more attractive. In the manufacturing process fabrics can absorb odors from their surrounding environment such as perfumes, air fresheners, pesticides, combustion gases, or tobacco smoke.

Always wash new clothing before wearing. Try adding one half to one cup of baking soda to each load of wash, rinse, then follow with another wash, this time adding one to two cups of white vinegar. If you still detect odors you can repeat this cycle several times until the odor is gone. It may be necessary to let your newly washed clothing air outside for a while as well.

I am particularly concerned about children's clothing. In addition to the chemicals already mentioned, they sometimes have fire retardant chemicals added to them. What are the effects of all these fabric chemicals on their young bodies? Children grow so fast they are constantly in need of new clothes. Their exposure levels can be much higher than adults. Passing down well-washed clothing from older siblings not only saves money but reduces the chemical exposure to your children. If you buy second-hand clothes, I would still suggest putting them through the new clothing washes just recommended to remove laundry detergent residues and washed-in fragrance from the previous owners.

Sinks

Having a sink in your laundry makes a lot of sense. As you return to washing more clothing by hand instead of dry cleaning delicate items, it is useful to have everything you need in one place. Your retractable clothes dryer can be used to dry delicates naturally. Sinks are also very useful if you need to soak something overnight.

Ideally you have a whole house water filtration unit installed in your home so that every room in the house has filtered water available. As laundries are extensions of the bathroom, the quality of the water you wash your clothes in is also important. Who knows what chemicals and substances you are washing into your clothing (which is your second skin layer) if you use unfiltered water.

If you don't have a whole house water filtration system at least purchase a point-of-source filter for the main tap in your kitchen. Besides having better quality water to drink and cook with, you will be able to use this filtered water to hand wash delicate items in your kitchen sink. You will need to wash in cold water if you use a filter with a carbon medium as they don't work as well if you run hot water through them. Be sure to thoroughly scrub your kitchen sink first to make sure there is no coating of grease on your sink that could get onto your clothes.

Ventilation

Always open a window when doing laundry to let the humidity and smells out. If you have an exhaust fan, run that too. If you don't have a window in the immediate vicinity, where is the closest one? Can you open that? It may be necessary to install a small exhaust fan (making sure it vents to the outdoors) to create the ventilation you need to make your laundry a healthier place.

Let's get organized

Changing over to a completely healthy laundry may take a while, so enjoy the small victories along the way. Every time you get rid of a toxic laundry product and replace it with a healthy store-bought one or your own homemade formula, that's cause for celebration. Every time you get rid of a synthetic piece of clothing and replace it with a natural one marks a personal victory.

So, let's get organized and figure out where to begin.

Most immediate gains

1. Decide how you can ventilate your laundry space.
2. Replace washer hoses every three years or upgrade to the stainless steel mesh reinforced variety.
3. Make sure your dryer vents to the outside of your home; make sure the vent is not blocked or obstructed.
4. Develop the habit of cleaning the lint from dryer filters or vents after each use. Your dryer will work more efficiently and you will reduce the amount of lint particles in the air.
5. Take an inventory of your current laundry products. Read labels and get rid of products that contain the words "warning" and "caution" or even "poison." Do not dispose of these products down the sink, on the ground, down a storm drain, or in your garbage can. Call your local Household Hazardous Waste facility for guidance.
6. Stop using fragranced laundry products. Healthy, freshly laundered items have no smell.
7. Replace toxic products with healthy alternatives that are kind to the environment. Start with your most used products first like laundry detergent and fabric softener. Stock your laundry with staples such as white vinegar and baking soda.
8. Put "Mr. Yuk" stickers (see Chapter 16) on all products and store away from where children and pets can get at them.
9. Use a little less detergent. According to *Consumer Reports* magazine, manufacturers recommend more detergent than necessary.
10. Washers use 32-59 gallons of water for each cycle. Save water and wait until you have a full load to run your washing machine.
11. Take a clothing inventory. Replace synthetic fabric underwear with organic cotton. Children's sizes are easily available through mail order catalogues and the Internet. Next replace your most frequently worn garments like trousers and blouses.
12. Wash synthetic fabrics separately from natural fabrics.
13. Replace your ironing board cover and pad with untreated, undyed, 100 percent cotton ones and upgrade your iron to one with a stainless steel sole plate.

14. Leave your washing machine door open after each use to ensure it dries out thoroughly. This will help reduce mold growth. If you have young children, you may have to keep your laundry door closed or put a child safe fence across the doorway to keep them out and prevent any accidents from children climbing inside the washer. Once your washing machine has dried out, you can close it up again.

CHAPTER 11

Home Offices

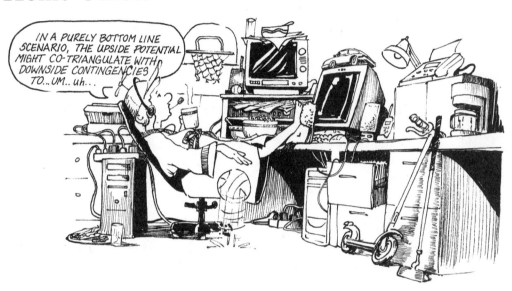

"How to survive Fridays," is the question on Mark's mind. Mark's new home office is a frenzy of activity and looks like a bomb has hit it.

"Damn it!" shouts Mark as his computer crashes for a third time. "I've got to get this report finished or I'm a dead man." With psychic precision the phone rings. It's Mark's boss, calling from head office. "Yes, I'm just finishing that report up. Having a few technical hitches today. Nothing to worry about. I'll have it to you by the end of the day. You'll be really happy with these figures."

As Mark slams the phone down he gives his computer a rude gesture and crawls under his desk to inspect all the electrical sockets, looking for a reason for his computer's erratic behavior.

The phone rings again, causing Mark to bash his head against the metal frame of his desk. "***@@!!" he curses. He grabs the phone while rubbing the sharp pain in his head. "Hello." Mark's boss has a couple more additions he wants him to make to his report. While they are still talking, Mark's cell phone rings. He puts his boss on hold and grabs his cell phone. A customer needs some technical advice. He puts his customer on hold. As he turns back to pick his cordless phone up the lights in his office suddenly go out.

There is a moment of suspended animation, while Mark's mind processes this new piece of information. Regaining his senses he grabs his cordless phone. The line is dead. His boss is gone. He grabs his cell phone. The customer has hung up. The stabbing pain in Mark's head is now accompanied by a throbbing pain in his temples. Blood pressure. "BE THAT WAY!" Mark yells at the top of his lungs. He looks around his state-of-the-art executive office. Maybe he won't be getting that promotion after all.

Regaining some of his composure Mark rummages around in his office closet muttering, "Houston, we have a problem," and retrieves a screwdriver and a flashlight. He grabs his cell phone as he heads towards the garage where the main panel is located. He presses #3 on his cell phone which automatically dials a pre-programmed number. "Uncle Joe, it's Mark. I'm going to need you to talk me through the electrical wiring in my house."

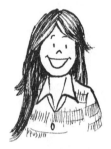

Commentary

Home offices are becoming increasingly popular as people seek more efficiency and convenience, and as their leisure interests change. These range from full blown state-of-the-art offices like Mark's through to a desk and computer contained within another room in the house. Many of our children now have mini-offices or "work stations" in their bedrooms. Home offices are definitely "in."

Building Biology perspective

One of the fascinating things about the study of Building Biology is that it is constantly evolving. Whether we are studying the health effects of new building materials or the possible effects of a new wireless technology that everyone suddenly wants to have in their home, humans are avid consumers and our homes constantly change as a result.

A great part of the popularity of home offices stems from the impact that modern technology, especially computers, has had on our life. Everyday activities such as e-mail and computer games now require that every home has a least one if not two computers and a designated place to put them. From a Building Biology perspective home offices, small or large, have become the next most used part of the home after bedrooms.

Let's look at the home office in layers.

The Third Skin Layer

Follow the basic checklist and then add the following ideal building features for a healthy home office:

1. Open windows or install an energy recovery ventilator for good ventilation. Ample supplies of oxygen and reduced carbon dioxide are needed for concentration and productive work. Good ventialtion also allows office VOCs from printers and photocopies to dissipate.

2. All office equipment is properly grounded and shielded.
3. Home offices should be separate from main living spaces and have a door that can be closed. Many pieces of office equipment such as printers and photocopiers will offgass chemicals when in use.

Your layer

Let's take a closer look at Mark's office.

Office equipment

By their very definition home offices usually contain a varied selection of office equipment. Mark has a computer, additional external speakers with a sub woofer, printer, scanner, photocopier, fax machine, CD player, desk lamp, standing lamp, cordless phone, and a cell phone all within easy reach of where he sits. He also has a wraparound desk, expanded work surface, and a matching bookshelf/cupboard system than spans a whole wall. His office chair was thrown in with the package deal he bought at the office supply store.

Mark spends from eight to ten hours a day in his office during the week working and several hours on the weekend playing computer games and surfing the Internet. He often spends more time in his office than he does sleeping in his bedroom, in which case, from a Building Biology standpoint, Mark's office would be very important to focus on and make healthy.

EMRs

As Mark is stationary and seated in his office chair most of the time, he is consistently bathed in high electromagnetic radiation from the plethora of electrical office equipment surrounding him. On the other side of the wall from where Mark sits is the kitchen refrigerator, another constant source of AC magnetic fields. If we were to test where he sits with a Gaussmeter and body voltage meter we would see both high AC magnetic and AC electric field readings. These fields, although invisible, disrupt the electrical messages in his nervous system and the chemical messages in his endocrine and immune systems. Mark attributes the regular headaches he gets and the tiredness he feels each day while working to hard work and stress. The truth is, nobody dies of hard work, but your own office might kill you!

Static electricity and air ions

While on the subject of EMRs we should also include a brief and simplified discussion of static electricity and air ions. Air ions are atmospheric molecules that have become charged by the loss or gain of an electron. They are constantly being formed and are constantly recombining to neutralize their charges.[1] Static electricity is created when electrons in the air we breathe become positively or negatively charged. In nature's normal balance there are more negative ions than positive ions. High negative ion concentrations are found next to waterfalls and in the mountains. These environments are considered beneficial to health. You may have noticed yourself how well you feel after a day's hike in the mountains.

This natural ion balance can be upset by a variety of things such as static electricity-generating materials, ungrounded electronic devices, air with less than 50 percent relative humidity, metal ducting (as in forced air heating), cigarette smoke, and general indoor air pollution. Negative ions become depleted and positive ions increase. Offices can generate high levels of static electricity because office equipment and furnishings, which are often made of synthetic materials such as plastic, deplete negative ions. This static electricity can be problematic when using sensitive electrical equipment and it also has an effect on our health.

Ions are biologically active and can affect the production of the powerful neurohormone seratonin. Tests show positive ions increase the production of seratonin, while negative ions decrease it. This disruption of normal seratonin production has profound effects on the nervous, glandular, and digestive systems. Positive ion excess has been shown to have three major effects: irritation and tension, exhaustion, and a hyperthyroid response. Common symptoms include dizziness, headaches, depression, anxiety, and a generally lower level of physical/mental function.[2]

Mark's office is crammed full of office equipment encasedin plastic as well as synthetic fibers in everything from his carpet to his office chair — and he never opens his office window.

Opening windows is a simple way to replenish negative ion concentrations and to offset the positive ions generated in daily office use. You can also use an electrical device called a negative ion generator. The quality of these varies a lot as do the results. See if you can try a model for a while before buying it. Look for one that comes with its own collection plates that can be regularly cleaned, otherwise the negative ions generated will attach to particles of dust and debris in the air and your walls and ceilings will steadily become dirtier. Remember to place it far enough away from you, as it will generate EMRs.

Computers

Computers have become the focal point of most offices. But did you know your computer could affect your health? Many studies in the past have linked video display terminals (VDTs) with a variety of health problems from eyestrain to irritability. The cathode ray tube (CRT) inside some models of computers emits radiation at various frequencies, in particular very low frequency (VLF) and extremely low frequency fields (ELF). The spot of electrons, which sweep the screen, generates what scientists call Pulsed Electro-Magnetic Radiation (PEMR), which, at close range, disturbs the balance of all living cells.[3] Of course this is the subject of heated debate between those who have experienced harm and those who manufacture these products. The precautionary principle would advise us to research what our options are and choose the safest alternative.

Liquid crystal display (LCD) screens have lower EMRs and are currently considered the best option available. Laptop computers or flat screen (thin) desktop versions are available. Unfortunately Mark has a monitor with a cathode ray gun that he faces all day long.

If you do have a CRT computer there are different shields you can attach to the screen that are supposed to offer some protection from AC electric fields but AC magnetic fields are more difficult to shield (see Appendix C). Keeping a distance of at least 30 inches from the front and 40 inches from the back and sides of computers is considered sufficient to protect yourself from electromagnetic radiation.

If you are looking to buy a new computer check to see if it complies with the "TCO" recommendations of the Swedish Association of Professional Employees, which has been a leader in the development of strict limits on VDT emissions. As the U.S. still has not set safe standards, the Swedish MPRII guidelines for emissions are very helpful: "Less than 2 milliguass at 30 centimeters of extremely low-frequency EMRs from the screen."[5] You can also contact the International Institute for Bau-Biologie and Ecology and request a copy of document SBM-2003 *Standard of Bau-biologie Methods* for their current recommendations.

Ask companies for their lowest-EMR models, and one with a power-down feature (after a specified period of time in which a computer is turned on but not used, the power is automatically reduced). Although this feature was designed for energy-efficiency, it also reduces EMRs.

Phones

Phones are another main feature of both homes and offices. Where would we be without them? Mark has a cordless phone and a cell phone in his office. In the rest of the house are two other cordless phones, one in the master bedroom and one in the kitchen. Liz has her own cell phone, for a grand total of five phones between the two of them.

Traditional or standard telephones connect directly to a telephone wiring system. These are the ones you have to plug into the wall and the handset is connected to the base with a curly cord. These phones are all wired, use low-voltage direct current and information comes and goes via a copper wire system that is connected to other systems throughout the country and the rest of the world. The handset of the telephone contains a microphone in the mouthpiece and a tiny speaker in the earpiece, which generates a small AC magnetic field.

Computers have revolutionized the lives of millions of people-but at what price? They generate ozone, positive ions, static electricity, and EMRs that can bother some individuals. The cathode ray tube behind the video display terminal can cause eyestrain, eye irritation, double vision, irritability, fatigue, stress, itchy skin, and chest, head, neck, and back pains.[4]

"Most people are stunned to learn about the volume of toxic chemicals that are used in the manufacture of computers, and that end up becoming a real problem when the equipment is obsolete," says Ted Smith, executive director of the Silicon Valley Toxics Coalition (SVTC), formed in 1982 following the discovery of local groundwater pollution from chemicals used to make semiconductor chips. "Every computer contains five to eight pounds of lead," he adds. Exposure to lead and other toxic ingredients, such as mercury, cadmium, brominated , flame retardants, and some plastics, may harm developing brains, disrupt hormone functions, cause cancer, or affect reproduction.[6]

These older models have been replaced in many homes with the cordless/wireless phone. These phones connect into the telephone wiring system through a base unit which remains plugged in while the handset can be mobile and used in other parts of the house, even outside, as long as it remains within a certain range of the base unit. These phones are popular because of the flexibility they provide. Wireless phones are similar to traditional phones with one exception: their sound signals are transmitted in the radiowave and microwave frequencies (RF). The transmitters which give out these frequencies in the handheld units are often very close to the user's head. Cordless phones that are linked to domestic lines through a base unit use relatively low power (less than one watt depending on the model).[7]

Cell phones are completely mobile (they are called "mobiles" in the U.K.) and are not linked to any lines. Of all three phones, they need more power to function (between one half and six watts of output). These phones also transmit in the radio frequencies. Many people do not realize that RF is a form of low-intensity microwave radiation and some cell phones can emit more radiation than the FDA allows for microwave ovens.[8] The close proximity of the antennae next to their heads is the primary health concern for users. Studies have shown that the RF radiation's heating effect on the brain can affect cognitive function, memory and attention, and can weaken the blood/brain barrier, whose function is to prevent potentially dangerous chemicals from reaching sensitive brain tissue.[9]

If you are interested in reading more about the studies that have been done around the world, Ellen Sugarman's book *Warning: The Electricity Around You May Be Hazardous To Your Health* is one of the easier ones to read.

Having read different research, and believing in the precautionary principle's guidelines, I have come to the conclusion that rethinking how we use our communication systems in our homes and offices is

The balance of current research evidence suggests that exposures to radio waves below levels set out in international guidelines do not cause health problems for the general population. However, there is some evidence that changes in brain activity can occur below these guidelines, but it isn't clear why. There are significant gaps in our scientific knowledge. This has led a group of independent experts, commissioned by the (U.K.) Government and headed by Sir William Stewart, to recommend "a precautionary approach" to the use of mobile phones until more research findings become available. If you use a mobile phone, you can choose to minimize your exposure to radio waves. These are ways to do so:

- Keep your calls short
- Consider relative SAR* values when buying a new phone.[10]

(*SAR values stand for Specific Absorption Rate, and are a measurement of how much radio wave energy your body receives from each model of mobile phone)

a really good idea. I decided to get rid of the cordless phones in my home and have gone back to traditional phones, which have lower EMRs, and no RF. In my office I use a traditional phone with a headset for optimum freedom, and because it significantly reduces the tension in my neck and head. I only use a cell phone for emergency use when driving or traveling and even then for the shortest time possible.

You must weigh up what is right for you and your family. The truth is, we are all taking part in a massive technological experiment and though there are already many suggestions, and in some cases solid proof, that byproducts of these technologies are bad for us, many people still resist accepting this evidence. But we really must consider the total costs in the choices we make and be willing to rethink our everyday realities to safeguard our family's future.

Printers, photocopiers, faxes, modems and other machines

The main considerations with these machines are:

1. They all generate EMRs. Photocopy machines can give off much higher EMRs than computers, depending on the model. In general the more capabilities a machine has, the higher the EMRs can be. If you can, step about three feet away from these machines when they are in use. Faxes also contain technology similar to photocopiers and therefore generate higher EMRs within one foot than a wired phone does.[11]
2. Printers, photocopiers and fax machines also emit VOCs from toners; photocopiers also emit ozone.
3. Most of these machines are made from or contain plastic which can emit more VOCs and chemicals that can get onto your skin from handling them.

Mark has so many pieces of equipment in his state-of-the-art office generating EMRs and emitting VOCs into the air he breathes, in addition to the carpet, wallpaper, paint, furniture, and soft furnishings, that it's no wonder he gets headaches and often feels tired. He would be wise to rethink his office and consider how much of this machinery is really necessary. If some items are not used very often, he could at least unplug them or consider placing some of them in a less used, well-ventilated part of his home. This way he would significantly reduce the overall chemical and pollution load on his body and probably find that his productivity increases substantially.

Office supplies

Every office contains a plethora of office supplies including permanent markers, dry erase markers and white board cleaner, correction fluid, various glues, PVC binders and clear sheet covers, and carbonless copy paper. The list is endless. Many of these contain toxic chemicals, some of which are known carcinogens. Unfortunately product labeling is often extremely lacking or inadequate. As many of these products also fall under the category of art materials and supplies we shall cover them in more depth in Chapter 12.

Suffice it to say here, that only non-toxic materials certified by the Art and Crafts Materials Institute (ACMI) should be used in a healthy office, and even then, products should be used sparingly in a well-ventilated space. Some products like PVC and carbonless copy paper should just be avoided altogether. The long-term effects of low-level exposures to many of these materials are still unknown.

Furniture

Mark's new office furniture is all made from particleboard with wood veneer. By now you will know what that means — yes, large amounts of formaldehyde! I recently came across an interesting piece of information making a very specific reference to formaldehyde levels in new homes:

Then there is the new chair that was a free gift with his office furniture. It looks like a regular office chair with its plastic frame, hydraulic system for height adjustment, and its synthetic fabric upholstery. But what Mark does not know is that many textile trimmings used in office fabrics are considered hazardous waste, as a result of the dyes and sealants used.[12] Architect and textiles expert William McDonaugh says, "Most people are sitting on chairs that are an amalgam of hundreds of chemicals that have never been defined in terms of their effects on human health, and the deeper we look, we find things that are cancer-causing chemicals."[13] Mark's chair also generates static electricity because of its synthetic content, to say nothing of the VOCs the chair offgasses.

When it comes to a healthy office, choose natural and non-toxic materials for furniture and furnishings. Full spectrum light fittings such as desk lamps or standing lamps give the best additional natural light to work with, reducing eyestrain, helping concentration, and boosting spirits in winter months when natural light is diminished.

> **"New Construction Residential Purchase Agreement (NCPA-1 Revised 1/01)" created by the California Association of Realtors:**
> "The United States Environmental Protection Agency, the California Air Resources Board, and other agencies have measured the presence of formaldehyde in the indoor air of homes in California. Levels of formaldehyde that present a significant cancer risk have been measured in most homes. Formaldehyde is present in the air because it is emitted by a variety of building materials and home products purchased by Seller from materials suppliers. These materials include carpeting, pressed wood products, insulation, plastics and glues."

Office set up

It has become popular to buy office furniture in sets, like Mark did. Sometimes this forces you into a predesigned horseshoe configuration where the work surfaces surround you on all sides and hence all your office equipment also surrounds you. From an organizational point of view this might be desirable as it puts everything only a fingers-reach away, but from a Building Biology stand point you are bombarding yourself on all sides with chemicals and pollution. In particular, EMRs from several different pieces of office equipment may converge, creating an augmentation effect in a particular spot, which could happen be your office chair where you sit for hours.

Try to arrange your office equipment in a row and create the maximum distance between where you sit and the bulk of your electrical equipment. The only thing that should be at your fingertips is your computer keyboard. If you have the space you could also put some items, such as a photocopier, in another less-used part of the home and keep it well ventilated. Just make sure it isn't near a bedroom.

At the end of your working day, close off your office space to contain any office smells from the rest of the house.

Children's offices

Children's bedrooms are often mini-offices with their computers, phones, and marker pens and deserve mentioning here. All the same considerations we have just discussed apply to your child's bedroom with a few more specific things to pay attention to.

If your child has a computer in their bedroom consider putting it in another part of the house away from where they sleep. If this is not possible, then make sure the computer is as far away from the bed as possible. Some modern bunk-bed designs have a desk under the top bunk bed, which encourages locating items such as computers there. I am concerned that by doing this your child is essentially sleeping on top of a large source of EMR. What will be the health consequences?

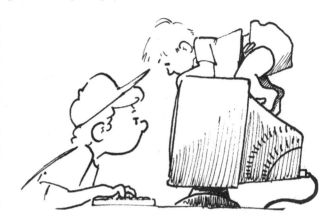

Also, if your child has a CRT monitor, shield the screen and teach them to keep a safe distance of at least 30 inches away from the screen, more if you can, and 40 inches away from the back or sides. This can be very challenging with children absorbed in computer games for several hours and if you are not around to observe their use. I recommend defining how much screen time your child is allowed per day and watching for any negative health signs associated with too much use.

Keep phones out of children's bedrooms at night too. If your child has a cell phone make sure they don't sleep near it or have it plugged in charging near them all night long.

Children's office supplies are also called school supplies, art and craft supplies, or hobby supplies (see Chapter 12). Teach your child to open a window when using these products in their bedroom and to put caps back on tightly. Sometimes keeping these kinds of supplies in their own tightly sealed container is a good idea because even with caps firmly back in place

Dr. Doris Rapp in her book *Is This Your Child's World?* gives the following advice: "Clues to Possible Electromagnetic Illness: Until more is known, you should be alert for signs that your child may have developed an illness in reaction to exposure to EMFs. If he experiences any of the following symptoms at school or home, EMFs might be the cause.

1. Chest pain, headaches, blurry vision, or any unexplained discomfort while sitting directly in front of a standard upright computer. (By contrast, laptops cause fewer health difficulties).
2. Looking, feeling, or behaving in ways other than normal after exposure to a computer, television set, or microwave oven.
3. Feeling ill or different just before or during a thunderstorm or certain other weather changes.
4. Not feeling right near high-power electric wires.
5. Tics or seizures."[14]

some VOCs can still be emitted into the air your child breathes. Always read labels before purchasing these products. Remember, "non-toxic" is not an absolute guarantee that these products will not harm your child's health.

Partial offices

Even a partial office in one part of your home can have health affects on your whole family. Until safer standards and guidelines are established we must be vigilant with what we allow into our homes and never be lulled by false assumptions that all these products must be safe, otherwise they would not be so readily available.

The radiation plume that emanates from a cell phone antenna penetrates much deeper into the heads of children than adults. And, once it penetrates children's skulls it enters their brains and eyes at an absorption rate far greater than it does in adults. A study done by Dr. Om Ghandhi in 1996 found that the radiation absorption rates inside the brain were:

- 7.84 milliwatts per kilogram (mW/kg) in an adult
- 19.77 mW/kg in a ten-year-old child
- 33.12 mW/kg in a five-year-old child.[15]

By now you have a lot more information to make even a tiny office corner as healthy as it can possibly be. By demanding computers with lower EMRs, choosing non-toxic office supplies, and not purchasing furniture made of particleboard and plywood, you can wield your consumer power to improve the quality of these products and pave the way towards a better future for our children and their children.

Most immediate gains

1. Choose an office chair made from natural materials such as wood or leather that provides good posture support.
2. If you have a CRT display, install a shield and sit a minimum of 30 inches away from the screen.
3. Arrange your office equipment in a row rather than a horseshoe configuration to reduce EMRs and chemical exposures on all sides.
4. Choose natural and non-toxic office furniture and furnishings. Replace particleboard furniture or seal it with a special sealant to contain its formaldehyde content. You will need to seal particleboard on all sides for this method to be effective.
5. Replace incandescent and fluorescent light bulbs with full spectrum bulbs.
6. Test office equipment with a Gaussmeter before buying to check the level of AC magnetic fields generated.
7. Having plants in your office will help reduce VOC levels (see Chapter 14).
8. Open windows and ventilate your office daily. If you can, place VOC-emitting equipment in another well-ventilated space in your home that is not used very often. If you have to keep your windows closed then run an air purifier that is designed to remove VOCs. Remember to place your air filter several feet away from you to reduce EMR exposure.
9. Replace toxic office supplies with ones approved by the ACMI.

CHAPTER 12

Other Rooms

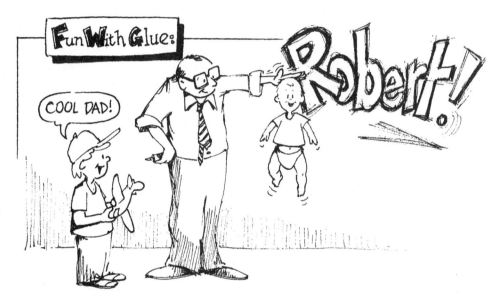

Bob, Tom, and Jack are spread out around the dining table engrossed in a project. Bob is teaching Tom how to make model airplanes like he used to make when he was a boy. Though Jack is a little young for such detailed hobbies he cannot be pried from the source of such activity.

"Right then Tom, read the next instruction," Bob says.

"Apply a thin line of glue along the entire left side of the wing." Tom grabs the tube of glue. No one reads the warning on the tube of glue saying the product is hazardous if inhaled or ingested, is an irritant to the skin, and is flammable.

With Bob overseeing his son's skills, Tom carefully applies a thin line of glue as instructed. The glue gives off a strong smell and Jack sneezes.

"Bless you," Bob says with a smile.

The glue tapers into a long string as Tom pulls the tube away from the wing. Tom promptly uses his fingers to detach the glue string, which he then wipes on his T-shirt.

He puts the tube of glue back down on the table without replacing the lid. Jack instantly seizes the moment to get his hands on the interesting prize and attempts to copy his big brother by squeezing the tube of glue. The glue dribbles out with an uncontrollable force and within seconds Jack has glue all over his hands. "Ooops!" is his only comment.

"Oh Jack, I told you not to touch anything." Bob scoops up Jack, holding him at arm's length, and heads for the kitchen.

While his father is gone Tom seizes his opportunity to test drive the soldering iron from his dad's toolbox he has not been allowed to touch yet. He plugs it in and waits impatiently for it to heat up. He has watched his Dad several times soldering electrical things in the garage. "It can't be that hard," Tom says to himself. In seconds the soldering iron is heated. Tom tests its readiness by quickly touching it with the tip of his finger.

"Ow! That seems ready." He grabs two pieces of electrical wire from the toolbox and some solder, places the two ends together on the table and presses down with the soldering iron. The metal melts instantly. "Cool," Tom says, as the strong smell of solder fills the living room.

Tom's dad runs back into the room shouting, "What are you doing?"

Tom drops the soldering iron onto the table, trying to act innocent. The soldering iron burns a hole in the dining table before their eyes. A clean Jack walks back into the living room and climbs back onto his chair ready for more action, "Poo ... stinky!" he says.

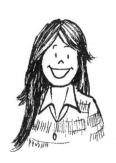

Commentary

Many homes have other spaces or rooms in the house beyond the main ones we have discussed so far. Homes tend to change and adapt to suit our ever-evolving needs. As a family grows a storage space may become an extra family room; as a family shrinks, a room or a whole section of a house may be shut off and neglected; a dining room may double as a place for hobbies and projects. For the sake of simplicity in this chapter we will group together some of the key considerations for the remaining rooms in a home and ask you to then translate these ideas to fit your individual needs.

Building Biology perspective

Your home is a living organism so no area or room in the house should be neglected in the overall picture of health. While the third skin layer may contain the same basic features in all these other rooms we need to consider what these spaces are used for, what they contain, who spends time in them and for how long?

The Third Skin Layer

These remaining rooms all follow the basic checklist from Chapter 7. Any specialized building features will depend on what these spaces are used for, what they contain, who spends time in them, and for how long.

Your Layer

Let's take a look at the other rooms in Jane and Bob's house.

The Basement

The previous owners of Jane and Bob's house had attempted to finish the basement by putting up sheet rock on some of the walls and paneling on others. The furnace and hot water heater had been partitioned off with some flimsy stick frame walls and more sheet rock, but no door. Bob always planned to finish off the basement some day, but in the years that followed the basement had only been used for storage. Now with a new baby on the way Bob has reclaimed the basement as his space calling it the "games room." He regularly retreats there to escape the bustle of remodels and family life.

He has put carpet on about two thirds of the bare concrete floor, added an old sofa, a reclining chair, coffee table, a TV, a scattering of toys, an old pool table, and now calls it finished. But is this a safe and healthy place for him or his family to be spending time in?

Mold

The basement has a musty smell and Bob sometimes notices a mild sore throat or develops a temporary cough after he has spent a whole evening there. His youngest son Jack does not like going in the basement at all, even with the lure of the TV, and when Bob can persuade him to spend some time there he often has an asthma attack. Though Bob has not yet made the connection, his basement has a mold problem. How has this happened?

Mold loves warm, damp, dark places to grow in and basements can provide the ideal environment. Bob's basement has only four small basement-style windows, positioned almost at ceiling level; on the outside of the house they are at ground level. Yard debris leans against these windows blocking some of the natural light and acting as a deterrent to opening them from the inside. Hence Bob never opens them. Poor ventilation is a classic problem in basements.

> There are no established standards for acceptable levels of indoor mold.[1]

The basement also has high moisture levels for a couple of reasons. The basement walls were not finished properly on the outside during construction, something that Bob would have no clue about, and this allows moisture from the ground outside to wick through the concrete walls to the inside. The sheet rock and paneling on the walls disguise the dampness in the wall, again leaving Bob with no obvious clue that there is a problem.

The other source of moisture comes from the kitchen above. The current remodel has uncovered a slow leak from the dishwasher, which has been quietly leaking water down through the kitchen floor into the basement ceiling and walls for some time.

The most immediate thing that Bob can do to help his basement is getting into the habit of opening the windows, even if just a little, whenever he is down there. He should also invest in a dehumidifier and run it in the basement to remove excess moisture. This unit will need to be cleaned out regularly, otherwise it too will grow more mold and bacteria.

On April 6th, 1998, the American Academy of Pediatrics Committee on Environmental Health released a statement concerning toxic effects of indoor molds and pulmonary hemorrhage (bleeding in the lungs) in infants. They recommend that until more information is available on this condition, infants less than a year old should not be exposed to any moldy or water-damaged environments.[2]

Hopefully, when the Indoor Environmental Professional comes to assess the water leak in the kitchen he will trace it to the basement, discover the mold problem behind the sheet rock and paneling, and include the basement in the overall remediation plan. The paneling and sheet rock will need to be removed, the walls will have to be properly sealed, and the carpet and other spoiled furnishings will all have to be disposed of professionally.

If you have a musty smell in your basement, try opening windows or running a dehumidifier and see if that gets rid of it. If the smell keeps returning or you find visual signs of dampness, condensation, or mold growth in your basement it is wise to have this professionally evaluated (see Chapter 4). Mold can be a serious health hazard.

Radon

Another important consideration in basements is radon. Radon is an invisible, odorless, naturally occurring, radioactive gas, which can seep from the ground into homes through cracks in the foundation, basement slab, or through mechanical openings (see Chapter 3). Closed spaces like basements can be hazardous because radon levels can build up to values many times higher than outdoor levels. Radon is the second leading cause of lung cancer after smoking.

The Environmental Protection Agency says: "Everyone should test their homes for one of the leading causes of lung cancer in the country: indoor radon gas. In some areas of the country, as many as one out of two homes has high levels of radon. Radon levels can soar during the colder months when residents keep windows and doors closed and spend more time indoors."[3]

The EPA says, "Radon is estimated to cause thousands of cancer deaths in the U.S. each year."

If you have a basement, it's important to test it at least once a year for radon, especially if your children use the space. Children's lungs are very delicate and may be affected at radon levels lower than currently allowed by the EPA (the current action level is set at 4.0 pico-curies of radon per liter of air). Home tests are simple, inexpensive, and come with easy-to-follow instructions. Basically, all that's involved is exposing a special filter medium in the form of a canister or sponge for a few days to the air in the basement, sealing this sample up, and mailing it to a designated laboratory that will analyze it and send you the results.

If you discover high radon levels, open windows and stop using your basement. Contact either the National Radon Information Line at 1-800-SOS-RADON (1-800-767-7236), or The Radon FIX-IT Program at 1-800-644-6999 <www.radonfixit.org> for guidance and advice. From a Building Biology standpoint we recommend reducing radon levels to 0.5-1.5 pCi/L[4] which is similar to what occurs in nature.

Mechanicals

Bob's basement also contains the mechanicals for his home which include the furnace and the hot water heater. In a healthy home, mechanicals are best kept in their own space outside the house. Another option is a room that is connected to the house but opens directly to the outside.

Here are some basic things for you to consider about these appliances:

Furnace

Bob has the same furnace that came with the house when he bought it. It's an old gas burning furnace and he knows it really should be replaced, but if it could just last through one more winter … The problem with gas burning furnaces is that they produce combustion by-products such as carbon dioxide, carbon monoxide, formaldehyde, nitrogen oxides, particulates, sulfur oxide, water vapor, and some hydrocarbons. Some by-products are worse than others. Carbon monoxide is one of the worst pollutants found indoors because it can be deadly at fairly low concentrations.

There are two main problems with Bob's furnace. First, it does not have a sealed combustion chamber. It works instead by drawing air from the living space (the basement) into an open combustion chamber, where the gas and air mix and are burned. Then the combustion byproducts rise out of the chamber up the chimney and leave

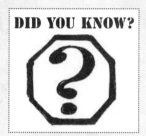

Several hundred Americans die each year from carbon monoxide poisoning. Fortunately, most cases are not serious enough to kill people. But low-level carbon monoxide poisoning seems to be a very common cause of flu-like symptoms such as nausea, malaise, headache, etc. In one study, 24 percent of people who thought they had flu didn't. They were actually being poisoned by exposure to low levels of carbon monoxide.[5]

Chronic exposure can result in multiple chemical sensitivities because carbon monoxide has the ability to interfere with the detoxification pathways in the liver, allowing the accumulation of toxic substances. Other effects of chronic carbon monoxide exposure include heart arrhythmia, decreased cognitive abilities, confusion, and fatigue.[6]

the house. As Bob never opens the windows in the basement the only air the furnace can draw on is whatever is in the basement. Bob does not realize that when he spends large amounts of time in the basement the furnace is quietly competing with him for the air and subsequent oxygen content. If Bob were to sleep overnight in his basement he would probably wake in the early hours of the morning with a terrible headache brought on by insufficient oxygen.

Second, the chimney, which is supposed to vent the combustion by-products, is prone to backdrafting. This happens when the normal draft pressure of hot air rising up the chimney and exhausting the contaminated air is affected by a negative pressure created within the house that wants to pull that air back in. This negative pressure can be created by something as simple as running a clothes dryer. If the force of the negative

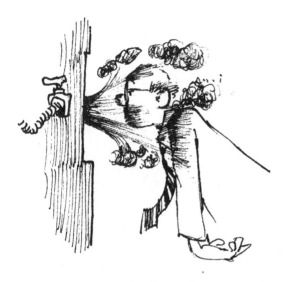

pressure is stronger than the force of the draft pressure, then the exhausted air will be pulled back into the house along with all the toxic combustion by-products. If Bob is playing pool with his son Tom while his wife Jane is doing laundry upstairs the air in the basement will steadily become polluted from the furnace back-drafting. How will that impact their health?

The best thing for Bob to do is invest in a new furnace. If you are looking to buy a new gas furnace choose one that is energy-efficient and has a totally sealed combustion chamber. In these units air is pulled from the outdoors through a sealed intake pipe into a sealed combustion chamber, where it mixes with the gas and burns. The combustion by-products generated are then blown outdoors by a fan through a sealed exhaust pipe instead of a chimney. In this way, combustion by-products never enter the home. The exhaust pipe for the furnace should be situated away from windows or places where fumes could re-enter the house, and away from where children play.

Hot water heater

Bob has an electric hot water heater that is only a few years old. It is situated next to the gas furnace. Electric hot water heaters do not generate combustion by-products and are therefore considered cleaner than gas hot water heaters. However they can generate strong EMRs. Check your hot water heater with your Gaussmeter and if you find high AC magnetic fields have an electrician look at the wiring.

Fortunately, Bob's hot water furnace is situated far enough across the basement and away from where he spends most of his time so that the EMR does not affect him. The furnace is also against an outside wall (below ground) so there are no risks to anyone else either.

Here are some general guidelines for mechanicals:

1. Ideally the mechanical room should be a dedicated room that is insulated and isolated from the rest of the living space. Outside the house is best. If it has to be inside then make it a well-sealed room that ventilates to the outside and is easily accessible for routine maintenance.
2. Ensure an adequate supply of combustion air to this room.
3. Do not locate this room adjacent to bedrooms or spaces where people spend a lot of time as some mechanical appliances generate large EMRs.
4. If there is water in the mechanical room, install a floor drain.
5. Install a fire alarm and a carbon monoxide detector.

6. Use sealed combustion appliances to prevent the leakage of combustion by-products.
7. Purchase equipment for backdrafting prevention if you have a chimney.
8. Plan a regular maintenance schedule including annual checks for the furnace and chimney and more frequent checks to clean components, purge any mold growth, and change filters.

Indoor air quality (IAQ)

Other things that can affect the air quality in your basement are termites (see Chapter 14), particles from any bare insulation such as fiberglass or asbestos, and VOCs or leaks from any stored materials such as paints, stains, pesticides, hobby and craft materials. What else do you have in your basement that could affect your family's health?

Some basements, such as conditioned basements, have been built with higher standards than others. Homes like Steph's healthy home (see Chapter 5) don't have a basement at all. If you do have one its important to ask yourself if it is safe. Was it built for people to spend time in, like a living room? What have you been using it for? Does it have a termite problem and have you or previous owners ever had a professional exterminator treat it? Is there anything strange or smelly about it? Does it feel damp? How do you feel if you spend a few hours down there? Sometimes you have to use your intuition to evaluate these situations as some things may not be visible to the eye or create a smell. If something isn't right about your basement have your family stop using the space while you do some detective work or bring in an environmental inspector to check it for you. Once your basement has been given the all clear, begin to practice healthy house maintenance in it, opening windows, removing anything toxic, and cleaning regularly. Enjoy the satisfaction of knowing that your family's health is not being harmed.

The Family Room

The family room is one of the most frequented rooms in the house and consequently often contains, and is used for, all kinds of everything. Jane and Bob's family room contains a TV, a Nintendo game, the family computer, a wood-burning stove, a large sofa, two reclining chairs, a large upright lamp, two small end tables with lamps, a folding table and several book cases containing books, toys, and sundry items. Let's look a little more closely at some of them.

Television sets

Today's home typically has several television sets: one in the family room, one in the kitchen, and one in the bedroom. The average viewing time is four to six hours a day.[7]

What you may not know is that TVs do a lot more than throw pictures up on a screen. They also give off small amounts of ionizing radiation in the X-ray band near the screen, and the entire set emits a broad band of non-ionizing frequencies including 60-Hertz power frequencies, radio frequencies, and light frequencies. As a general rule, the larger the screen, the stronger the fields will be, unless you have a large projection-screen model, in which case the stronger fields will be near the projection unit.

People tend to think that most of these emissions come from the front of the screen, but in fact the entire set gives off varying fields. AC magnetic fields easily penetrate through walls, so be sure not to place the back of the TV against a wall that has a bed, crib, frequently used chair, or workspace on the other side.

As different models vary in their field strengths, use your Gaussmeter to find a safe distance to sit from your television set. To help children remember this distance, place a small piece of tape on the floor or position their favorite chair at a safe distance for them. Children often sit too close to the screen, especially when playing television games, so they will need to be taught to sit further away. Some sources recommend at least three feet but Dr. Doris Rapp, an environmental medical specialist and pediatric allergist, recommends more than nine feet from the front of the television set, even when it is turned off. Remember to check the safe distances and positioning of all the television sets in your home, particularly bedrooms.

It's where computers end up that could eventually create the most widespread health threats. Since manufacturers don't accept most computers for recycling, only 14 percent of the over 24 million computers that were thrown away in the U.S. in 1999 were properly disposed of or recycled. The rest are releasing toxins as they decay in landfills or are burned in incinerators. By the year 2004, the National Safety Council estimates, the U.S. could house around 315 million old computers. If discarded, they would contribute a total of roughly 1 billion pounds of lead, 4 billion pounds of plastics, 1.9 million pounds of cadmium and 400,000 pounds of mercury to the environment.[8]

Computers

Computers can emit strong EMRs like television sets (see Chapter 11). The biggest difference is that computer users usually sit within a foot or two of the screen, especially if the keyboard is attached.

If you have a computer in the family room or other rooms in your home, use your Gaussmeter to discover the safe distance to keep from the screen, back, and sides and also pay attention to where you place it. If it is against a wall, what's on the other side? Is your computer close to a sofa or chair where people often sit? Remember to keep at least 30 inches from the front of a screen and at least 40 inches from the sides or back of the computer. Pay particular attention to children, they may become engrossed in a computer game and sit too close or sit close to the side while someone else plays.

Lamps

If you have upright lamps or table lamps, check to see if they have three-pinned plugs or not. If your plugs have only two pins they are ungrounded and can emit strong AC electric fields when plugged in as well as AC magnetic fields when switched on. As we often sit close to our lamps to read, we come in contact with these fields. The simplest solution is to move your lamps three to six feet away from where people sit, as the strength of fields diminishes with distance. If you need a lamp to read by, try to find one that has a three-pinned plug that is grounded and will not emit AC electric fields.

Another alternative is to have an electrician rewire an existing lamp and ground it. When lamps are not in use unplug them to eliminate AC electric fields. What other electrical appliances or gadgets do you have in the room? How many can you eliminate? How many can you at least unplug when they're not being used?

Fires

For additional warmth many homes also have woodburning stoves and gas fireplaces in different rooms in the house. Both of these units need to be carefully maintained; otherwise they can be huge sources of indoor air pollution.

Gas fireplaces.

Concerns around gas fireplaces are the same as previously mentioned for gas furnaces. Because of the combustion byproducts they produce choose a sealed combustion model. Sometimes these are called "direct-vent fireplaces." If you have an older model that is not sealed, have the chimney cleaned and checked regularly and install equipment to prevent backdrafting. This will force combustion by-products up and out of the chimney. It's a good idea to keep a carbon monoxide detector in any room with a fuel-burning appliance and also keep a window slightly open to replenish oxygen levels, which may diminish over time.

Wood burning stove

Loose stovepipe joints, leaky door gaskets, and backdrafting can all allow significant amounts of pollutants to escape indoors. If the chimney is too short it will allow smoke from the outside to reenter your home at windows, doors, and air vents. As some of these pollutants are carcinogenic, this is an important health consideration for the whole family. Fortunately with the advent of secondary combustion chambers and the catalytic converter, woodburning stoves are less of a pollution problem than they once were.

If you already have a wood-burning stove, are thinking of purchasing one or are about to start using a different space in your home that contains one, here are some reminders and guidelines for clean operation:

1. If you are purchasing a new woodburning stove, choose one with a secondary combustion chamber and/or a catalytic converter to reduce emissions of hydrocarbons.
2. Make sure your stove is carefully installed. Periodic inspections for possible air leakages and regular cleaning to ensure a proper draft will help to exhaust combustion by-products efficiently.

Wood smoke is a complex mixture of substances produced during the burning of wood. The major emissions from wood stoves are carbon monoxide, organic gases (containing carbon or derived from living organisms), particulate matter, and nitrogen oxides. Wood smoke contains many organic compounds known to cause cancer (such as benzopyrenes, dibenzanthracenes, and dibenzocarbazoles), and other toxic compounds (such as aldehydes, phenols, or cresols). The particulate fraction is composed of solid or liquid organic compounds, carbon char (elemental or soot carbon, similar to charcoal), and inorganic ash.[9]

3. Install a fresh-air duct directly to the firebox, and close the fireplace opening itself with glass doors. This will alleviate pollutants and make your fireplace more energy efficient.

4. Be careful with what you burn in your stove. For example, do not burn coated-stock paper or colored-print paper such as magazines and newspaper comics. Arsenic vapor and volatile chemicals in the inks can cause acute respiratory problems in poorly ventilated spaces.[10] Burning plastics can create toxins such as dioxins.

5. Avoid synthetic fireplace logs. These are basically wood pulp bound with highly flammable resins and alcohols and impregnated with various chemicals to give off bright colors when burned. Traces of all these chemicals can persist in the air and cling to carpet and furnishings.

Tobacco smoke

Another source of indoor air pollution is environmental tobacco smoke (ETS). This is the smoke given off by the burning ends of cigarettes, pipes, and cigars, or exhaled by smokers. A 1997 report published by the Natural Resources Defense Council entitled *The Five Worst Threats to Children's Health* states that lead, air pollution, pesticides, environmental tobacco smoke, and drinking water contamination are the worst offenders.

Reducing or eliminating environmental tobacco smoke in your home is the simplest and easiest strategy to prevent this pervasive and dangerous form of pollution. I've worked with many people over the years who wanted to stop smoking, and the single

Environmental tobacco smoke is a known cause of lung cancer and hence is classified as a Group A carcinogen.[11]

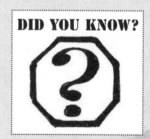

DID YOU KNOW?

One half to two thirds of all American children under five years of age are exposed to cigarette smoke in the home.[12]

A 1992 report by the EPA entitled, *Respiratory Health Effects of Passive Smoking: Lung Cancer and Other Disorders*, estimates that passive smoking causes approximately 3,000 lung cancer deaths among nonsmokers each year, and that children exposed to environmental tobacco smoke are more likely to suffer an increased prevalence of respiratory symptoms such as coughing, sputum, and wheezing; an increased prevalence of middle ear effusions, or presence of excess fluid in the middle ear; a small but statistically significant reduction in lung function; exacerbation of asthma and long-term lung deficiencies (e.g. cystic fibrosis); and increased prevalence of lower respiratory infections including pneumonia, bronchitis, and bronchiolitis.

The same report also says that environmental tobacco smoke contains some 4,000 substances, more than 40 of which are known to cause cancer in humans or animals.

Cigarette smoking is the leading known cause of avoidable death in the United States.[13]

deciding factor between success and failure was having a strong enough reason. I hope the statistics on children's health effects has provided you with a multitude of strong reasons.

Here are some suggestions and strategies to help you in your home:

1. Don't smoke in your home and don't allow others to do so. Place signs around your home and at the front door where people enter. Tell babysitters and anyone else who works in your home not to smoke in the house or around your children.
2. If someone insists on smoking in your house increase ventilation in that area. Open windows, use exhaust fans, and run an air purifier that can remove chemicals.
3. Store cigarettes and other tobacco-related products out of the reach of children. Put "Mr. Yuk" stickers (see Chapter 16) on any containers and teach your children to stay away from anything with this picture on it.

Hobby, art and craft supplies

Indoor hobbies and the use of art and craft materials at home are a source of enjoyment and pleasure for many. They express our creativity and personality and can reduce stress in our busy lives. Some hobbies are quite benign and don't pollute our homes or cause us harm. But some hobbies expose us to dangerous and toxic substances such as asbestos, heavy metals, and organic solvents that can have profound health consequences on the whole family.

Many people believe that art and craft materials, like personal care products, must be safe to use or they would not be available to buy off a store shelf. Unfortunately this is not true. For the purposes of this discussion we will focus on the health threats posed to children by products used in the home. In taking extra precautions to protect our children's health we will protect the rest of the family at the same time. If you or another adult in

WHY CHILDREN ARE A HIGH-RISK GROUP.

Up until their late teens, children are still growing. Their body tissues are metabolizing faster than those of adults and, as a result, are more likely to absorb toxic materials that can result in body damage.

First, the brain and nervous system of young children are still developing, making these organs a prime target for many toxic materials. This is why children are especially susceptible to lead poisoning.

Second, infants' lungs are immature at birth and develop slowly. They have smaller air passages, poorly developed body defenses, and inhale more air than adults in relation to their body weight. All these factors make young children more susceptible to inhalation hazards.

Third, children absorb more materials through their intestines than do adults. Therefore, they are more susceptible to poisoning by ingestion. What increases the risk even more is that children weigh much less than adults. The smaller the body weight, the greater the effect of a given amount of toxic material, since there is a higher concentration of the material in the body. Thus, the smaller and the younger the child, the greater the risk.[14]

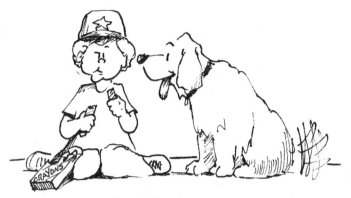

the family are an artist and have a workshop inside or attached to the home, Michael McCann's book *Artist Beware* is an informative resource for hazards associated with different art and craft materials.

One of the main problems with art and craft materials is labeling. Even though laws have been passed, such as the 1988 Labeling of Hazardous Art Materials Act, requiring all chronically hazardous art materials to carry state which are inappropriate for children's use, many art products are still not properly labeled.

The Art and Creative Materials Institute (ACMI) attempts to fill these gaps. The ACMI is considered the leading authority on art and craft materials. All products in their program undergo extensive toxicological evaluation and testing before they can bear the ACMI certification seals. Look for ACMI seals on materials when shopping for art and craft supplies, but be aware that this does not guarantee that the product is 100 percent safe. For a free listing of products tested by the ACMI call 781-293-4100 or use their online database at <www.acminet.org>.

Let's review the earlier story about Bob and his two sons building a model airplane. First of all, Bob has no idea that children's hobby materials can be toxic and dangerous. Though he has Tom read the instructions on how to assemble the airplane, no one reads the label on the glue. If they did they would see that it contains solvents and a warning that the product is hazardous if inhaled or ingested, is an irritant to the skin, and is flammable. Definitely not something you want your children inhaling or your toddler grabbing hold of and getting all over his hands.

> Young children cannot be expected to follow instructions for the proper use of art and craft materials; it is only reasonable to expect that the use of these materials by children will result in contact with the skin, eyes, mouth, hair, and clothing. Such contact provides ample opportunity for inhalation, ingestion, or skin absorption of potentially toxic compounds.[15]

Then there is the soldering iron Tom experiments with. Young children should never use soldering irons and even older children should be under strict supervision. Soldering irons can inflict serious burns. Then there is the material used to solder with. Older lead solder, that many people still have around, produces toxic lead fumes when heated. Given how close to these fumes most people work when soldering, inhalation poses a potent health hazard. Fortunately, the solder Bob has in his toolbox is a more recent version made from tin, copper, and silver and is lead-free. Even this releases noxious fumes, and as Bob has not opened any windows while they work on their project, these fumes quickly fill the house. Noxious fumes can be very irritating to young eyes and lungs.

So what makes an art or craft material safe?

Knowledge of materials and their proper use makes them safe. Before buying, read the label on all products you plan to use. Only purchase products with the ACMI non-toxic seals for young children, so you will know the product has been evaluated by a qualified toxicologist for both acute and chronic hazards. Or, look for indications that the product conforms to ASTM D 4236, the chronic hazard labeling standard that is now part of U.S. labeling law.

When you are ready to use the product, follow all safe use instructions carefully such as ventilating the space by opening windows or wearing personal protective gear if necessary. Listen to your children. If they say something stinks and they don't like it, or they suddenly get a headache or stomach ache or start complaining they feel sleepy, stop what you are doing and get them outside for some fresh air and remove the materials from the home.

Here are some basic guidelines to follow for healthy, happy hobbies:

1. Only purchase art and craft materials with an ACMI seal.
2. Before starting any project read labels carefully and follow any instructions to ventilate the space or use personal protective gear.
3. Even if ventilation is not suggested, always open windows anyway so that contaminants may be diluted and eventually removed from the air.
4. Refrain from eating or drinking while engaged in art projects.

ART AND CRAFT MATERIALS TO AVOID AND RECOMMENDED SUBSTITUTES

1. Avoid: Products that may generate an inhalation hazard. Examples include clay in dry form, powdered paints, glazes, pigments, wheat paste, and aerosols (for example, spray paints, fixatives).
   Substitute: Wet or liquid non-aerosol products. (If dry products are used, they should be mixed while young children are not present.)
2. Avoid: Hazardous solvent-based products. Examples include rubber cement and its thinner, turpentine and other paint thinners, and solvent-based markers.
   Substitute: Water-based glues, paints, markers.
3. Avoid: Materials that contain lead or other heavy metals. Examples include some paints, glazes, and enamels.
   Substitute: Products that do not contain heavy metals.
4. Avoid: Cold water dyes or commercial dyes.
   Substitute: Vegetable dyes (onion skins and so forth).
5. Avoid: Instant papier-mâché, which may contain asbestos fibers or lead or other metals from pigments in colored printing ink.
   Substitute: Papier-mâché made from black and white newspaper and library or white paste (or flour and water paste).

Some art and craft projects involve processes that are inappropriate for young children. Some examples are airbrushing, enameling, photo developing, and soldering. Instructors are encouraged to avoid projects that would involve these processes.[16]

5. Thorough cleanup after use of art and craft materials will help prevent exposures.
6. Make sure children wash their hands thoroughly with soap and water when finished.
7. Store art and craft supplies safely and make sure materials are properly labeled. Keep the wrapper to a product if it contains special instructions or warnings.
8. If an art material has been transferred to an unlabeled container and its identity is unknown, it should be disposed of appropriately.
9. Store art and craft supplies in closets or storage rooms that have good ventilation or an exhaust fan.

Other rooms

When it comes to the other rooms in your home, remember they are all interconnected. There may be some rooms in your house you need to reacquaint yourself with. Take a walk around your home and look at each room with fresh eyes. Is it safe for the purposes it is being used for? Allow your intuition to guide you. You may want to make a list of things that you have questions about now that you know more. What needs to be checked or replaced? If you have teenagers who have taken over the basement as their personal space, have you any idea what the air quality is like down there? Visit and find out. What kind of products do your children use on a regular basis in their bedrooms? Again, visit and find out. The more time you invest into your detective work the safer and healthier your home will become.

Most immediate gains

1. If you plan to spend time in your basement then treat it with the same health considerations as the rest of the house, i.e. open the windows, ventilate the space, and clean it regularly.
2. If your basement contains the mechanicals for the house make sure they are maintained regularly. It's best if you can contain them in their own sealed room.
3. Have your main mechanicals checked annually including your chimney if you have one.
4. Create a home maintenance plan for optimum mechanical room health including cleaning, checking for mold, checking for carbon monoxide and gas leaks, and replacing filters. (See Chapter 17).
5. Upgrade to energy efficient units when possible. If gas appliances are cheaper to use where you live, purchase sealed combustion units.
6. Use your Gaussmeter to find the safe distances from all your main EMR sources like TVs and computers.
7. Have your gas fireplace and wood burning stove checked for leakage and consider fitting additional backdrafting equipment to assist the exhausting of combustion by-products.
8. Keep environmental tobacco smoke out of your home and away from your children.
9. Follow the guidelines listed above for healthy, happy hobbies.

CHAPTER 13

Garages

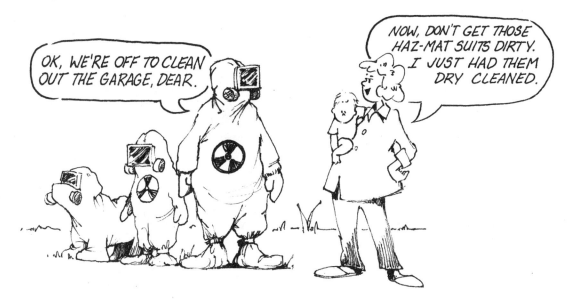

"**Y**ou're not serious about cleaning this garage up are you?" Mark asks, as he stands in the connecting doorway between the house and the garage.

"I promised Jane I'd get it done before the baby comes. Actually, I promised her I'd do it eight years ago when we first moved in, but as you can see, I never got to it." Bob scratches his head nervously as he surveys the magnitude of his project.

"Well I think you're having an attack of Jane's hormones. She's in there cleaning like a maniac!"

"I like the garage this way it is dad, it's full of cool stuff," Tom adds, showing some moral support.

"Yes, well your mother doesn't, so we'd better get to work or I'll be in the doghouse tonight." Bob smiles, giving Tom a pat on the back. "Come on Mark, roll up your sleeves and give us a hand."

"I can't believe I'm giving up an afternoon of golf to do this. You're going to owe me big-time," Mark says in a threatening tone of voice, shaking his head.

"BIGTIME!" repeats Jack enthusiastically, as he climbs down the step from the kitchen doorway into the garage ready to join everyone.

"Now Jack, I need you to stay OUT of things OK?" Bob emphasizes the word "out" in a firm voice.

"OK," says Jack as he toddles off looking for something interesting.

"What do you want me to do with all these?" asks Mark holding a large box he has filled full of old paint cans and various half empty bottles including degreasers, windshield wiper fluid, and motor oil. "Should I dump them down the drain outside?"

"Just set them down on the drive and I'll go through them, I seem to remember some of those need to be disposed of a certain way," Bob says, trying to remember what he did with the list Jane cut out of the newspaper on household hazardous waste material.

"Really? I put everything down the drain at home," shrugs Mark.

"Yuk," Jack says, walking towards his dad holding a tin of something, with grease smeared all over his face.

"Oh Jack!" yells Bob. "What have you got into now?"

The sound of glass shattering makes everyone jump. "Sorry!" Mark shouts from behind a pile of boxes. A noxious smell fills the garage.

"This is going to take a long time," Bob sighs, as he scoops Jack into his arms and heads for the kitchen.

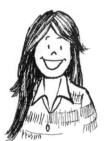

Commentary

Garages were originally small, simple structures designed to house and protect a car from the elements. These structures were always separate from the home. Today garages for multiple cars are attached to houses and are often the most pronounced feature at the front of any home.

Building Biology perspective

Would you ever dream of parking your two cars in your living room or spare bedroom and living around them? Hopefully not. Yet attached garages are just that. They are another room of the house, separated by a door, from our living spaces. An average family loading and unloading children, dogs, and groceries back and forth each day can make garages one of the most used and heavily trafficked rooms in the home. But garages are also homes for our fuel-burning cars and storage space for a whole host of other hazardous products.

If you are building a new home, a detached garage is the healthiest choice, as it will keep the many sources of pollution associated with a garage out of your home. However we will focus our attention in this chapter on attached garages as this is what most people have today and there are a multitude of health considerations to be aware of.

Third Skin Layer

The basic building features for a healthy attached garage are:

1. All connecting wall surfaces in the garage are sealed to prevent leakage of vapors or fumes into the living space.

2. Non-toxic finishes are used.

3. Low EMR design.

4. Energy efficient fluorescent lighting with good color value.

5. Doors that connect from the garage into the living space must be air tight to prevent entry of any garage pollutants into the home.

6. If mechanicals must be placed in the garage, they are placed along an outside wall, are easily accessible and are away from where people spend time sleeping, working, or relaxing.

7. An exhaust fan is installed with a timer that turns it on automatically when the garage door is opened. The fan should run for 30-45 minutesto fully exhaust all fumes from the area.

Your layer

Bob and Jane are a typical modern family. As Bob works away from the home and Jane has two children to take care of, they both require cars. Besides housing the cars, their garage is also home to Bob's workbench and tools, gardening tools and gardening products, household cleaning and maintenance products, two shelves full of car-related products, cans of paint and solvents, camping gear, some old furniture in need of repair, several bikes, and many columns of boxes containing old clothes, toys, bedding, and other miscellaneous stuff.

Let's take a closer look at some of the things in their garage:

Cars

We usually think of vehicle exhaust as an outdoor pollutant, but an attached garage regularly fills with exhaust fumes and gasoline odors which can easily find their way into your home and become a significant indoor pollutant.

Car exhaust contains many kinds of gases and chemicals including carbon monoxide, nitrogen oxides, sulfur dioxides, and particulates. On the chemical front, gas can contain benzene, cadmium, chlorine, formaldehyde, toluene, xylenes, and additives such as MTBE (methyl tertiary butyl ether) which is a suspected carcinogen.[1] Asbestos brakes generate dust as they wear, releasing asbestos fibers into the air. Despite the EPA's attempts to get auto manufacturers to voluntarily remove asbestos from brakes many old cars and trucks still have them, and asbestos brake pads are being used on new cars. There is still no known medically safe level of asbestos exposure.

On winter mornings Bob often starts his car engine and lets it run in the garage to warm up before heading off to work. The car's exhaust fumes easily enter the house even though the connecting door between the garage and the kitchen remains closed. As this is often happening when his wife Jane and the boys are having breakfast they all receive a significant dose of toxic fumes to start their day off. What are the health affects of this regular exposure, especially to Jack who already has asthma?

When Bob returns home from work he uses his garage door remote and always closes the garage door behind him. This traps car exhaust fumes inside the garage and when he opens the connecting door into his kitchen another large dose of pollution follows him inside his home. When you add to this Jane's daily trips taking Tom to and from school plus trips to run errands, the combined effect of pollution generated by their two cars is staggering. If this scenario sounds like your household let's look at a couple of simple ways to make some improvements.

Try these safer strategies:

1. Never leave your car idling in the garage. If you want to warm your engine up, pull it out of the garage and a little away from the house to do so.
2. Move other have fuel-burning machines, like lawnmowers, outside the garage before starting their engines.
3. Don't leave young babies and toddlers sleeping in the car while the engine is still warm and parked in a closed garage.
4. Leave your garage door open for a while after parking to help your car engine cool and to allow exhaust fumes to escape, or else park your car outside to cool off and then bring it into the garage.
5. Keep connecting doors between garages and living spaces tightly closed at all times.

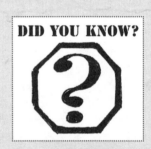

DID YOU KNOW?

Shipments to U.S. ports of potentially hazardous asbestos brake material have increased 300 percent in the past decade.[2]

Scientific Instrument Services (SIS) identified over 100 volatile organic compounds (VOCs) in the air inside a brand-new Lincoln Continental. The chemicals in the fumes include toluene and styrene, which can damage the human brain and nervous system and liver, and benzene, a known human carcinogen. SIS found that the high concentration of VOCs — long with the new car smell — declined after two months, but the chemical levels rose when the temperature increased.[3]

MTBE (a gas additive) is a suspected carcinogen that doesn't break down in water. As a result, MTBE is now the most common contaminant in ground water in the United States, the National Exposure Research Laboratory (NERL) reports. "As little as a tablespoon in an Olympic-sized pool makes water taste and smell like turpentine," reported the Associated Press in January 2001.

Carbon monoxide is a colorless, odorless, and tasteless gas that suffocates the body by replacing oxygen in the bloodstream. Symptoms of carbon monoxide poisoning are headache, dizziness, confusion, nausea, and shortness of breath. Pregnant women, developing fetuses, and newborns absorb carbon monoxide into their bloodstream at even higher rates than others, according to the Carbon Monoxide Medical Association and Carbon Monoxide Safety & Health Association (COMA-COSHA). Oxygen deprivation can impact brain development of fetuses and newborns.

Ventilation

Garages need to be well ventilated and well sealed at the same time. The best way to ventilate the space is to install a mechanical exhaust fan to force pollution out of the garage. Make sure it has enough CFM (cubic feet per minute) of air movement to effectively remove polluted air from the whole garage. You will need to keep a window slightly open all year round to bring in fresh air to replace the vented air.

There are also two choices when it comes to installation. The exhaust fan can be electrically connected to the garage door so that it is automatically triggered whenever the garage door is opened. Or you can use an automatic timer or a spring-wound crank timer that you manually turn to run for 30-45 minutes. This will air out the garage while the vehicle cools down and then shut off automatically. The only challenge with this second method is to remember to crank it.

Sealing

To prevent the passage of contaminated air into living spaces your garage must also be well sealed. On a larger scale, this means sealing the entire common wall between the home and garage and making it airtight so that fumes do not seep from the garage through the wall into your home. If you have a bedroom or living space above a garage you will need to seal the garage ceiling too. There are special products that can be painted onto these surfaces to seal them (see Appendix C).

There are several other common air infiltration points including electrical outlets, lighting fixtures, air vents, the juncture where sheetrock meets the floor, poorly sealed plumbing, and electrical and ductwork penetrations. These all need to be sealed.

Other things to look for are:

1. The fresh air intake vent for central heating or air conditioning. If this is located in the garage it will be supplying heavily polluted air into your home.
2. The vent from your clothes dryer. This is supposed to be vented to the outside of the house. If this is located in the garage lint will accumulate, creating more debris to be tracked back into the house. The high amounts of humidity generated from the dryer will encourage mold and mildew growth. Anyone coming into the house through the garage when the dryer is running will let any heavily fragranced laundry product smells back into the house, increasing indoor pollution levels. And finally, when the dryer is not in use, exhaust fumes from the garage have an open pathway directly back into the home.

Weather stripping doors

The connecting door between the garage and your home must be airtight. This is a primary pathway for pollutants to enter your home even when the door is closed. Place weather stripping around the door and install a sealed threshold. Most available weather strips are made of synthetics, including silicone, urethane foam, polypropylene nylon, and neoprene. Some will outgas. Brass and stainless steel is also available at hardware stores. Choose the least odorous weather stripping that accomplishes the job.

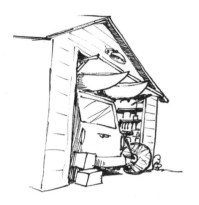

Storage

What else do garages contain? Bob and Jane's garage is the household overflow space used to store everything that either cannot fit or does not belong in the house. But most people don't know that some of these things can outgas, leak, and emit toxic chemicals and pollutants that can find their way into the home.

Take an inventory of products in your garage. Read the labels. Many of these labels will contain the words "warning," "danger," "caution," "flammable," "combustible," "pesticide," "corrosive," "toxic," and "poison." These products are considered household hazardous waste products. Simply storing them in your garage is no guarantee of safety or protection for your family's health. Many of these products may no longer be needed or used. If that is the case, get rid of them. Reducing the sheer volume of hazardous products in your garage is a great start to making your garage a healthier place. Never dispose of household hazardous waste in your garbage can, down the sink, on the ground or down a storm drain. Call your local Household Hazardous Waste facility for advice.

Here are some guidelines for the remaining products:

1. Are they safe or could they be replaced with healthier alternatives? Many products are now available such as non-toxic pest and garden products that work great, are gentle on the environment and will not hurt your family's health (see Chapter 14).

TOP TEN HAZARDOUS PRODUCTS IN THE HOME

1. Paints and stains
2. Pool and spa chemicals
3. Pesticides and other poisons
4. Household cleaners and disinfectants
5. Aerosol spray products
6. Art and hobby chemicals
7. Batteries
8. Automotive products
9. Solvents and thinners
10. Sharp instruments such as medical syringes and lancets

2. Experiment with home recipes and replace toxic car and home cleaning products with safer alternatives (see Chapter 16).

3. Any hazardous products you have to keep around should have "Mr. Yuk" stickers placed on them to show children they are dangerous (see Chapter 16). Ideally, storing them in a securely locked shed outside creates the most distance between any odors and fumes and the inside of your home. If any products have to be kept inside the garage they should be stored in a

locked, fireproof, sealed container, which can be independently vented to the outdoors. Never underestimate children's or pets' curiosity or how easily they can be poisoned.

4. Keep all substances in their original containers.
5. Whenever possible, handle volatile solvents, fuels, oils, or paints outside the garage. At least make sure the garage window is open and the exhaust fan is working. Keep children away.
6. For accidental spills or leaks, ventilate your garage well and use nontoxic, unscented, undyed detergent or absorbents to remove them. Avoid toxic solvents and always use heavy-duty gloves to protect your hands while cleaning (see Chapter 16). Keep children away from the area until the problem is resolved.

Keeping the rest of your garage organized and uncluttered will make it easier to cleanand reduce the temptation for termites to set up residence there.

> Americans generate 1.6 million tons of household hazardous waste per year. The average home can accumulate as much as 100 pounds of household hazardous waste in the basement or garage and in storage closets.[4]

Mechanicals

Mechanicals located in the garage can add to pollution levels depending on whether they are gas or electrical units. Gas units generate combustion by-products and electric units generate EMRs (see Chapter 12).

If you are building a new house the best-case scenario is to situate the mechanicals in their own room outside the house. If they must be contained in the house somewhere and you have an attached garage, then put them in the garage and locate them as far away as possible from any door that connects into the house and along an outside wall away from any space where people spend large amounts of time. Choose energy efficient, electric units and have them properly installed. These are considered cleaner units. If electricity is too expensive where you live then choose sealed combustion fuel-burning units and be diligent in maintaining them regularly.

Rooms above garages

If you have a room over the garage such as a bedroom or an office, keep in mind that garage pollution will easily find its way inside through the garage ceiling if it is not properly sealed, and through any opened windows. This can pose significant health problems, particularly if this is a child's bedroom.

It is simple to seal the garage ceiling, but closing windows whenever someone goes in or out of the garage or leaves the car idling on the drive under a bedroom window is a little more challenging. If there is an alternative window to open that is not directly over the garage door, use this for fresh air. If you don't have that option you may need to run an air purifier in the room that can remove gases and VOCs and only open windows during periods of the day or night when no cars are around.

The healthy garage

The truth is, most attached garages were not designed or built to prevent garage-generated pollutants from passing indoors, regardless of the age of the house or how much it cost to build. Even with all the recommended strategies that have been suggested, whenever the connecting door from a garage into a home is opened, pollution will enter your home.

If you are building a new home or adding on to an existing home and have to have an attached garage, then follow the guidelines in Chapter 5.

Detached garages need to be designed back into new homes, along with simple breezeways for weather protection between the garage and the home. Use your consumer power to insist that your new home is built that way. If necessary, educate your architect or builder about the health concerns associated with attached garages.

Most immediate gains

1. If you have a window in the garage, keep it slightly open all year round to help vent exhaust fumes and odors that build up there.
2. Install an exhaust fan, vented away from the house or any windows, and set it on a timer to run for 30-45 minutes after a car leaves or parks in the garage.
3. Don't let your car idle in the garage, especially with the garage door closed.
4. The exhaust fumes from gasoline powered yard equipment can be even worse than from cars. Replace them with manual or electric models. Until they can be replaced always start these pieces of equipment outside the garage and let them cool off outdoors after use before bringing them back into the garage.
5. Seal common walls and ceilings and other common air infiltration points including electrical outlets, lighting fixtures, air vents, the juncture where sheetrock meets the floor, and any poorly sealed plumbing, electrical, or ductwork penetrations.
6. Weather-strip any connecting doors to make them airtight.
7. Get rid of as many hazardous household waste products as possible and dispose of them safely.
8. Any hazardous products you want to keep should be stored either in an outside shed which is securely locked or in a locked, fireproof, sealed container, which can be independently vented to the outdoors.
9. Don't let children play in garages.
10. Make sure your garage is equipped with a multi-purpose fire extinguisher and store it somewhere easily accessible and prominent. Check the gauge occasionally to see that it's properly charged.
11. Organize your garage and get rid of as much clutter as possible. It will be easier to keep clean and will help deter termites.
12. Don't air things like dry-cleaning in the garage; it will just become more contaminated.

CHAPTER 14

Yards, Plants, and Pests

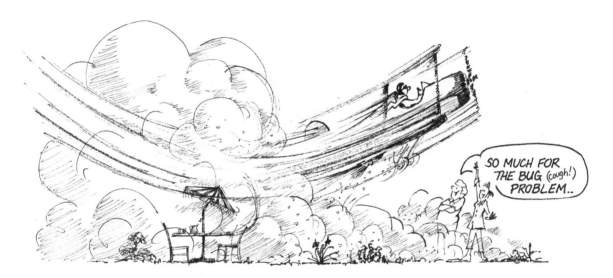

The lawn care truck pulls away from the house and Mark waves cheerfully. "What a great deal!" Mark enthuses. "These guys do everything." He looks at the assortment of products sitting on his driveway. Two large plastic sacks — one says "weed killer" and the other says "lawn food" — a large plastic container with a hose and spray attachment which is another brand of weed killer, and a cardboard box containing an assortment of sprays, aerosols, and cans of household products. He consults the invoice in his hand to see what all this has cost him and then flicks through the accompanying brochure.

"Greens Customized Lawn and Landscape Services. A perfect lawn and beautiful landscape says a lot about you and your home. Our professionals are specially trained in numerous application techniques designed to optimize the health and beauty of your lawn and landscape. We offer a full array of services to make your lawn its absolute best, including: Weed and Insect Control, Disease Control, Fertilization ..."

"Wait till I tell Liz about the special price I got on this introductory one year package." With that he disappears into the house.

Liz is unloading the dishwasher in the kitchen when Mark walks in waving the invoice as though he's just won the lottery.

"Well, that's one less thing to worry about."

"What is?"

"I just signed us up for customized lawn and landscape care. Every two weeks they send their guys out and they do whatever needs to be done. I feel like that lawn guy really understood how much I hate weeds, he had that look in his eye like he really hates weeds too, and he kept nodding his head, he even gave me some professional-strength stuff to use whenever I need to kill a few weeds myself. And he gave me some stuff that he says kills any kind of indoor pest like ants or flies instantly. You can even spray a fly from three feet away, in mid flight, and it'll drop down dead like that." Mark slaps the kitchen counter top with his hand to emphasize his point, making Liz jump.

"Great, knock yourself out. You know how much I hate any creepy-crawly things in my kitchen," Liz says with a little shudder.

"Well, I think I'll have a go with that new weed killer and see if it's any good. It's supposed to kill dandelions and about 200 other things. Just call me 'Arnold the exterminator.' Hasta la vista, baby ... I'll be back!"

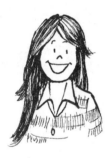

Commentary

Our homes extend beyond the boundaries defined by the walls of our home to connect with the elements and nature outside. Even the tiniest piece of property is required by law to have a certain amount of space between any two houses. These spaces include simple walkways, yards and gardens, and in some cases vast acres. But whatever the amount of outdoor space you have, it is intimately connected to the overall health of your home.

Building Biology perspective

Building Biology also includes the study of "Building Ecology." Building ecology focuses on how buildings interact with and affect the environment and seeks to maintain the best balance and harmony between the two. Minimizing any damage to the earth and surrounding environment in the building process and retaining as much of the original vegetation are some of the guidelines this field of study promotes.

The Third Skin

There are several ideal outdoor building features that are part of the overall picture for a healthy home:

1. The driveway should be made of the least toxic material such as concrete, pavers, or gravel over a well-drained and compacted base.
2. Any attached decks, wooden structures, or walkways should contain no Copper Chromated Arsenic (CCA) pressure-treated wood.

3. Any landscaping should be organic and follow Integrated Pest Management (IPM) guidelines.

Your Layer

What people do to their yards, gardens, and the property surrounding their homes varies considerably. In this domain you must also consider what your neighbors do. If their property joins yours, you are intimately linked and directly impacted by the choices they make.

Yards

Mark is delighted to employ the services of a customized lawn and landscaping service. Like many other people today, Mark wants his lawn and yard to look good, but he's too busy to work on it himself. However, the convenience offered by these home-visiting lawn and landscaping companies needs to be considered in a little more detail. Unless you know exactly what products the company uses on your property, you could unwittingly expose your family and pets to a vast array of toxic chemicals.

Even if you care for your own yard and garden, how much do you know about the products you use?

Pests

Pest problems are a fact of life. If you have a home, a yard, cultivate a garden, or have a pet, sooner or later you will have to confront termites, cockroaches, mice, slugs, weeds, fleas, or ticks, to name but a few of the most common pests. Most people respond to pests by reaching for a pesticide. This may seem to work well at first, but these products can also damage beneficial insects, food crops, the environment, and our own health. Some authorities claim that over half of the insect pest species are now pesticide resistant.

Pesticides

Pesticides are among the most commonly used lawn, garden, and household products. But as we've seen with other common products, just because they are readily available does not mean they are safe for human health. And don't be fooled by the smiling lawn and landscaping professional who assures you their products do no harm.

Pesticides are designed to attack and kill living cells and organisms. The suffix "-cide" comes from a Latin word meaning "to kill." But aren't humans, pets, and wildlife also made from living cells? Yes. So how does a pesticide know to attack only a bug or a plant and not your child? It doesn't. Pesticides don't know when to stop killing. These designer poisons can cause tremendous harm.

The national pesticide law is called the Federal Insecticide, Fungicide and Rodenticide Act (FIFRA). FIFRA defines a pesticide as "any substance or mixture of substances intended for preventing, destroying, repelling, or mitigating any pest." This definition includes: insecticides (used on plants and animals such as insects), herbicides (used on weeds), and

A new study of the health histories of 948 male Kansas farmers who had cancer and an equal number of non-cancer victims for comparison, points at 2,4-D as a cause of cancer. 2,4-D is found in many lawn-care products commonly used around suburban homes.[1]

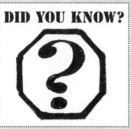

DID YOU KNOW?

Today, one in ten single-family American households uses commercial lawn care services, and one in five applies the chemicals themselves.[2]

2,4-D is the most widely used herbicide in the world. Almost 60 million pounds are used annually in the U.S. An estimated 35 million lawn and garden applications are made each year.[3]

fungicides (used on molds and fungus), rodenticides (used on rodents), and antimicrobials (used on bacteria and viruses), as well as plant growth regulators, defoliants, and desiccants. The term "pesticide" is commonly used as a synonym for "insecticide," a substance that targets insect pests.

All pesticides must be registered with the EPA in order to be legally sold in the U.S. But the EPA does not view registration as a guarantee of safety. In fact EPA regulations specifically prohibit manufacturers of pesticides from claiming that their product is "safe," "harmless," or "non-toxic to humans or pets" with or without accompanying phrases such as "when used as directed." While the EPA requires pesticide manufacturers to submit test data for registration, their full products, including both active and inert ingredients, are tested only for short-term toxic affects resulting from a single exposure. Long-term testing for cancer, birth defects, and neurotoxicity (affects on the nervous system), are required only for the active ingredients. Effects on the endocrine system (hormones) are not tested for at all.

This leads us to another interesting point. Pesticide products consist of both active and inert ingredients. The active ingredients are the chemicals designated to actually kill, and these must be named on product labels. This much is quite straightforward. Inert

Everyone wants the best for their children and to protect them from danger. Why would anyone knowingly allow their children to be exposed to toxic pesticides when effective alternatives already exist? Rachel Carson Council

ingredients however, are where pesticide formulations become quite convoluted. Despite their misleading name, inerts are neither chemically, biologically, or toxicologically inert in their effects. These ingredients, which are sometimes listed as "other" ingredients can include solvents, detergents, propellants, carriers, or other ingredients intended to make the product more potent or easier to use. Many of these chemicals can themselves cause cancer, reproductive harm, nervous system damage, and other health effects. Some can be even more toxic than the active ingredients. The identity of these inert ingredients often remains a secret to the general public because manufacturers classify them as trade secrets and because the EPA only requires that 0.3 percent of these chemicals be disclosed on product labels.[4] When you consider that pesticides designed for home use often contain a mere one percent or less of active ingredients, wouldn't you want to know what's in the other 99 percent?

Most pesticides are synthetic chemicals made from petroleum. Many of the most harmful pesticides fall into three categories: organochlorides, organophosphates, and carbamates. Pesticides can be absorbed through the skin, inhaled, or swallowed. They pose significant threats to the individuals applying them if they are not wearing appropriate personal protective gear. Pesticides can also attach to whatever they come in contact with and have far-reaching health affects on people indirectly exposed to the original application.

Pesticides used outdoors

In Mark's case, although he reads the basic instructions on the pesticide product he is about to apply to his lawn, he does not heed any of the warnings and goes about applying these chemicals wearing open-toed sandals, shorts, and a T-shirt. As he liberally sprays his lawn with the liquid pesticide only a small percentage of the product is actually delivered to the one or two young dandelions attempting to grow on his lawn. The rest of the product becomes airborne, coating him in an invisible layer of pesticides which adhere to his shoes, clothes, and bare skin, where it is immediately absorbed into his body. He also inhales the product delivering a dose of pesticides to his sinuses and lungs.

It simply does not register with Mark that he is being exposed to toxic chemicals that will directly affect his health as well as kill a few dandelions. When he returns indoors the pesticide residue on the soles of his shoes is quickly deposited onto the carpeted surfaces in several rooms of his home. He washes his hands as a gesture of cleaning up, then goes to relax and watch TV, promptly distributing more pesticides from his clothes onto the sofa. In less than five minutes he has added an invisible layer of contaminants that can quietly affect the intimate world inside his home.

He also does not realize that his liberal and frequent use of pesticides outdoors impacts other people because pesticides do not stay where you put them. Pesticides can become airborne and drift long distances from their origi-

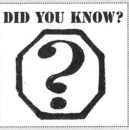

DID YOU KNOW?

Pesticides with significant health hazards are applied in startling quantities. For example, looking at just the 26 most widely used pesticides, Americans annually apply about 380 million pounds of pesticides classified by the EPA as carcinogens. About 650 million pounds of pesticides that cause reproductive problems are used annually, with hundreds of millions of applications in our homes, on our lawns, and in our gardens.[5]

Recent epidemiologic studies have shown that as children's exposure to home and garden pesticides increase, so does their risk of non-Hodgkin's lymphoma, brain cancer, and leukemia. Yet right now, you can go to your hardware store and buy lawn pesticides, paint thinner, and weed killers, all containing toxic chemicals linked to these diseases.[6]

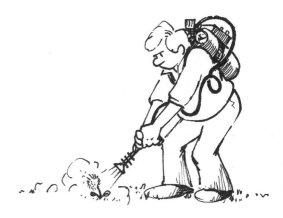

nal application site, leaving residues for neighbors, including children and pets, to come in direct contact with. Again, these residues can be inhaled, absorbed, ingested, and tracked into other homes on shoes (or paws), leading to contamination of carpet and furnishings, where they can remain imbedded in fibers for years and become part of other people's household dust.

An EPA study in Florida found the highest household pesticide residues in carpet dust.[7]

Health effects of pesticides

So what do pesticides do to our health? Pesticides can cause both acute and chronic health effects. Acute health effects appear shortly after exposure, within a few minutes to a few hours. These can include irritant effects such as stinging, burning, and itching of the eyes, nose, and throat; skin effects such as rashes, blisters, and skin burns; eye effects such as chemical conjunctivitis; and a long list of systemic effects including headaches, vomiting, jerky muscle movements, and seizures.

Chronic health effects generally result from long-term, low-level exposures to these toxic chemicals and may not be apparent until months or years later. These delayed effects pose the greatest problems to human health. Many pesticides are fat-soluble and accumulate in tissues where they can exert prolonged effects on the immune, endocrine, and nervous systems. Children are most susceptible because their developing organs and nervous systems are more easily damaged. Infants and small children are more likely to come into direct contact with pesticides on household surfaces such as carpets and by playing on lawns or with pets with flea collars. Besides causing cancer, pesticides have the potential to cause infertility, birth defects, learning disorders, neurological disorders, allergies, and multiple chemical sensitivities, among other disorders of the immune system.[8]

Do pesticides work?

Another problem with pesticides is that they kill pests, but they don't solve pest problems. Pest problems are solved when the cause of the problem is addressed. Simply killing pests, instead of solving pest problems, leads to routine and repeated use of pesticides because pests will need to be killed over and over again. Many lawn and landscaping companies spray on a calendar cycle whether there is a pest problem or not. If pesticides really worked why would the sale of pesticide products keep increasing? There are over 800 different pesticides and over 20,000 products currently registered for use in the U.S. The estimated total U.S. pesticide use in 1998 and 1999 exceeded 1.2 billion pounds.[10] (These are the most current figures available as of December 2003.) An estimated 4.4 billion applications are made annually in homes, yards, and gardens.[11] If pesticides really solved pest problems, these enormous numbers would be declining.

Children eat, breathe and drink far more than adults based on proportional body weight. For example, they drink seven times more water and take in twice as much air than adults on average. They also ingest half of their lifetime pesticide intake mostly through food by the age of five.[9]

Pesticides used indoors

Not only does Mark attack pests with a vengeance outdoors, he and Liz attack them indoors too. Not even a pesky indoor fly is to be tolerated. The new fly spray he just purchased is worth considering because many people use these kinds of products without hesitation. But based on what you now know about pesticides, do you think it's a good idea to regularly add uncontrollable amounts of pesticides to your indoor air, for everyone to breathe? If a product can instantly kill a fly, what might it do to a baby or small pet?

Other common products for indoor pests include mouse and rat poison, flea foggers, pet shampoos and collars, sprays for roaches, ants and spiders, and lice shampoos. All of these contain toxic ingredients, but the toxicity of the products varies. Older products that have been around for a number of years can be particularly toxic: some of them may even have been banned. Newer insecticides are more likely to be water-based and use shorter-lived ingredients such as pyrethrins. Many aerosol spray pesticides now use flammable propellants such as propane, which can ignite if used near a flame, such as a pilot light or gas stove. Read product labels carefully for specific information.

All these indoor pesticide applications add up. What might seem like a little spray at the time is another drop in your home's barrel of toxic pollution and subsequently yours. Sometimes the combined effects of many different products and the repeated and varied applications from different family members can create a completely unmonitored situation with staggering levels of pesticides being used. Pesticide residues persist much longer indoors than outdoors, where sunlight, flowing water, and soil microbes help break them down or carry them away. Yard chemicals tracked indoors on the bottom of shoes can remain impregnated in carpet fibers for years.

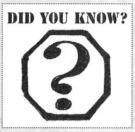

DID YOU KNOW?

Pesticides were first developed as offshoots of nerve gas during World War II. [12]

A series of studies have shown that women who have been exposed to higher levels of the organochlorine insecticide DDT have a risk of breast cancer that is between two and four times the risk of cancer in women with lower exposures. [13]

A recent study found that combining pesticides can make them up to 1,600 times more potent. [14]

A National Cancer Institute study indicated that the likelihood of a child contracting leukemia was more than six times greater in households where herbicides were used for lawn care. [15]

According to a report in the *American Journal of Epidemiology* more children with brain tumors and other cancers were found to have had exposure to insecticides than children without cancer. [16]

According to the New York State Attorney General's office, the EPA considers 95 percent of the pesticides used on residential lawns probable carcinogens. [17]

Integrated Pest Management

Hopefully by now you are convinced that using toxic pesticides in and around your home is not an option. But what do you do about pests and how will you care for your lawn?

What are the safer alternatives? Fortunately, there are many non-chemical methods for controlling indoor and outdoor pests. In addition, less toxic and highly selective chemicals are also available. The best way to manage pest problems is a strategy called Integrated Pest Management, or IPM. An IPM approach seeks to avoid pest problems through good design and maintenance practices.

Insects and weeds are two of the most common outdoor pest problems that people are concerned about. One IPM strategy for insects is to allow some level of pest damage in order to maintain predators that help control pest populations by preying on them. When and if damage becomes excessive, a combination of tools can be used, with priority given to non-chemical methods. With regard to lawns, getting your lawn off toxic chemicals is a great place to start; it just requires a little patience. How quickly your lawn returns to an environmentally sound and healthy state depends on how toxic and exhausted the soil is from past chemical use and how willing you are to change your thinking and behavior. One IPM strategy is to stay away from chemical fertilizers that green up a lawn quickly at the expense of good root development. Shallow roots mean more pest and disease problems. This will allow your lawn to green up nicely without adding toxic chemicals and stressing it.

Most indoor pest problems can be solved using the preventive strategies outlined in Chapter 9. If necessary, powders, dusts, and baits that do not give off vapors or leave residues can be used selectively. A good resource for more extensive information about IPM and safer alternatives for all your home and yard needs is Dr. Marion Moses' *Designer Poisons: How To Protect Your Health and Home from Toxic Pesticides*. The Internet also has lots of resources and there are some great organizations such as the Northwest Coalition for Alternatives to Pesticides and another group called Beyond Pesticides that provide a lot of free information and are happy to brainstorm and help you over the phone (see Appendix C). You can also find a local pest control company that uses natural or organic methods and avoids the use of toxic pesticides and chemical fertilizers.

It is never too late to change toxic pest control practices over to non-toxic alternatives and least toxic methods. Declare your yard a pesticide free zone. Washington Toxics Coalition has a colorful "Pesticide Free Zone" sign you can place in your lawn or garden or attach to a fence (see Appendix C). This lets neighbors know that you don't use pesticides. You can also be a resource for friends, neighbors, and relatives who use pesticides and want to learn how to stop.

Disposing of pesticides

Although local practices may vary somewhat, generally speaking all unwanted pesticides are considered hazardous waste and must be disposed of carefully at a household hazardous waste site. Pesticides should not be discarded in the trash or flushed down the drain. For information about disposal of household hazardous waste in your community, call your local solid waste utility, household hazardous waste facility or health department.

Fertilizer

Another thing to look for is toxic waste in fertilizer products. A July, 1997 Seattle Times investigative series entitled, "Fear in the Fields: How Hazardous Wastes Become Fertilizer" revealed that toxic wastes from steel mills, paper mills, and other major polluting industries are being turned into fertilizer and spread onto food-producing lands. As a result, poisons such as lead, cadmium, mercury, and dioxin also wind up in fertilizer products used for farms and peoples' backyard gardens. These toxins build up in the soil over time and can pose serious health risks.

No thorough study has ever been done to determine whether adding wastes to fertilizer is a safe method of disposal. Right now, the EPA is considering regulations on metals and dioxins in zinc fertilizers.

In the meantime, give composting a try. Using your everyday vegetable and organic waste scraps you can create compost rich in nutrients that will fertilize your soil and allow plants to grow stronger and be more resistant to disease (see Chapter 9). Landscaping with native plants and trees also helps to ensure trouble-free gardening. These plants usually require less water and care because they are accustomed to your particular climate. If you can't make your own compost, look for organic fertilizers at your local stores and, if you need to use chemicals, try the least toxic product you can find. Try some natural approaches; they might just grow on you!

Chromated Copper Arsenate (CCA) pressure-treated wood

Mark and Liz also have a wooden deck at the back of the house that looks out on their lawn and garden. Although Mark knows that the wood has been treated with a preservative to prolong the wood's life, he does not know what the preservative is made from or that he should be concerned about it.

Arsenic treated lumber is also known as "pressure-treated" wood and is used to build more than 90 percent of all the outdoor wooden structures in the United States. Actually, the term pressure-treated is misleading because it hides the fact that this kind of wood is injected with vast amounts of toxic compounds to preserve the wood and kill termites.

Pressure-treated wood can be found in decks, fences, building foundations, boat docks, playground equipment such as climbing frames and sandboxes, picnic tables, or anywhere wood needs to be protected from decay. The most common arsenic formulation used in the United States is Chromated Copper Arsenate (CCA). CCA consists of chromium (a

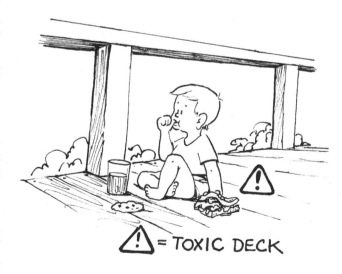

⚠️ = TOXIC DECK

bactericide), copper (a fungicide), and arsenic (an insecticide). The standard formulation of CCA used in wood contains 22 percent pure arsenic.

The EPA and the World Health Organization classify arsenic as a "known human carcinogen," and children are at greater risk from arsenic than adults because their growing bodies are less able to metabolize this contaminant. Other health effects include acute poisoning resulting in seizures or permanent nerve damage, immune system suppression, as well as increased risks of high blood pressure, cardiovascular disease, and diabetes.[18]

Children can be exposed to the arsenic in CCA-treated wood by coming in direct contact with it. Arsenic sticks to children's hands when they play on treated wood such as play structures, and is absorbed through the skin and ingested when they put their hands in their mouths or when they touch food or toys, which are then placed in their mouths.

> "We know that arsenic in drinking water is dangerous for children, but what we found was that the arsenic in lumber is an even greater risk," said Environmental Working Group Analyst Renee Sharp, principal author of the report *Poisoned Playgrounds*. "In less than two weeks, an average five-year-old playing on an arsenic-treated play set would exceed the lifetime cancer risk considered acceptable under federal pesticide law." [19]

When Mark's nephews, Tom and Jack, come over to visit they often play on the deck. Tom likes to climb on and off the structure and Jack in particular crawls around on it when playing with his dog or anything else he can find. These seemingly harmless acts of fun expose them to high levels of arsenic. The constant back and forth between indoors and out also deposits traces of arsenic indoors onto carpet and other furnishings. What are the long-term effects of these exposures on their health? And what is the chemical status of Mark's carpet from regular chemical deposits from the outdoors?

Numerous laboratory and field studies clearly show that potentially hazardous amounts of arsenic leach out of pressure-treated lumber, even though the wood preservation industry argues that the arsenic remains fixed in the wood. One study by the University of Florida showed the surface soil arsenic levels below CCA wood decks had elevated soil concentrations that on average were elevated by 2,000%.[20] Unsafe levels of arsenic can still be detected on the surface of arsenic treated wood after more than 15 years of outdoor exposure and use.

If you have wooden structures outdoors, here are some guidelines to follow:

1. It can be difficult to distinguish CCA-treated wood from non-CCA-treated wood. If you are not sure whether your wood is treated you should test it. Purchase an inexpensive home test kit to find out (see Appendix C).
2. Replace arsenic treated decks, swing sets, and picnic tables with safer alternatives. There are two alternative pressure treatments:
   ACQ: Ammoniacal Copper Quaternary is an alternate wood pressure treatment widely marketed as ACQ Preserve and ACQ Preserve Plus by Chemical Specialties.
   CBA: Copper Boron Azole a newer alternate wood pressure treatment just becoming available in the US lumber yards.

According to a November, 2001 report by the Environmental Working Group and the Healthy Building Network entitled *The Poisonwood Rivals* "We estimate that one out of every 500 children who regularly play on swing sets and decks made from arsenic treated wood, or one child in an average size elementary school, will develop lung or bladder cancer later in life as a result of these exposures".

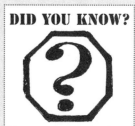

DID YOU KNOW?

Another of their reports, from May 2001, entitled *Poisoned Playgrounds* says, "All other uses of arsenic as a pesticide are banned by the EPA. But under a special federal exemption, millions of pounds of CCA a year are injected into wood that is then sold to families all across the country."

Arsenic is on the EPA's very short list of chemicals known without question to cause cancer in humans. The National Academy of Sciences (NAS) and its National Research Council (NRC) have concluded that arsenic causes lung, bladder, and skin cancer in humans, and may also cause other cancers including kidney, prostate, and nasal passage cancer. NAS and the EPA's Science Advisory Board (SAB) also have concluded that arsenic may cause high blood pressure, cardiovascular disease, and diabetes.

A 12-foot section of pressure-treated lumber contains about an ounce of arsenic, or enough to kill 250 people (*Poisoned Playgrounds*).

You can also choose naturally pest resistant woods such as redwood and cedar. If you can find certified sustainably harvested wood that helps the environment too. Playground equipment made of other non-arsenic containing components is also available such as cedar and redwood and non-wood alternatives such as metals and plastics.

3. Avoid Ammoniacal Copper Zinc Arsenate (ACZA). It is a very similar arsenic formulation. ACA and ACC are two more arsenic treatments that are less widely used.

4. Read labels and ask questions. Despite a voluntary EPA/manufacturers labeling agreement, pressure-treated wood is often unmarked or poorly labeled in stores. If you're not sure or the label is unclear, ask if the lumber has been treated with CCA, ACZA, or another arsenic compound. If the store clerks can't tell you exactly what it is, don't buy it.

5. If you can't replace the structures you have, then seal the wood at least once a year with polyurethane or an oil based penetrating sealer. Do not use acid deck wash or brighteners as these are suspected of accelerating the release of arsenic from the treated wood. Test the structure regularly to ensure it is definitely not leaching. Some sealers only slow the release and do not stop it.

6. Remember the soil around arsenic-containing structures will probably contain high amounts of arsenic. You may want to remove this and replace it with uncontaminated soil.

7. Never burn treated wood. Arsenic treated wood is hazardous and should be disposed of properly according to local environmental regulations. Contact your state or local solid waste management offices for advice. Burning CCA wood creates a highly toxic ash. One tablespoon of ash from a CCA wood fire contains a lethal dose of arsenic.[21]

8. Do not store children's toys under decks. Rainwater could leach arsenic off the wood leaving a toxic coating on the toys.

9. Arsenic treated picnic tables should be avoided and children should be discouraged from eating while on CCA-treated playgrounds.

10. Anyone who comes in contact with arsenic treated wood should wash his or her hands afterwards, particularly before eating. Young children will need to be helped or reminded.

Sandboxes

Another thing to pay attention to is the play sand used in sandboxes, around swing sets, and in play pits. Some sand contains asbestos or very fine crystalline silica. Crystalline silica and asbestos are known human carcinogens.

If you already have play sand that is very fine in texture, check with the supplier you purchased it from to see if it contains crystalline silica or tremolite asbestos. Even though the Occupational Safety and Health Administration (OSHA) has exempted tremolite asbestos from its own asbestos standard for another year, asbestos is still asbestos. Are you willing to experiment on your child in the meantime?

For years, manufacturers of toy sand have successfully lobbied the Consumer Product Safety Commission (CPSC), the agency that is supposed to be watching out for children's health, persuading them not to require labeling of sand to indicate its source. As a result, consumers are unable to tell by looking at the sand whether or not it contains asbestos. Do not purchase sand for a sandbox unless the manufacturer can assure you that it consists of beach or river sand and/or that it is not quarry rock.[22]

If you inherited the sand you have and don't know where it came from, you may want to have it tested to find out what's in it or simply replace it with washed beach or river sand, which is fairly granular, not powder-fine. Ask the supplier or phone the manufacturer to verify the source before buying. If in doubt, don't buy it.

One last thing to consider with sandboxes is to locate them at least five feet away from your home if your house was built in the 1970s or before. The outside of your home may contain lead paint, which could flake or generate dust that falls into your child's sandbox exposing him to yet another serious poison.

Driveways

Asphalt is one of the most common materials used for driveways and pavements. In other parts of the world it is called bitumen. Petroleum tar, which is the main component of asphalt or black top paving, is carcinogenic and should be avoided. Not only does it emit harmful vapors during installation, but it will also volatilize when heated by the sun. In the National Institute for Occupational Safety and Health (NIOSH) book entitled the *NIOSH Pocket Guide to Chemical Hazards*, asphalt fumes are listed as irritating to the eyes and respiratory system and as being carcinogenic.

If you are building a new home or are faced with resurfacing an older driveway, healthier options include pavers, and or gravel over a well-drained and compacted base.

Indoor plants and fresh air

Many people appreciate the aesthetics of bringing nature indoors. Plants add color, vitality, and interest to indoor spaces and provide a much-needed connection with nature to compensate for the minimal time we spend outdoors. But did you know that plants have health promoting aspects too?

Bill Wolverton, Ph.D., conducted some interesting research for the National Aeronautics and Space Administration (NASA) in the 1970-80s. NASA was looking for ways to treat recycled air and wastewater in an effort to create life-supporting systems for planned moon bases. One of their primary questions was: how does the earth produce and sustain clean air? The answer, of course, is through the living process of plants.

> "Heredity is nothing but stored environment."
> — Luther Burbank (1849-1926)

Dr. Wolverton measured how well a single plant works to clean the air in a sealed chamber of common pollutants such as ammonia, formaldehyde, and benzene. His findings were later made available in a book entitled *How To Grow Fresh Air*, which focuses on 50 common plants that can be cultivated in your home or office to help naturally clean the air. Extrapolating from these results, Dr. Wolverton says that three plants per 100 square feet in a home or office will improve air quality.

If you have allergies, Dr. Wolverton suggests putting a layer of aquarium gravel on the surface of the soil to reduce mold growth. Do not let houseplants stand in water, this attracts pests. If you don't have any houseplants consider growing some organic ones yourself or purchase some from an organic supplier. If you purchase houseplants that are not organic they will contain pesticides. Organic plants can actually be purchased through mail order companies on the Internet and delivered promptly to your home. Let your children participate and learn alongside you. Children love to grow and care for plants because there is something intrinsically good about it. You are also teaching them an important life skill that they can pass on to their children one day.

Organic yards, gardens and plants

The only real way to know that the outside of your home is safe for your family and pets is to adopt an organic mentality. Doing this will assure you of a healthy, outdoor space that complements your indoor healthy home.

Those of you starting from scratch may have some clean up work to do first, such as getting rid of any CCA-treated wood and replacing pesticides with organic products or non-toxic IPM strategies. Follow the guidelines in "the most immediate gains" to help you get started. Some of you will already be further along and need only slight improvements. Either way, one thing I highly recommend is to make your home a "no shoes" zone. If everyone who enters your home removes his or her shoes at the door you will drastically reduce the amount of contamination brought indoors. Placing small but easily visible signs around your home at all the entry points will help remind everyone of this new family strategy. These may need to be placed both at adult and children's eye levels.

ATHENA'S TOP TEN HOUSEPLANTS

Bamboo palm (Chamaedores seifrizii

Rubber plant (Ficus robusta)

English ivy (Hedera helix)

Dwarf date palm (Phoenix roebelenii)

Boston fern (Nephrolepis exaltata "Bostoniensis")

Peace lily (Spathi hyllum sp.)

Corn plant (Dracaena fragrans "Massangeana")

Kimberly queen (Nephrolepis obliterata)

Florist's mum (Chryanthemum morifolium)

Gerbera daisy (Gerbera jamesonii)

Most immediate gains

1. If you currently use pesticides in or around your home, switch to an Integrated Pest Management approach. Get help from recommended books and organizations. Consider subscribing to newsletters that focus on these issues to keep you informed and updated.

2. If you have a lawn care service, discontinue any calendar spray programs and request a maintenance program without regular pesticide use. When pests are found in excessive numbers, ask for a report and proposal before any pesticides are considered. You can also find a local pest control company that uses natural or organic methods and avoids the use of toxic pesticides and chemical fertilizers.

3. Take an inventory of any pesticide products you have. Which of these can you do without? What kind of non-toxic products could you replace them with?

4. Pesticides are household hazardous waste and need to be disposed of appropriately. Keep any pesticides in their original containers and make sure they are sealed tightly. Put "Mr. Yuk" stickers on them and store them safely away from children until they can be disposed of.

5. Build healthy soil with organic homemade compost. This also saves a lot of food waste ending in up in landfills.

6. Follow the guidelines for dealing with Copper Chromated Arsenate pressure-treated wood.

7. If you have a sandbox in your yard make sure it's filled with washed beach or river sand.

8. Take an inventory of any houseplants you already have. Are any of them listed in the top ten houseplants for improving indoor air quality? Check existing plants for mold growth and consider adding a layer of aquarium gravel on the surface of the soil to reduce further mold growth.

9. Make your home a "no shoes" zone. This simple, no cost strategy will drastically reduce the amount of contamination that enters your home.

CHAPTER 15

Pets

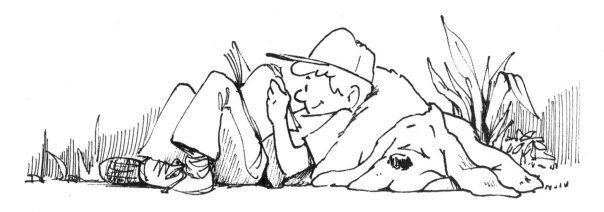

Pretending to be a Special Weapons And Tactics soldier, Tom sneaks down the garden sliding along the grass on his belly and hiding in flowerbeds and bushes, planning his surprise attack on his favorite friend, Mac, the family dog. Mac is completely oblivious to the impending ambush as he vigorously digs for a bone he buried some time ago. As the dirt flies in all directions, some is propelled over the mesh garden fence and hits Mr. Robbins, their elderly neighbor, on the back of his head.

"What was that!" he exclaims, turning around.

Tom stifles a roar of laughter by placing his hands over his mouth adding a layer of genuine camouflage dirt to his face.

"Oh, its you Mac. What are you up to then?" Mr. Robbins enquires kindly.

Mac's concentration is broken and he runs over to the fence hoping for some friendly attention. As Mr. Robbins reaches over the fence to pet Mac, they are both startled by a load war cry from Tom who has decided to take advantage of this moment and complete his surprise attack.

"Good heavens Tom, you nearly gave me a heart attack," says Mr. Robbins, clutching his chest.

Mac of course is delighted by the surprise and responds with loud barks of approval and lots of leaping.

"Hello Mr. Robbins. Sorry about that, I didn't see you there," Tom lies, completely satisfied with the outcome. "What are you doing?"

"Well, I just got this new spray to kill the bugs that are spoiling my roses. It was on sale, two for one, at the hardware store. Mrs. Robbins loves fresh roses in the house so I thought I'd better do something about them."

"Can Mac and I watch?" asks Tom intrigued.

"Of course you can, just stand back a bit." Mr. Robbins gets to work liberally spraying the solution.

Tom sneezes and Mac begins to bark at Mr. Robbins. "It's OK Mac, it's just a little spray, it won't harm you," Mr. Robbins tries to reassure the dog. But Mac simply turns and runs away.

Tom decides he has seen enough and runs after Mac, shouting good-bye over his shoulder to Mr. Robbins.

Tom catches up with Mac in the kitchen where he is thirstily drinking water from his bowl. He sniffs his bowl of new food but doesn't eat. "What's got into you then?" Tom asks. Mac lifts his paw to Tom for him to shake and wags his tail. Tom shakes his paw and gives Mac a big hug.

"Hello, hello, anybody home!" bellows the friendly voice of Uncle Joe, as he appears through the kitchen door.

"Hello Uncle Joe," Tom says, as he runs to give his uncle a big hug.

Uncle Joe is carrying his trusty toolbox and a brown paper bag tucked under his arm. "Let's see then. Do I have a little something for my favorite six-year-old?" He produces a large bar of chocolate out of the paper bag.

"Thanks Uncle Joe," Tom exclaims with obvious delight.

"And let's see. Do I have something for my favorite canine friend?" Uncle Joe fishes in his paper bag again and pulls out a new dog collar for Mac. "A brand new flea collar for you Mac," he says, shaking it in front of the dog as though it were a tasty piece of fresh meat. "This'll keep those horrible fleas away from you." Uncle Joe sets down his toolbox and reaches over to fasten the new flea collar around Mac's neck. Mac shakes his head and sneezes. "Right then, where's your dad? I believe we have a few jobs to do around here."

"I think he's in the basement watching TV," Tom says.

As Uncle Joe disappears out of the kitchen, Tom turns to Mac. "Come on then, want me to read to you?" The two of them race each other through the house into Tom's bedroom. Tom climbs onto his bed and grabs a book, followed by Mac who snuggles next to him ready for a story. Tom unwraps the bar of chocolate, takes a bite, then breaks off a large piece and gives it to Mac. "You're my best friend Mac," Tom says giving Mac a big hug around the neck and Mac licks Tom's face in agreement.

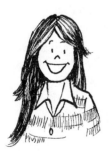

Commentary

Throughout history pets have been great companions to humans and today many people look on them as extensions of their family. I've met several people who care more for their pets than their fellow humans. Whatever your preference, pets that live indoors with you need to be considered in the overall picture of a healthy home.

For the purposes of this discussion we will focus our attention primarily on cats and dogs. These furry friends can present several health challenges in the home, including dander that triggers breathing problems and allergies, pesticide exposures from flea and tick products, and transportation of various outdoor contaminants indoors. Pets are also vulnerable to the same toxic chemicals in and around the home that we have already discussed.

Pet dander

Animal dander can trigger many kinds of adverse health reactions. Allergists usually recommend getting rid of pets if someone in the family has breathing problems or allergies. This is easier said than done. If you have a much-loved pet, getting rid of them can be a traumatic experience.

According to C.J. Puotinen in *The Encyclopedia of Natural Pet Care,* "Animals that lived to an average age of 15 or 16 in the 1960s now die at seven or eight."

Here's some information that might prove helpful in reducing the overall amount of pet allergens in your home.

Pet dander is more of a problem in carpeted homes than homes with bare floors, although rugs and other fabric furnishings can harbor dander too. What causes the problem isn't the actual hair your pet sheds but proteins in their saliva and flakes of their skin. Young puppies and kittens don't usually trigger allergies because they have no old skin to shed and therefore no dander. That's why a new pet may pose no problems for the first few weeks but then someone suddenly develops a breathing problem or allergy as the pet matures.

If you have a child with breathing problems or allergies who likes to sleep with their pet, negotiate a trial separation, explaining that you are working hard to help improve their health and keep their pet. Try a surrogate pet in the form of an organic cotton stuffed toy at bedtime. The immune system needs to recover and strengthen itself during the night, and simply removing your pet at night from the bedroom may allow your child's tolerance to strengthen to the degree that he or she can still have some access to their pet in the daytime without experiencing problems.

Tom's little borther Jack has asthma. Fortunately, Mac sleeps in Tom's room at night, but if Jack and Tom have pillow fights in Tom's bedroom, or if Jack lays around on Tom's bed long enough, his breathing is often affected.

It's important to remove dander regularly from bedding, carpet, rugs, and any furniture your pet likes to spend time on. A HEPA vacuum cleaner is necessary to trap fine particulates and prevent them from just being recirculated. Occasional steam-cleaning with non-toxic products helps to clean the deeper layers of any carpet. Whenever you clean carpets avoid fragranced products and ventilate the space well to allow the carpet to dry thoroughly, otherwise you may create a mold problem.

Washing pets themselves is also important. Research has shown that airborne allergens are drastically reduced if a cat is washed once a week. Young pets will soon get used to this. If you have older pets that are not accustomed to being bathed and are particularly resistant, try a sponge bath. You can use plain water or chamomile tea, or try one of the products designed for allergy sufferers now found at pet stores. They contain enzymes to digest the proteins in dander, rendering them harmless. Cats, dogs, birds, and rabbits can be cleaned this way. Avoid fragranced products and don't use soap for weekly washings because it strips away the natural protective oils and can leave irritating residues on the skin. Whichever method you choose the important thing is to clean down to the level of the skin.

Another approach is to remove dander at the source. Animals with dandruff or flaky skin problems are often reacting to something in their diet. Giving your pet a natural diet of raw food, filtered water, and nutritional supplements usually results in glossy fur, healthy skin, and reduced flaking and dandruff.

Brushing your pet outdoors will also reduce the amount of pet dander indoors. Forced air heating systems are notorious for blowing around pet dander and circulating it to all parts of the house. Installing a high efficiency filter in your furnace and changing it every two to three months is an important part of healthy house maintenance (see Chapter 17). Running a free-standing HEPA air filter in specific rooms where your pet likes to spend time can also help to trap dander.

All these suggestions may be enough to reduce the total allergens in your home and allow you to keep your pet.

Pesticides

Each year, pet owners apply vast amounts of toxic chemicals to their pets to kill fleas and ticks. Dipping, spraying, dusting, powdering, and securing flea collars around their necks are just some of the most popular ways we attempt to protect our pets and ward off home infestations. But these designer poisons not only kill the targeted pests, they can also poison the pets themselves and the people that handle them, including children.

Studies done with laboratory animals have raised concerns among scientists that children exposed to certain pesticides in common pet products, even at levels considered safe for adults, have higher risks, not only for acute poisoning, but also for longer-term problems affecting brain functions and other serious diseases.

Uncle Joe's attempts to prevent Mac from getting fleas by giving him a flea collar is a choice many people make, not realizing the toxic effects these synthetic chemicals have on their beloved pets. In the previous chapter we talked about how pesticides can't distinguish between an insect and a child. Likewise they cannot distinguish between a pest and pet. Pesticides are designed to kill.

Pets accumulate toxic chemicals in their bodies the same way humans do. Using the analogy of the "barrel effect" discussed in Chapter 1, it comes as no surprise to realize that our pets are also being bombarded with daily, low-level (sometimes high-level) amounts of deadly chemicals. The massive rise in cancer in pets speaks for itself. We must stop poisoning our pets with unnecessary pesticide products.

Then there are the toxic exposures that pet owners themselves receive while chemically treating their pets. The simple acts of petting and hugging your pet or allowing

Childhood brain cancer has been linked with flea collars on pets and home pesticide "bombs."[1]

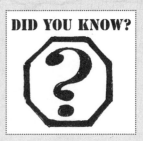

DID YOU KNOW?

The pesticide carbaryl, commonly used in pet flea and tick killers, has been shown to cause birth defects in dogs.[2]

People applying flea and tick dips can suffer muscle weakness and tingling of extremities.[3] People who dust pets with powders are likely to suffer nausea and headaches. People who chemically sponge pets may suffer convulsions and mental confusion.[4]

Limonene (also known as d-limonene) in flea sprays can cause vomiting, nausea, salivation, muscle tremors, staggering, imbalance, and other symptoms of nervous system poisoning. It is especially hazardous when used on cats,[5] but should not be used on dogs either. Also, limonene is suspected of causing cancer, birth defects, kidney damage, and harm to the immune system.[6]

Cats constantly lick their fur and, if treated with chemicals, can consume a lot more poison than dogs.[7]

One study that looked at, among other factors, pregnant women who had been exposed to flea and tick products, found that their children were 250% more likely than those in a control group to be diagnosed with brain cancer before their fifth birthday.[8]

Another study showed that pet dogs living in households whose lawns were treated with 2,4-D were significantly more likely to be diagnosed with canine lymphoma than dogs whose owners did not use weed killers. The risk rose with number of applications. Lymphomas doubled among pet dogs whose owners applied lawn chemicals at least four times a year.[9]

your pet to sleep near you, or sit on your lap can expose you to lingering pesticide residues. How much toxic pesticide is Tom exposed to when he hugs his dog with its new flea collar? And how much pesticide residue is deposited onto Tom's bedding where he and his pet like to hang out? Wherever pets roam around the house their chemically contaminated bodies can deposit residues into carpet, bedding, furnishings, and other surfaces they come in contact with. Cats in particular will wander over kitchen counter surfaces, across pillows, and often lay on top of clothes. But who is measuring the health effects of these additional everyday layers of chemicals in the home? What happens when they combine or interact with other pesticides or chemicals used in the home? Some pesticides increase in potency when mixed together.

Its not Tom's fault, its not Mac's fault, and its not Uncle Joe's fault. The responsibility ultimately lies with the manufacturers of these products. Their inadequate safety testing is biased towards company profits and away from the much needed research into acute and chronic health affects posed to young, elderly, or immune-compromised pet owners.

The EPA calculates that a child's exposure to individual organophosphates (OP) in pet products on the day of treatment alone can exceed safe levels by up to 500 times, which equals 50, 000 percent.[10]

Fortunately, safe alternatives do exist for all your pet product needs. Next time you encounter a flea problem, consider these safer guidelines:

1. Groom your pet daily with a flea comb and place any fleas in soapy water to kill them. If you cannot groom your pet daily, then do so at least twice a week.
2. Wash your pet with a non-toxic flea product such as LiceBGone (see Appendix C) and follow directions closely.
3. Spray your pet daily below the neck (to avoid eyes) with half white vinegar and half water to help control fleas between treatments.
4. Wash your pet's bedding at least once a week in hot water and dry on high heat.
5. Keep your pet's area clean. Vacuum regularly. Remove vacuum bags outdoors after each vacuuming and seal with tape before putting them in the trash. There are also special non-toxic enzyme products available to clean floors and other surfaces with.
6. There are many herbal products and different supplements that claim to help prevent flea infestations. Check with your vet, local health food store, pet store, or the Internet. Read labels and understand that even natural ingredients may be irritating or not agree with some pets or their owners. In general, fleas are not attracted to well-fed, healthy pets.

Poisoning

In humans, the symptoms of short-term acute poisoning from organophosphate pesticides found in some pet products look very much like the flu, and include nausea, vomiting, diarrhea, sweating, lightheadedness, and shortness of breath, and in the most severe cases, seizures, coma, and death. In pets, symptoms can be difficult to identify. Look for watery eyes, lack of appetite, excessive salivation and urination, nervous signs such as tremors, and behavioral changes such as hyperactivity or anything unusual.

Long-term effects are harder to identify. Young children exposed to organophosphates might develop asthma but the damage these products do may not appear for decades, and may never be traced. It may include increased incidence of cancer.[11]

If you think you or your pet have been affected by a pet product containing pesticides call your local poison control center immediately. Also report the incident to the EPA's National Pesticide Telecommunications Network at 1-800- 858-7378. The EPA needs to be made aware of any product that causes harm.

What do pets bring indoors?

If your pet stays indoors 100 percent of the time you can skip over this section and move on to the next section on how homes affect pets. For those with pets that get to wander outdoors there are a few additional considerations when it comes to your healthy home.

Fresh air, natural light, and exercise boosts pets' health and well being as well as ours. However, we humans don't tend to dig around in dirt or find rotting or decaying things as fascinating as our pets do. Nor do we go to the bathroom outside in places we might later casually walk around in. We also have outer clothing and shoes that we can remove when we return indoors.

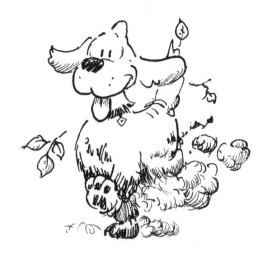

A microscopic look at what our furry friends bring indoors with them on fur and feet would reveal more than just obvious pests like fleas and ticks. Common garden dirt can contain pesticide residues, lead from the paint on older homes, arsenic from CCA pressure-treated lumber, mold spores, microbes, and a miscellaneous variety of other chemicals and heavy metals from whatever is in the ambient outdoor air where you live. Combine this with lawn pesticides and chemical fertilizers and probably a percentage of pet excrement and you have a dizzying concoction being trafficked into your home each day. Now don't get me wrong, I'm not advocating quarantining pets indoors all day long. I think the benefits of the outdoors are a valuable part of having happy, healthy pets. But this knowledge does require we do a little rethinking about what enters our home and how best to deal with it.

As part of this rethinking process, ask yourself the following questions: Does your pet wander freely in your home? Where does your pet spend the most time? Do you know where your pet hangs out while you are at work? Are you sure about that? Where does your pet sleep? Where does your pet go to the bathroom? Does your pet have any secret places it occasionally uses as a bathroom or to store things? Once you have these answers, ask yourself if you are comfortable with the picture you now have in light of what your pet could be bringing indoors each day. If you are, that's great. If not, what needs to change?

Here are some suggestions to reduce the amount of unknown substances coming into your home with your pet.

1. If you allow your pet to sleep on your bed with you, at least wipe your pet's fur and paws down each evening with a damp cloth. Even if your pet doesn't sleep with any family member, wiping them down whenever you can remember helps.
2. Have your pet sleep on a towel or its own sheet on your bed that you can change each day.
3. If your pet has its own bed, remove the covers and wash once a week in hot water and dry on high heat.
4. Consider restricting your pet's access to certain rooms of your house where you are more concerned about contaminants being deposited, such as children's bedrooms. Simply keeping doors shut usually works. The trick is training yourself and other family members to remember to do so.

5. Thoroughly vacuum any carpeted areas or furniture that your pet is partial to with a HEPA vacuum cleaner at least twice a week, or clean hard surface floors with a damp cloth soaked in a non-toxic cleaner.

6. Wash your pet once a week with a non-toxic, fragrance-free shampoo and be sure to rinse out all residues so your pet's skin won't be irritated.

How your home affects your pet

All the preceding information about toxic chemicals and polluters in the home applies not only to your family, but equally to your pets. In fact, their exposures may be higher. Many pets spend long periods of time indoors in homes that are tightly sealed with little to no fresh air. Some pets never leave the house.

Pets are also more likely to spend time in close proximity to sources of toxics: lying around on new carpet or on a floor with a toxic finish. They may experience symptoms from poisonous fumes long before their owners do, but how would you know if your pet was being harmed? Pets can only tell us they don't feel well through their behavior. Look for signs such as anxiety, breathing problems, coughs, depression, irritability, nausea, excessive thirst, loss of appetite, skin rashes, or general uncharacteristic behavior. These can be precursors to more serious problems later like cancer. For a more detailed discussion of symptoms and specific sources of pet poisoning in homes see *Are You Poisoning Your Pet?* by Nina Anderson and Howard Peiper.

Here are some other considerations:

1. Fresh air. If your pet is left indoors for long periods of time leave a window open to allow fresh air in. If this is a security risk, consider installing an energy recovery ventilator (ERV) to mechanically bring in fresh, filtered air and remove stale air (see Chapter 5).

2. Drinking water. Give your pet ample supplies of good quality, filtered drinking water to avoid exposure to chlorine and other toxic contaminants now found in most water supplies.

3. Cleaning and laundry products. Avoid toxic, fragranced cleaning and laundry products. Make sure any lids or openings are sealed tight and store these products away from where pets can get into them.

4. Natural light. If your pets stay indoors all day make sure they get good quantities of natural light. When pets are exposed only to artificial light they can develop a variety of health problems as well as become depressed.

5. Carbon monoxide. Combustion by-products can produce invisible, odorless carbon monoxide, which is deadly. Install a carbon monoxide detector and check levels regularly. Good maintenance checks on all fuel burning appliances, combined with ample supplies of fresh air is the best form of prevention.

6. Poisonous plants. Though some houseplants improve the quality of indoor air, some are poisonous to pets who may decide to nibble on them in a bored or

curious moment. Some of these include dieffenbachia, philodendron, daffodils, and Indian rubber plants. The ASPCA Animal Poison Control Center has a helpful book entitled *Household Plant Reference*, which lists many household and garden plants that are harmful to pets.

The bottom line

If your pet becomes sick or you are interested in prevention, always consider environmental factors. Have you changed anything in your home recently such as adding a new piece of furniture, applying fresh paint, or having your carpets cleaned? If your pet spends time outdoors, have you used pesticides or chemical fertilizers in your yard or garden recently? Have your neighbors? Also consider if your pet has been to the groomer's recently or if you have used any new product on your pet, or changed its food or water. Sometimes manufacturers change formulations so that a product you have used without problems suddenly becomes problematic.

The bottom line is that the estimated 235 million pets in the 58 million U.S.

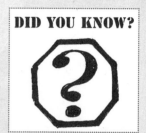

One of the most common vet emergencies is antifreeze poisoning. It only takes half a teaspoon per pound to poison a dog, even less for a cat.[12]

DID YOU KNOW?

Light enters the eyes not only to facilitate vision but to activate the hypothalamus, which in turn controls the nervous and endocrine systems, which regulate functions throughout the body. The pineal, pituitary, adrenal, thyroid, thymus and sex glands are all directly or indirectly dependent on the eyes' exposure to natural light. Their health in turn affects body temperature, sleep patterns, growth, the immune system, emotions, fluid balance, energy balance, circulation, blood pressure, breathing, reproduction and aging. Exposure is crucial to the health of your pet's hormone and immune systems.[13]

homes depend on us to care for them safely and provide homes in which they, like our children, can thrive. Is that really so much to ask for when you consider what they provide us in return? Researchers have shown that people who own pets, enjoying their companionship and love, live longer and enjoy better health. It's all connected!

Most immediate gains

1. Follow the guidelines suggested to reduce animal dander in your home.
2. Have pets sleep in one place (preferably not on anyone's bed with breathing problems or allergies). Choose bedding that has removable covers made from organic cotton or 100 percent cotton (see Appendix C). Wash their bedding weekly in hot water and dry on high heat to reduce flea infestations.
3. Vacuum frequently around pet sleeping areas, floors, upholstered furniture, and draperies to minimize flea infestations. Vacuum the inside of your car if your pet travels with you. The flea cycle from egg to next generation egg is about two weeks. Remove vacuum bags outdoors and seal the bags with tape before disposal to prevent flea eggs hatching in your trashcan.

4. Groom pets regularly with flea combs dipped in hot soapy water. This is especially important if your pet is often outside or has a long coat.

5. Children should never be allowed to apply flea shampoos, dusts, or dips containing organophosphate and carbamates pesticides to their pets. Also keep children away from other people's pets whose owners use these kinds of toxic products.

6. Don't "free feed" pets, it attracts pests. Put their food out and remove it when they have finished eating.

7. Many pesticides are toxic to pets. Slug bait is hazardous to dogs and cats, especially if spread on the ground. Animals may think they are being fed.

8. Pay attention to cats walking on kitchen surfaces. Be sure to thoroughly wipe down surfaces before preparing food.

9. Keep pets away from the dirt beneath and immediately surrounding any CCA-treated wood structures.

10. Spray predatory nematodes in lawn areas where your pet goes. The worms prey on flea larvae and pupae.

11. Stop using pesticide products on your pets and choose safer alternatives. Shampoos and fatty acid soaps, purchased at pet shops or garden nurseries, are safest. Leave the soap on your pet's fur for half an hour, suffocating the fleas, then rinse.

12. Store pet food in a non-toxic, airtight container. Avoid storing food in the garage where toxic garage fumes can contaminate it food.

13. Develop the habit of wiping pets' fur and paws with a damp cloth after they have been outdoors.

14. Follow the additional guidelines to make your home safe for your pet, such as giving them good quality, filtered water to drink.

13. Chocolate contains theobromine and is invariably toxic to dogs, especially semi-sweet and dark baker's chocolate. A six ounce dose of dark chocolate can kill a 60 pound dog.[14]

CHAPTER 16

Cleaning

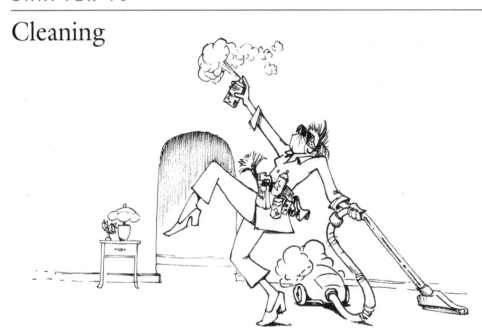

One month after moving into her new home, Liz decides she really must give her home a good cleaning. Especially now that she's hired a lady to professionally clean the house each week, starting on Monday. "I can't have her thinking we're dirty people," Liz thinks to herself, as she heads upstairs with her arms full of cleaning products.

In the master bedroom Liz selects a favorite CD from her kick-boxing exercise class. She cranks up the volume and joins in singing, "I've got the power!" with attitude, as she squirts some glass cleaner at the mirror.

In a flurry of squirts, the mirror and several glass surfaces are cleaned. Liz sneezes three times in a row. "Oh for goodness sake ... now I'm allergic to cleaning!" she yells above the music. "Looks like I hired Edith just in the nick of time."

As she walks into the ensuite bathroom she looks at the glass cleaner bottle. "What's in this stuff anyway? Ammonia. Is that it, pure ammonia?" Liz turns the bottle over looking for more information. "Oh, that's clever! Put the writing on the back of the label facing inside the bottle. What are you supposed to do, empty the contents of the bottle out so you can read what it is they have to say? I bet that was a man's idea!"

Liz selects another product from her arsenal and climbs into the shower cubicle to

239

clean the glass shower panels from the inside. "I'm every woman, it's all in meeeee," she sings with enthusiasm in another flurry of squirts. Suddenly she is short of breath and grabs for the handle of the shower door to steady herself. "Now what?" She carefully climbs out of the shower and staggers over to the window, opening it and sticking her head outside gasping for air. Her chest feels weird and constricted. After a few minutes her breathing returns to normal. Still clutching the spray bottle in her hand, she turns it over.

"What's in this product?" She reads the front of the bottle: "'All purpose cleaner,' that's good. 'Natural lemon scent,' that's good. 'Kills 99.9% bacteria,' that's good. Ingredients, 'dimethyl ... benzyl ... ammoni ... um ... chloride,' what the heck is that? Honestly, they should be advertising 'free chemical dictionary with purchase,' and look at that, 99.5% inert ingredients, but there's no mention of what they are. So is this stuff good for me or bad for me?" Turning it over Liz reads the back of the bottle: "'Caution, causes eye irritation. Do not get in eyes, on skin or clothing.' What's the point of cleaning your shower with something you're not supposed to get on your skin? 'Wash thoroughly with soap and water after handling. Avoid contact with foods,' but I clean my kitchen counter tops all the time with this stuff! Oh this is hopeless, what's a woman supposed to do?" Liz fumes.

"I wonder what Steph cleans her healthy house with? I think I'll call her."

Liz sits on the edge of her bathtub, waiting while the dial tone rings. She absently chews on the acrylic nail she just broke picking the phone up. "Hello Steph, it's Liz. What kind of cleaning products do you use?"

"Let's see, I mostly use regular kitchen stuff," Steph begins.

"You mean like 'Windex' and '409'," Liz says, feeling hopeful.

"Gosh no, that stuff drives my allergies nuts."

"Oh," Liz says, crestfallen, and continues apprehensively, "did they ever make you sneeze or short of breath?"

"Yes, on both counts. I haven't used that stuff in years. When I say kitchen stuff I mean things like vinegar and baking soda."

"Really, but those are things you eat or cook with. How can they clean your house?" Liz asks incredulously.

"That's what our grandmothers used years ago and it still works great today," comes Steph's simple reply.

Feeling the first stabs of a headache Liz's exasperation gets the better of her, "Then what's the point of all these cleaning products I've got, with all these chemicals I can't even pronounce?"

"That's exactly the point," Steph replies "there is no point!"

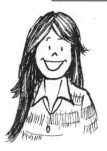

Commentary

Cleaning your home is a vital part of maintaining a healthy indoor environment, so a whole chapter has been dedicated to this subject. For those of you that flat-out hate housework, please don't skip this chapter. And for those of you who have a cleaning service that comes into your home to clean for you, the following information may be an eye-opener that generates some new curiosity and ideas about taking care of your home.

Cleanliness is part of good health, everyone knows that much. The days of the bubonic plague have long passed (thank goodness!) mostly because of the massive improvements made in sanitation. But the pendulum has swung from one extreme to another. Today, in our attempts to sanitize our homes we have become ensnared between our lack of time and the use of toxic cleaning products that allow us to wipe this or spray that, and get the job done quickly. As a result, these chemical concoctions are creating a new kind of plague, one that robs us of our energy and ability to think clearly, one that makes our joints ache or gives us headaches, one that makes our children hyperactive or have problems breathing. I call it the all-new "chemical convenience plague".

Building Biology Perspective

Let's go back to the idea that your home is its own living organism. Like us, to stay healthy homes need fresh air, sunlight, and regular cleaning to remove the daily accumulations of dirt and debris,. It's really a simple formula. So how has something so simple become so complex and dangerous? Let's take a closer look.

What exactly is "clean"?

I had to smile when I looked up "clean" in the dictionary; it said, "free from dirt, marks and stains." It sounded so calm, civilized, and straightforward. Given the strength and toxic nature of so many of the cleaning products commonly used in homes today it would seem more appropriate to see a description that says "annihilate, destroy, and kill at all costs."

Cleaning is really just about lifting the dirt, debris, and microbes generated as a result of daily living, and removing them. In most situations, heavy-duty chemicals are really not necessary. But here's an important consideration. It's so simple, but most people don't recognize the consequences. Do you clean a little each day and take care of spills when they happen; do you wait and do things later, all at one time; or do you let your cleaning person deal with it?

Daily cleaning and taking care of accidents when they happen is actually less time-consuming and requires less effort. When everyday grime is allowed to accumulate, when stains are not thoroughly removed, and when food is allowed to harden onto surfaces over several days, what results is the need for harsher and more caustic products to do the job. A classic example is the oven. If you wipe it down after each use or sprinkle a little baking soda onto any spills, it comes clean in minutes. If you don't do this and let it go for weeks on end, like many people do, then you may turn to some of the most toxic chemical cleaning products on the market to prize away partially incinerated food and layers of grease. It's not that we need more professional strength cleaners; we just need to change our cleaning habits.

Another benefit of small, daily cleanings is that they allow you to keep an eye on your home, as you do with the rest of the family. A mother is always the first to notice when her child has started to sniffle or run a temperature. Bestowing this watchful eye on your home will help ward off many of the problems that usually stem from neglect. Noticing the first visible signs of mold growth can lead to discovering a slow water leak. Caring for your home this way builds a relationship that leaves you feeling empowered and with the peace of mind that comes with knowing your family is safe.

Ventilation

Cleaning the air in your healthy home is rather like making sure your lungs are working properly. The clean, fresh air goes in and the stale, used air goes out. Opening windows each day is a simple way to create this exchange. One of the simplest improvements Liz could make to her home and her health would be to always open windows when cleaning, to let additional fresh air in and any polluted air out. If you live in an area where outdoor air quality is poor or fluctuates you will need to do a little detective work to discover the least polluted periods of time to have your windows open. If you absolutely can't find any, then seriously consider moving to a better location.

There are also two mechanical ways to provide clean, fresh air. One is to install an energy recovery ventilator (ERV) that will bring in fresh air and vent stale, concentrated air out on a timed cycle whether you are home or not. These systems are very convenient for people who are away at work for long hours of the day. The other method is to have an upright, mobile air purifier that can be placed wherever it's needed in your home. These machines mostly "polish" the air and can remove certain contaminants but are not a complete replacement for fresh air coming in from the outdoors. Remember, the EPA says that indoor air can be many times more polluted than outdoor air.

Sunlight

Natural sunlight is also important for a clean, healthy home. Sunlight is made up of many different rays and contains large amounts of ultraviolet (UV) radiation. There has been a lot of debate in the last few decades about UV light. Is it good or bad for us? To avoid generalities, it's helpful to look at the individual effects associated with the three components of UV light. UV-A is responsible for the tanning effect in humans, UV-B seems to activate the synthesis of vitamin D and the absorption of calcium and other minerals, and UV-C which is mostly filtered out by the Earth's ozone layer, is germicidal, killing bacteria, viruses, and other infectious agents.[1]

Dr. John Ott, in his book *Health and Light,* offers clarifying insight, saying that UV light in large amounts is harmful, but that in trace amounts, as found in natural sunlight, it acts as a "life-supporting nutrient." Bacteria, viruses, and mold can proliferate in homes where natural sunlight is blocked out by curtains, blinds, shutters, or furniture. People and pets who live in homes like these can develop the medical condition known as seasonal affective disorder (SAD) resulting in depression, mood swings, and lethargy.

Simply allowing natural sunlight into your home and supplementing with full spectrum lighting in darker rooms is equivalent to giving your home a tonic.

The many ways to clean

Keeping your home in good health requires a variety of different cleaning techniques and products.

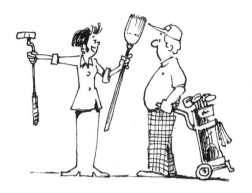

Vacuuming

If you are building a new house I recommend installing a central vacuum system (see Chapter 5). It's the cleanest way to remove dirt and debris completely out of the house. If this is not an option, then a HEPA vacuum cleaner is essential. Before I got my first HEPA vacuum cleaner I could never stand the smell generated while vacuuming, it was always so stale and would often make me sneeze. Not surprising, really, when you consider that regular vacuum cleaners generally regurgitate about 70 percent of the dust they collect, back into your home.

If, like Liz, you have a cleaning person do your vacuuming, make sure they use your vacuum. Otherwise their vacuum will spew out dust and particles collected from other people's homes, exposing you to possible pet dander and other unknown contaminants.

Ideally, high traffic areas in a carpeted home should be vacuumed daily. The rest should be vacuumed twice a week, especially in bedrooms. In order to properly clean any section of carpet I have read that anything from six to eight passes back and forth is needed to clean down to the deeper layers. Vacuuming alone will not remove pesticide residues or other chemicals embedded in the carpet. Hard surfaced floors still benefit from regular vacuuming to remove debris before wiping them down. Modern vacuums also have an assortment of attachments that make it easy to vacuum furniture, drapes, and in tight spaces such as under box spring beds that tend to harbor a lot of dust.

Dusting

There are many fancy new products available to dust with, including impregnated sheets, pieces of fabric that can grab dust, and mitts that fit your hand. Of course good old-fashioned versions such as pieces of retired cotton clothing and feather dusters still work great too.

I have been quite impressed with the dusters that can grab dust and even get grime off glass because they allow you to clean without any solutions at all. These dusters are made of a synthetic material called microfiber and rely on their own innate static-electric charge to attract and hold onto dust, grime, chemical residues, and most bacteria. Household cleaners can leave a residue that traps bacteria and dirt, actually leaving the surface more contaminated over time. With repeated use, microfiber cloths supposedly can remove 99 percent of this bacteria-filled residue. They can be used dry for dusting or wet for tougher jobs (see Appendix C).

Mopping

For me, mopping conjures up childhood memories of my mother down on her hands and knees cleaning the kitchen floor. Today we use cellulose sponges and cotton strands on long sticks. No kneeling required! When cleaning with these kinds of mops, be careful not to use too much water, otherwise it can slip into cracks and under joints where the floor surface meets a cabinet or baseboard, creating conditions for mold growth. If you are using a 100 percent cotton dust mop you need only lightly mist it with water. Cellulose sponge mops usually need to be wet through to activate their gripping qualities and so will need to be squeezed out thoroughly before using.

Other cleaning accessories

Other cleaning accessories most people have in their homes include hand size sponges and waterproof gloves to protect hands while cleaning. It's interesting to note that both of these items now commonly contain added antimicrobial chemicals. Antimicrobials are pesticides, added to protect the life of the product, not the health of the user!

Look instead for natural cellulose sponges which can be found in health food stores and some kitchen accessories stores. When new, these sponges are compressed flat and expand to their full size when water is applied. Remember to replace sponges regularly as bacteria and mold can grow in them. Cotton cloths work just as well as sponges and are easily cleaned; just throw them in the laundry at the end of each day.

As for waterproof gloves, your choice will depend on whether you have a latex sensitivity or not. If you are not latex-sensitive choose latex gloves without antimicrobials. If you are sensitive, try some of the other alternative synthetic products such as neoprene. Like latex, synthetic gloves can still cause allergic reactions because they may contain chemical additives similar to those found in latex. Some people find using thin cotton glove liners inside latex gloves helpful.

Cleaning products

How and what you clean your home with can make the difference between a healthy and not-so-healthy home. The average household contains anywhere from 3-25 gallons of toxic materials, most of which are in cleaners. Some of the worst offenders are drain cleaners, oven cleaners, furniture and floor polish, and glass cleaners with ammonia. No law requires manufacturers of cleaning products to list ingredients on their labels or to test their products for safety. That leaves the responsibility with us to make sure our homes are not only clean, but non-toxic and safe for our families.

In our earlier story, Liz has some very obvious reactions to the cleaning products she uses: sneezing, breathing problems, and headaches. But she still wants to believe that these products are safe; after all she bought them off the store shelf. Liz does not know that federal laws require only that products carry warnings if they are immediately harmful or fatal if swallowed or inhaled. No warnings are required on products that can affect your health more slowly, over time. No one really knows the

One of the most common chemicals found in household cleaning products is butyl cellosolve, which is toxic to the blood cells, kidneys and liver. It is absorbed through the skin. The nation's most popular brand of window cleaner, Windex, contains butyl cellosolve, but it's not on the label.[2]

long term health effects of exposures to all these chemicals, but what you can do is decide whether you and your family want to participate in these experiments or not.

Hopefully you will choose health over possible harm. There are many safer alternative cleaning products to choose from today. You can choose from common ingredients found in your kitchen such as vinegar and lemon juice, or you can choose from some of the ready made preparations found at some natural food stores and supermarkets. Making the change need not be difficult. It just requires a little basic information followed by some detective work and non-toxic experimentation.

As a side benefit you will also be saving money. Homemade products are usually cheaper to make than buying a commercial product. But let's consider other costs you will be saving, even when comparing a store bought product that is healthy to one that contains toxic chemicals. What is it worth to have one less headache or one less asthma attack for your child? What is it worth to have your child consistently healthy with no absenteeism from school? What is it worth to be productive and not hampered by general feelings of fatigue or irritability? What is it worth to reduce your family's impact on the planet's resources? What is it worth to you to protect your family's and future grandchildren's health and well being? These are the total costs to keep in mind next time you need a cleaning product.

> If every household in the U.S. replaced just one 28 ounce bottle of petroleum-based dishwashing liquid with an alternative vegetable-based product, we could save 118,700 barrels of oil, enough to heat 6,800 U.S. homes for a year.[3]

Here's a list of some of the most common hazardous chemicals found in household cleaning products. Avoid these:

- Alcohols such as ethanol, methanol and isopropyl alcohol
- Ammonia
- Butyl cellosolve
- Chlorine bleach or sodium hypochlorite
- Dye
- Formaldehyde
- Glycols
- Hydrochloric, hydrofluoric, phosphoric and sulfuric acids
- Hydrocarbons or petroleum distillates
- Lye or sodium hydroxide
- Naphthalene
- Paradichlorobenzenes (PDCB's)
- Perchloroethylene (PERC)
- Phenol or carbolic acid
- Propellants such as butane, propane and CFC's
- Synthetic fragrance
- Trichloroethylene (TCE)

Now it's time to walk through your house again and retrieve all your cleaning products and read their labels. As you know by now this is just the first disqualifying round. Set to one side all obvious hazardous products with labels that say "Warning," "Danger," or "Poison." Next, look for any of the ingredients on our list. Any products containing these are the next to go. Of the remaining products, how many do you absolutely know are non-hazardous? Set those aside in a separate area from the rest. These products you can keep. Any products in the twilight zone can be further qualified by looking in *The Safe Shoppers Bible* by David Steinman and Samuel Epstein, M.D., which lists many of the commercially available products and their associated hazards.

Contact your local Household Hazardous Waste facility for guidance in disposing of the toxic products you have identified. Do not empty them down the drain or put them in the garbage. If you need to store hazardous products until they can be collected or disposed of, make sure all are sealed tightly, kept in their original containers, and locked away somewhere where children and pets will have no access to them. Poisoning is a preventable cause of harm.

With the toxic stuff out of the way, it's now time to decide whether you want to try your hand at following some basic recipes to make your own non-toxic household cleaners, or whether you need to buy some ready-made products, or a combination of both. Whatever you decide, the place to begin is identifying what your cleaning needs are. Many people keep far more cleaning products around than they ever use.

If you decide to go for ready-made products, arrange for some free time to visit your local health food store or supermarket without hungry children swinging on your arms or when you're rushing to get somewhere else. Invite a friend to join you to make it more fun. Take this book, a pen, and some paper, or take a clipboard if you really want to get the store employees' attention. I don't know what it is about clipboards, I guess they look official, but carrying one will often get you that special attention from the shop assistant and even a visit from the manager, if you're lucky. It's a great way to make your concerns known, to make requests, or ask for additional information from your captivated, and usually somewhat nervous audience. All this because you used a clipboard!

You can also shop through certain mail order catalogues and the Internet if your local resources are not very good (see Appendix C). Have this book handy if you are on the Internet and look at the list of ingredients to avoid as you read labels.

Look for products that fulfill the following criteria:

1. They use natural, non-toxic ingredients.
2. They use non-petroleum-based surfactants that are chlorine and phosphate free.
3. They use no synthetic fragrance.
4. They claim to be non-toxic and biodegradable.
5. They list all their ingredients on the label.

A note of caution: some cleaners may advertise that they are "environmentally sound" but fail to provide a full list of ingredients. As a general rule, the manufacturer that gives you the most information about its product is usually the manufacturer you can trust (see Appendix C).

Homemade cleaners

Learning to clean from scratch by making your own home-made recipes is a wonderful way to know exactly what you are using, rather like knowing what you are eating by cooking from scratch instead of buying a TV dinner. Many of the common kitchen cupboard ingredients used in these recipes are generally regarded as safe (GRAS), because they have been around and used by people for many years without causing harm. That cannot be said of many commercial synthetic ingredients.

But do these homemade cleaners really work? Yes and no. Some recipes such as vinegar and water to clean windows, work equally as well as their chemical counterparts, whereas for others, it can be very hard to match the hyperdissolving power of toxic chemicals. For instance, when it comes to cleaning an oven that has been left to burn on grease and food debris for several months, it may take longer and require a little more elbow grease to get the results you are looking for, but at least elbow grease is non-toxic.

Asthma among women has skyrocketed in recent years. Some doctors now suspect a connection between this rise and household cleaning products. The link is the subject of an on-going medical debate. But one thing is certain, women get asthma more often than men, with more severe, sudden attacks, more hospitalizations, and more deaths. Medical professionals say females over 30 are prime targets. "The rates have gone up 105 percent for females over the past 15 or so years, compared to about a 41 percent increase for males," says Dr. Stephen Redd, of the Centers for Disease Control.[4]

Getting started

All you need to get started are some basic ingredients, many of which you will probably already have in your kitchen, and some containers. Here's a shopping list of items you will need to make the suggested recipes that follow:

- Baking soda
- Borax
- Organic essential oils (optional, if you like some natural scent)
- Filtered water
- Liquid Castile soap
- White distilled vinegar
- Four 16 ounce clean, empty squirt bottles
- One 22 ounce squirt bottle
- One shaker container (plastic or stainless steel)
- A couple of natural cellulose sponges
- Some cotton cleaning rags
- A cotton mop
- A squeegee

- A measuring cup and measuring spoons
- A glass or ceramic bowl

I personally prefer larger size containers to mix and store recipes in because they don't need to be refilled as often. You can use smaller containers if you like. I also don't recommend reusing older containers if they previously contained a product with toxic chemicals in it. Sometimes residues remain in the plastic that can then pollute your new, non-toxic recipe.

If you decide you want your cleaning products to have an aroma, then pure essential oils are the best way to achieve this. All essential oils however, are not equal. When choosing essential oils, look for brands that don't use harsh solvents in their extraction process. Organic and wildcrafted varieties are best (see Appendix C). Though these purer varieties cost a little extra, essential oils last a long time. Lavender, lemon, and peppermint oil will be the most versatile to begin with.

It's also important to understand a tiny bit of chemistry before you start mixing your own cleaners. Even mixing non-toxic ingredients should be treated with care. All chemicals have what's called a "pH" that identifies whether a substance is acid, alkali, or neutral. A pH of 1 is highly acidic, a pH of 14 is highly alkaline, a pH of 7 is in the middle and called neutral. Neutral is usually considered safe whereas the extremes of acid and alkali can cause serious harm from burning or their ability to dissolve matter. Drain cleaners can be as corrosive as pH 14, a toilet bowl cleaner can be as acidic as pH 2, and a mild soap can have a pH of 8.

When mixing different substances it's important to know their pH value so you can anticipate the results. When an acid is mixed with an alkali they react and neutralize each other, developing a more neutral pH of seven. A good example is mixing baking soda, which is mildly alkaline, with vinegar, which is mildly acidic. These two neutralize each other forming carbon dioxide gas and water with a neutral pH of seven. This is a safe combination and their combined properties help to clean and remove dirt from surfaces, brighten glass and metal, unblock drains, and so on.

To ensure your safety, here are some general guidelines to follow when making your own cleaners:

1. Label all products you make on the actual container. List everything.
2. Follow recipes closely. Don't substitute ingredients. Use common sense.
3. Never mix commercial products with homemade products. You don't know what you could create.
4. Keep products away from your eyes. Liquid soap, detergent, and vinegar are all irritants if they get in your eyes. Also avoid breathing in powders like baking soda. Any particulate can be an irritant to sensitive lungs.
5. I prefer squirt bottles rather than spray bottles. Spraying aerosolizes products into the air we breathe. An alternative method is to pour solutions directly onto a cloth and wipe.

5. Add "Mr. Yuk" stickers to your containers and explain to children that they are not food or drink. Store them in locked cupboards away from where children and pets can get into them.

Recipes

The following recipes have been chosen for their simplicity and because they take next to no time to mix. They are a good place to begin your less toxic cleaning endeavors:

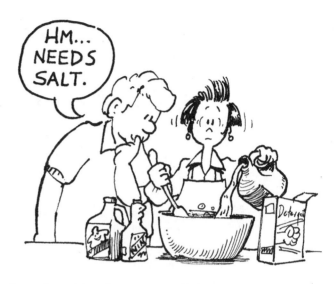

Kitchen cleaner

> Baking soda
> Essential oil (optional)

Half fill a plastic flip-top or stainless steel shaker with baking soda. Add 15-20 drops essential oil (try lemon). Stir. Fill the shaker almost to the top with more baking soda. Put the lid on tightly and shake to mix.

To use: sprinkle on kitchen counters or sink, then wipe with a damp rag or cellulose sponge. Rinse well. Don't use too much or you will need to keep rinsing and wiping. There is a great little book called *Baking Soda: Over 500 Fabulous, Fun and Frugal Uses You've Probably Never Thought Of* by Vicki Lansky that will give you lots more ideas.

Floor cleaner

> White distilled vinegar   Essential oil (optional)
> Filtered water

Fill a clean 16 ounce squirt bottle with equal amounts of white vinegar and filtered water. Add 15-20 drops essential oil (try peppermint). Shake to mix.

To use: squirt directly onto the floor and wipe with a clean rag or cotton mop. This cleaner can be used on wood, tile, or linoleum floors. For extra cleaning power on smudges and scuff marks, add a little baking soda from your kitchen cleaner recipe and rub. Follow with your vinegar floor cleaner. It may fizz a little, but that's fine, it will just help to lift the dirt off. Wipe over with a rag or mop.

All purpose cleaner

> 2 tbsp white vinegar   16 ounces hot, filtered water
> 1 tsp borax   1/4 cup liquid soap

10-15 drops of essential oil such as lavender or lemon (optional)

First, mix the vinegar with the borax in a 16 ounce clean spray bottle. Fill with hot, filtered water and shake until all the borax has dissolved. Next add the liquid soap, followed by the essential oil. Shake again to mix.

To use: spray and wipe, the same as you would any other all-purpose cleaner

All purpose glass cleaner

If you are changing from commercial window cleaners to non-toxic homemade recipes use this recipe first. The added soap helps remove the wax residues left behind by commercial brands. Otherwise windows will dry streaky.

1/4 cup white vinegar	2 cups filtered water
1/2 tsp liquid soap	5 drops essential oil (optional)

In a 16 ounce clean squirt bottle, add the soap to the water. Mix. Then add the vinegar and optional essential oil. Shake well.

To use: squirt on your window and either squeegee off or use a paper towel. I no longer recommend newspaper because of all the chemicals contained in the inks. Once you have cleaned your windows a couple of times with this formula you can switch to one half cup of vinegar in two cups of water alone to do the job.

Tub and tile cleaner

1 2/3 cups baking soda	1/2 cup filtered water
1/2 cup liquid soap	2 tbsp white vinegar

Mix the baking soda and liquid soap in a bowl. Dilute with one half cup of water. Add the vinegar last. Mix with a fork until any lumps are gone. It should have a pourable consistency; if not, add more water. Pour into a 16 ounce squeeze container (the kind with a squirt flip-top cap). Keep the cap on, as this mixture will dry out easily. Shake well before using. Add more water if it dries out.

To use: squirt onto tile, tub, sink, or toilet bowl and scrub. Rinse well. If any baking soda residue remains (which will look like powder), use a little vinegar and water to rinse, and next time use less baking soda in the recipe.

Antibacterial spray

Researchers from Tufts New England Medical Center now think that disinfectants are not effective in the first place, and that they simply lead to the development of more resistant strains of bacteria. Here is a great non-toxic and very effective way to rid your bathroom (or any room) of germs.

1 cup filtered water   1 tsp pure essential oil of lavender

Place water in a 16 ounce clean squirt bottle, add lavender oil, and shake vigorously to mix.

To use: squirt on surfaces and allow to stand for at least 15 minutes, or don't rinse at all.

This makes one cup of solution. To make larger batches, simply double the quantities. This recipe keeps indefinitely. Use on toilet seats, countertops, doorknobs, cutting boards — anywhere germs like to lurk. Lavender is more antiseptic than phenol, which is the industry standard.

Specialized cleaning situations

If you get the non-toxic cleaning bug and decide you want recipes for more specialized jobs I highly recommend *Better Basics for the Home* by Annie Berthold-Bond and *Clean House, Clean Planet* by Karen Logan. Both books are full of every conceivable solution for household cleaning challenges.

Cleaning companies

If you use a cleaning company or an independent person to clean your home have them provide you with a list of all the products they use and their Material Safety Data Sheets (MSDSs). Take some time to look over this list and highlight any products that are hazardous to health. If you can find any non-toxic products on their list, specify that these are the ones to be used in your home. If you find you are left with nothing to chose from, request that they do some research and provide healthier, alternative products. You would think that companies or individuals that provide such a personal service would take great care to ensure that the products and equipment they use do no harm to their client's health. Unfortunately many of them still do not realize the impact toxic chemicals have on health or what they are being exposed to themselves each day by using hazardous products. There is a huge market for anyone that can provide healthy house cleaning services.

You may need to educate your cleaning person a little to help them get started with their research. A good place to begin is with how to read labels. As you know by now, when a product says it's "non-toxic," it does not mean the product contains no hazardous ingredients whatsoever or that it is safe if ingested. By law, some toxic substances don't have to be listed at all in the ingredients if they are in small enough quantities or considered by the manufacturer to be proprietary (trade secret) information. Washington Toxics Coalition has an informative article entitled *Researching Household Products* that can be downloaded at <www.watoxics.org> or by phoning them (see Appendix C).

Another approach is to have your cleaning person use only your own cleaning supplies, vacuum, dusters, etc. This way you can exert the most control over what happens in your home.

The *2002 Annual Report of the American Association of Poison Control Centers* states that on average, U.S. poison centers handle one poison exposure every 13 seconds. Of the reported poison exposures, 39.1 percent are children younger than three years of age, and 51.6 percent occurred in children younger than six years.

Accidental Poisoning

As household cleaning products account for a high percentage of accidental poisonings in children, let's go over some of the most important points. The most dangerous poisons for children include the following common household items:

1. Cleaning products that cause chemical burns: these can be just as bad as burns from fire. Products that cause chemical burns include drain openers, toilet bowl cleaners, rust removers, and oven cleaners.
2. Nail glue remover and nail primer: some products used for artificial nails can be poisonous in surprising ways. Some nail glue removers have caused cyanide poisoning when swallowed by children. Some nail primers have caused burns to the skin and mouth of children who tried to drink them.
3. Hydrocarbons: this is a broad category that includes gasoline, kerosene, lamp oil, motor oil, lighter fluid, furniture polish, and paint thinner. These liquids are easy to choke on if someone tries to swallow them. They can go down the wrong way, into the lungs instead of the stomach. If they get into someone's lungs, they make it hard to breathe. They can also cause lung inflammation (like pneumonia). Hydrocarbons are among the leading causes of poisoning death in children.
4. Pesticides: chemicals to kill bugs and other pests can harm humans too. Many pesticides can be absorbed through the skin. Many can also enter the body through breathing in fumes. Some can affect the nervous system and make it hard to breathe.
5. Windshield washer solution and antifreeze: small amounts of these liquids are poisonous to humans and pets. Windshield washer solution can cause blindness and death if swallowed. Antifreeze can cause kidney failure and death if swallowed.

The best way to address the possibility of household poisonings is to take a preventative approach. Contact your regional poison control center and request their poison prevention package. They will often have "Mr. Yuk" stickers or their own equivalent that you can stick on any products at home that pose a poisoning threat. Sit down with your children and discuss what these stickers mean and what poisons are. Post the phone number for your regional poison control center or the national hotline number 1-800-222-1222 prominently near all phones.

The American Association of Poison Control Centers (AAPCC) has a specific website you can visit to read, print, or download helpful information such as the *Babysitter Phone Sheet* and *Poison Prevention Tips,* go to <www.1-800-222-1222.info/poisonHelp.asp>.

Some general guidelines include:

1. Lock up medicines and household products and store them where children cannot see or reach them.
2. Store poisons in their original containers. Should you need to go to hospital with someone who has been poisoned, always take the poison's container.
3. Use child-resistant packaging. But remember – nothing is childproof.
4. Teach children to ask first. Poisons can look like food or drink. Teach children to ask an adult before eating or drinking anything
5. If you have a poisoning emergency call 1-800-222-1222, available 24 hours, 7 days a week. If the person has collapsed or is not breathing call 911.

Making a difference

Cleaning your home with non-toxic products is one of the single most important changes to make in creating a healthy home. You now have enough basic information to get started. Whether you throw yourself in and make these change quickly, or you pace yourself and do it over time, the rewards are instant when it comes to your family's health. My basic philosophy is, if you can't change everything all at once, then at least work on changing something each day. Every toxic chemical you eliminate is one less drop in everyone's barrel, pets included. May you never know what you have prevented!

Most immediate gains

1. Open windows daily to let fresh air in and pollutants out; especially when cleaning your house.
2. Allow the health promoting qualities of natural sunlight into your home, at least for a few hours each day.
3. Purchase a HEPA vacuum cleaner and if you have a cleaning person come into your home, make sure they use your vacuum.
4. Try some microfiber cleaning cloths and see if you can reduce the amount of cleaning products you need to use in your home.
5. Avoid sponges, waterproof gloves, and any other cleaning accessories that are treated with antimicrobial chemicals.
6. Take an inventory of all your current cleaning products. Use this chapter's guidelines to eliminate those that are hazardous to your health.
7. Dispose of hazardous products properly.
8. Replace toxic products with either store-bought healthy alternatives or try making the recipes above suggested to get started.
9. Always clearly label any product you make and what it contains.
10. Store all cleaning products, including non-toxic ones, in a locked cupboard out of the reach of young children and pets.

11. Educate your cleaning person and ensure they use only non-toxic products in your home.

12. Request a poison prevention package from your regional poison control center. Post the national hotline number, 1- 800-222-1222, next to each phone in the house.

CHAPTER 17

Home Maintenance

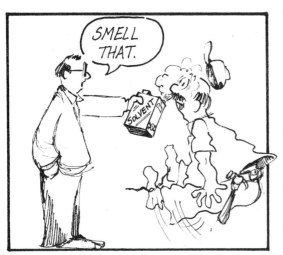
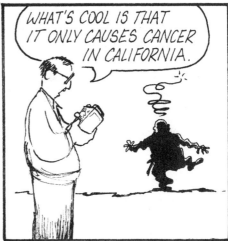

"Hello, hello … burglars!" calls out Uncle Joe with a chuckle as he descends the basement stairs.

Mark is slouched down low in his reclining chair watching TV in a vegetative state. "Hello Joe," Mark says, straightening himself in his chair with great effort.

"Well you look like the life and soul of the party, don't you?"

Uncle Joe punches Mark lightly on the shoulder and shuffles his feet on the floor in a pseudo-boxing style. "Float like a butterfly, sting like a bee." Another punch strikes Mark's shoulder. "They don't make them like Mohammed Ali anymore." Uncle Joe sighs as

he drops his fists realizing Mark is no sparring partner today. "What's up with you lad?"

"Oh, Jack was wide awake at four again this morning wanting me to read Winnie the Pooh to him. He's got my number right now. Every morning he's doing this. It's as if he knows he can get away with it. Jane needs her rest so I have to get up before he makes a fuss and wakes her. I tell you, she better have this baby soon or I'm going to loose my marbles." Mark scratches his head nervously.

"Little Jacky," Uncle Joe says with adoration. "How could anyone say 'no' to that angel face boy?"

Mark rolls his eyes, "Well, while the little

'angel' is taking a nap, let's fix that shower shall we? I see you've got your trusty toolbox."

"Oh yes, I never go anywhere without it." Uncle Joe gives his toolbox a friendly pat.

Upstairs the two men are on their hands and knees inspecting the shower floor.

"I don't know why it's leaking again. When I fixed it last week, I used extra caulking around that seal just to make sure. Maybe you didn't let it dry long enough." Uncle Joe pushes his glasses back up his nose and rubs his chin thinking what to try next.

"And look at the floor boards. The warping is getting worse." Mark lifts up the small rug and points to the section of floor immediately outside the shower stall.

"Well, we'll at least get that fixed today. I brought a couple of pieces of wood with me, and some stain. And look at this stuff I found at the hardware store." Uncle Joe rummages in his toolbox and produces a long tube of glue and shakes it at Mark. "'Screws-in-a-Tube,' this is what the professionals use." He throws the tube to Mark.

Catching the tube in mid-air, Mark turns it over in his hand and begins to read. "It says here 'Danger! Extremely flammable. Harmful or fatal if swallowed. Harmful if inhaled. May cause central nervous system effects, including dizziness, headache, or nausea. Causes eye, skin and respiratory tract irritation. May be harmful if absorbed through skin. Use only with adequate ventilation.' Then listen to this, 'This product contains a chemical known to the state of California to cause cancer, birth defects, or other reproductive harm.'"

"Well we're alright then aren't we? It only affects people who live in California," Uncle Joe says matter-of-factly. "Pass me that hammer will you and let's get to work!"

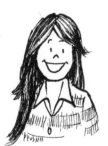

Commentary

All that remains to be discussed is how to maintain your healthy home. After the initial thrill and discovery of all these simple ways to transform your home into a place that nourishes everyone's health, comes the long-term commitment of ensuring that it remains that way.

Building Biology Perspective

Healthy home maintenance is equivalent to keeping your immune system in good condition with daily care and by planning ahead. Think of it this way: giving your child a little vitamin C each day helps boost her immune system, as does keeping her away from refined sugar. When the first child starts coughing and sneezing it's time to add a little echinacea or zinc to your children's breakfast meal. It's the same with our homes. Daily care entails not slipping back into toxic chemical convenience because you're pushed for time. Planning ahead means getting the furnace checked and installing a new filter before turning on your heating system as the cooler weather looms on the horizon.

Homes are not static, unchanging things. They constantly evolve to accommodate our needs and desires. Besides cleaning and maintaining our homes we often want to change something about them. Decorating, exchanging something old for something newer, and remodeling are inevitabilities if you stay in your home long enough. In these situations careful planning will allow these events to happen in the healthiest way possible.

Regular Cleaning

Part of maintaining your home involves regular cleaning. Once you've made the transition to healthier, environmentally friendly cleaning products, all that remains is consistency. There may be challenges at times that tempt you to reach for something with a powerful chemical punch, but if you use the resources at the back of this book you should never exhaust your options for non-toxic solutions. Living in a less toxic home, free from neurotoxic chemicals, improves sleep and concentration, makes babies less fussy, and gives a sense of well being. The benefits far outweigh any perceived inconvenience.

Home Maintenance

An ounce of prevention is worth a pound of cure. Maintenance is nothing more than remembering and following through with lots of little details. Occasionally something big will come along that requires professional help, but for the most part all that you need is right at your own fingertips.

Let's divide maintenance into categories.

1. Bite-sized daily maintenance

A lot of maintenance can be easily taken care of each day along with doing other household activities. Here are just a few examples:

1. If you get in the habit of cleaning the lint out of your dryer before each use, not only will your dryer work more efficiently, it will last longer.
2. Checking your washing machine for mold before each use is another simple habit to develop. Look in the rubber folds of the seal around the door of front loaders and under the upper edge of top loaders for slime or discoloration. Wipe this out with a cloth to prevent it being washed into your clothes. To prevent mold build up, leave your washing machine door open between uses or at least until it has dried thoroughly.
3. Cleaning the hair out of the shower drain after each shower will save your drains from getting blocked.

What else does your home need on a daily basis? Write down any maintenance ideas in the back of this book or in a special notebook.

2. Weekly, monthly, and annual maintenance

Some maintenance jobs need to be performed regularly but less frequently. Here are some more examples.

1. If you use a humidifier, clean it out weekly with hot, soapy water. Do the same if you use a dehumidifier. Make sure these units dry thoroughly after cleaning.

2. Empty your refrigerator tray (drip pan) at least once a month. It can start looking rather swampy in there, and the fridge fan blows the moldy air right into your home. Clean the interior of your fridge to prevent mold build up. Take an inventory and throw out anything that's gone bad.

3. Once a week wipe down vents on forced air heating systems and make sure the return vent is unobstructed and clean.

4. When doing general house cleaning, look around for any signs of moisture problems such as condensation marks on bathroom ceilings or drips under any sinks or washbasins. Find the source and fix these problems as soon as you notice them.

5. Depending on whether you have an active family, pets, a lot of carpeting, or have done any home improvements, forced air heating systems will need their ductwork cleaned every one to three years . Find a professional who cleans for people with allergies. They usually take more care. Don't forget to request that they not use any fragrance.

6. Have your furnace professionally maintained once a year to ensure it's working efficiently and there are no leaks. Clean your oil burner. A dirty furnace doesn't function as well and can emit more harmful carbon monoxide and other undesirable compounds.

7. If you have other kinds of heaters, dust them every week; otherwise the dust fries and can be an irritating indoor pollutant.

8. Find the source of any unusual smells. Running air purifiers are only temporary measures.

9. Clean chimneys once a year to help prevent chimney fires and toxic combustion by-products from entering your home.

10. Once every couple of weeks, run your washing machine while empty and add one to two cups of white vinegar to help clean it out.

11. Replace tile grouting in bathrooms as soon as you notice it's starting to erode. Use a non-toxic product.

12. Install carbon monoxide detectors outside all bedrooms and next to all heating and combustion appliances. Check these each week to see if there has been any change. If there is, bring in a professional immediately to find the source and fix it. Carbon monoxide will quickly diffuse throughout the entire house.

13. Have all accessible gas appliances and piping checked for leaks at least once a year. Report any noticeable gas leaks immediately.

14. Check your smoke detectors once a week to ensure they are functioning properly.

15. Crawl spaces should be inspected every few months for signs of mold growth or termites.

What else does your home need on a weekly, monthly or annual basis? Write down your maintenance ideas in the back of this book or in your notebook.

3. Replacing things

Another aspect of maintenance involves replacing things. This includes planning ahead to replace things after a certain amount of time has elapsed and also being ready to replace things that wear out spontaneously. Here are some examples:

1. Light bulbs. Its good to have a few spare full spectrum, energy efficient light bulbs around in an assortment of sizes. Light bulbs always seem to blow at the least convenient moment. Having the right kind of light bulbs in stock will ensure the continued benefits of healthier light and better efficiency.
2. Water filters. In general, the larger the filter the less often it needs to be replaced. Whole house water filters are large and often have a pre-filter and a main filter (models vary). Pre-filters will need to be changed about once a year, and main filters about three to five years depending on use and water quality. A point-of-source drinking water filter in your kitchen, depending on its size, how many people use it, and how often, will need to be changed anywhere from every couple of months to once a year. Shower filters vary and need replacing anything from every two to six months. It is false economy to try and make water filters last beyond the date recommended for replacement. Though you may not taste any difference filters lose their filtering capacity with age.
3. Furnace filters. Install a HEPA pleated media filter on your furnace and replace it regularly, every two to three months, whether it looks dirty or not. Many household pollutants are invisible to the naked eye.
4. Vacuum cleaner bags. Always keep a good supply of vacuum cleaner bags available. Vacuums loose their efficiency quickly when the waste bag becomes too full. Replace vacuum HEPA filters as per manufacturers recommendations. Replace vacuum HEPA filters according to the manufacturers' recommendations.

What other replacement items does your home need to have available? Write down anything you need to order or purchase in the back of this book or in your notebook.

4. Repairing things and trouble shooting

In the event that something in your home breaks down, it's an important judgment call to know whether to try to fix it yourself or bring in a professional. In our earlier story Uncle Joe considers himself able to fix just about any household problem. The trouble is that he's not really getting at the source of the problem, he's only focused on patching things up on the surface. Mark and Uncle Joe have no idea how long the shower has been leaking or how far the leaking water has traveled. Remember, it only takes mold 24-48 hours to start growing. A leak like this needs to be fixed at the source. Any surrounding materials need to be thoroughly dried out or carefully removed if spoiled. Otherwise you can have a major health hazard growing silently in your home.

Uncle Joe also does not read labels. When he shops at his local hardware store he looks for the strongest glue he can find, overlooking the fact that his choice comes with several health warnings including that it contains known carcinogens. There are many people out there like Uncle Joe and although they may mean well, these are not the people you want repairing things in your healthy home.

Doing your own home repairs requires thinking things through in advance. Are you really equipped to find the source of the problem? Do you have the time? Do you have the tools? And what will you do if you discover the problem is much bigger than you thought? What often starts out as a simple way to save a little money can turn into a much larger and more expensive project than was anticipated.

If you decide to bring in a professional, choose one who comes highly recommended by someone you trust, or interview two or three people and have them evaluate the problem and submit bids. Always look for professionals with appropriate training and experience to deal with the specific problem you have, not a "jack-of-all-trades." Always check credentials. Look for builders who understand that building materials can affect health or are willing to address your concerns and use only non-toxic materials. Toxic products affect their health too, very directly. If none are available where you live, you may have to do the research and educate an open-minded builder yourself. Monitoring the situation to make sure they follow through with all your requests is another precautionary measure to take.

> Knowing what is *not* the solution is sometimes the most important first step in confronting a problem.

Maintenance charts

Remembering what to do when is the trickiest part of any maintenance program. Our busy lifestyles keep us spread thin and constantly on the run. But having worked with a lot of people over the years I have found that where there's a plan there's a way.

To help people remember and be able to evaluate their progress I created some *Maintenance Charts* (see Appendix C). By simply planning ahead, filling in your chart with the relevant information and then displaying the chart somewhere prominent so that you will see it regularly, a lot of the remembering is eliminated. It's a great way to remind yourself about the little tasks that need to be done, such as "change the filter on the furnace and buy a replacement one to have in stock," or "clean the humidifier." I have mine on the wall of my laundry room, my central headquarters for anything to do with cleaning and maintenance. Sometimes it helps to have a designated space in your home to organize your cleaning and maintenance efforts from. To preview these charts and see if they would be helpful for you, visit my website at <www.homesthatheal.com>.

You can also design your own system using a calendar or daytimer if that's a better reference point.

Decorating

Sooner or later most people are faced with decorating their home. Even the smallest of projects such as repainting trim requires using products that can have the potential to instantly pollute your healthy home.

Again, advance planning makes all the difference. Knowing what you want to achieve is the place to begin. Do you simply want to repaint a wall or do you want to strip down old wallpaper and replace it with new? Next, are you planning to do the decorating yourself or are you bringing in a professional? Either way you will need to educate yourself to know what's involved, what your options are, and what product choices you have.

If you decide to hire a professional decorator or interior designer, unless you can find one who specializes in healthy products and practices, you will need to take the lead and maybe even provide the actual materials yourself to be sure that what is used in your home is healthy. Beware of professionals who may try to "greenwash" you by telling you they use "green" or "environmentally friendly" products. All that is green or environmental is not necessarily healthy. Ask to see the MSDSs on any products they think will be suitable to use in your home, including anything they may need to use if there is an accident, such as a paint spill. Insist that they use no- or low-VOC products without toxic chemicals and pesticides.

When tackling a painting project yourself, there are several things you can do to save money, avert waste, protect the environment, and safeguard your health. First, do a little research before purchasing any products. Choose low or no-VOC paint. Some companies have MSDSs on their products that you can read or download from the Internet. There are a lot more choices in low- or no-VOC paints than there used to be, so you shouldn't have to choose between aesthetics and health (see Appendix C). Don't forget to research products to clean up accidents. If you go to a paint store, ask them to help you calculate the right amount of paint. Also, choose water-based products such as latex paint.

Though most new paint no longer contains lead (since 1977) or mercury (since 1990), it can still contain toxic volatile solvents like toluene, xylene, and benzene, as well as poisonous fungicides and mildewcides. Such compounds can have many serious health effects, especially on the central nervous system. Other symptoms found in painters include nausea, dizziness, headache, disorientation, and increased violent behavior.[1]

Once you have purchased your products and are ready to begin, try to choose a day and time that you can work with the windows open wide to ventilate the space. Winter months are generally not the best time of year to do projects like this as people like to keep windows closed and run heating systems, resulting in heightened VOC levels trapped indoors for everyone to breathe. When you have to close windows for security reasons, run a HEPA air filter that is designed to filter out chemicals. As a paint job puts a lot of demand on an air purifier and will probably exhaust the filter capacity, you will need to replace the filters after such heavy duty use. Never allow pregnant women to do painting projects.

Any leftover paint that you do not use needs to go to your local Household Hazardous Waste facility. If the can contains only a thin skin of paint, take off the lid, let it dry out (outside, away from children, pets, and windows) and recycle both the lid and can with your scrap metal.

Larger projects such as removing and replacing wallpaper require extra considerations. If you plan to remove vinyl wallpaper it must be done carefully in case mold has been growing behind it. You may want to seal off the room from the rest of the house including any vents, and remove any furniture as a preventative measure. If you do discover a mold problem enlist the help of a an Indoor Environmental Professional to thoroughly evaluate the situation (see Chapter 4). When choosing a new wall covering avoid vinyl wallpaper and find the least toxic adhesives. You could also consider low- or no-VOC paint instead of wallpaper. Always ventilate the space well while decorating and keep children away from materials.

All of this will require a little extra effort in advance but the benefits are the pleasure of a new look or better functionality without harming anyone's health.

Remodeling

Often the largest maintenance project a home faces is remodeling. There are many things to consider before deciding on an architect, builder or whether to take the project on yourself. Chapter 4 provides a lot of this preliminary information. To maintain the health of your home be sure to choose non-toxic building and decorating materials and seriously consider removing your family while the work is being done. Even if you are using healthier building products you don't know what you will encounter when you open up the structure of your home. Exposing your family to a possible mold problem, lead dust or asbestos could have very serious consequences.

And Finally

Now you can anticipate the different needs and the long-term maintenance your home will require to function well and stay healthy. It's really not that complicated if you take a little time to make a plan and then follow through. It's rather like making a weekly menu so you don't have to wonder what to cook every day or making a shopping list to remind you what you need from the store.

We have now covered all the main aspects of a healthy home. Take a few minutes and go back over the Healthy Home Quiz and circle any items you now know need to be removed, improved, or checked by a professional.

Most immediate gains

1. Create a maintenance plan for your home to remind you what needs to be done when. Display this in a prominent place as a visual reminder.
2. Always keep a supply of replacement items available such as light bulbs and water filters. Store these products in their original containers and write down manufacturers' or suppliers' phone numbers in case you have questions later.
3. If you are planning any decorating do some research to find out what your healthiest options are.
4. Read up on healthy home construction. See Appendix C for "Books to Build a Healthy Home Library."

CHAPTER 18

Living Happily Ever After ...

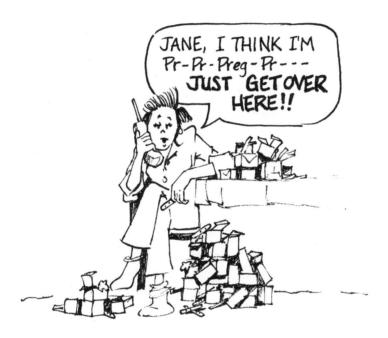

Liz sits on the edge of the bathtub staring transfixed at the white pen-like object in her hand. She checks her watch. Thirty seconds have passed. She looks back to the white object and focuses on the small window in its center. A pale pink line has formed at the lower edge of the window and another pale pink line is forming above. Beads of perspiration form on Liz's forehead as her mouth opens involuntarily into a gasp. One minute and 30 seconds. "That can't be right," Liz says to herself.

She reads the instruction leaflet for a third time. "See, it says wait for five minutes. Maybe it will change back." Liz tries to shut all thoughts out of her mind and focuses on regulating her breathing, which keeps trying to speed up.

One more look at her watch confirms that time is up. No more waiting. The results are in. Liz moves the wand-shaped proclamation back and forth attempting to bring it into better focus. "I don't know," she says exasperatedly. "Maybe it's faulty. That second line's not as strong as the first." She places it on the bathroom counter top next to two other identical pen-like objects and compares them. They all show two distinct pink lines. She reaches for the instructions one last time and reads. "Positive Result: Distinct color bands appear on the control and test regions. The presence of both test and control lines indicate possible pregnancy." Liz chews nervously on her acrylic fingernail. "Maybe I should do another test, just to make sure."

The phone rings, startling Liz out of her deliberations. "Hi sister, I've got some good news for you. Guess what? You have a beautiful little niece who's waiting to see you." A long pause follows while the news sinks into Liz's confused mind. Jane continues on enthusiastically, "You and Mark really should think about having your own some time soon. Then our children can grow up together." Liz moves her lips in an attempt to say something but words fail her.

"Are you all right? You're very quiet," Jane says.

"Me, oh yes, I'll be fine. I'm just a bit under the weather. That's great news Jane. I'll be over there in twenty minutes. Oh, and Jane, what's it like having a baby?"

"It's hard work, but it's the best job in the world!"

.... To be continued in Book 2.

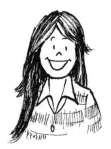

Commentary: Is it still possible to live happily ever after?

Inside many people's hearts is a deep desire to live happily ever after. Isn't that what you really want? To live out the rest of your days in good health, surrounded by those you love, having contributed something worthwhile back to your community, seeing your children grow into healthy, productive adults, raising their own children and being decent members of society?

But have you noticed how this simple desire has become so elusive to so many people? How everyday living seems to continually morph into ever-increasing layers of complexity leaving us with a hazard-filled existence? Today, if we want to give birth to a child without birth defects or a life-long neurological disorder such as autism, or a child who can grow through childhood without a learning disability or asthma, or a teenager who can make it through to adulthood without debilitating depression or cancer, we must educate ourselves in a variety of sciences and social studies such as the emrging field of preconception care (preparing to become pregnant and have a healthy baby) , early childhood neurological development and toxicology, whether we see ourselves as capable of this or not. Only when we are in full possession of the facts can we know how to proceed or who to trust in our increasingly chemical world.

> Science is fragmentary, incomplete; it progresses slowly and is never finished; life cannot wait.
> — Emile Durkheim,
> The Elementary Forms of Religious Life, 1912

For too long we have been lulled into believing that someone else is watching out for our health; that we are protected; that we can build or buy a new home or shop for everyday products without any consideration that these things could cause us harm. But as you now know from reading *Homes that Heal*, this is simply not true. There are tremendous gaps between the findings of science and what the public is allowed to know.

While our government and large corporations simultaneously battle with each other, make financial deals, and tell us that toxic chemicals and pollution are at safe levels, more and more parents are finding they have to assume the responsibility for ensuring proper health decisions for their children.

> "Ultimately, if we fail to use chemicals properly, we will injure deeply all nature and mankind."
> — Senator Abraham Ribicoff, Foreword to *Basic Guide to Pesticides*, 1992.

Cutting at The Root

The root of the problem is that we are dealing with a flawed system. Government and the private sector continue to rely heavily on risk assessment for making decisions. But risk assessment *always* fails with regard to children's health, because it assumes that there is some level of a toxic chemical that is safe. In reality, no one knows that level.

For instance, there is no safe level of dioxin, yet every child (indeed every living being) is currently being exposed to this lethal poison. Among other effects, dioxin alters fetal development and compromises the immune system. So, what is the "safe" level of yet another toxic chemical in a child whose immune system has already been compromised or whose development has been more subtly altered by dioxin? It's the same with combinations of toxics. Literally *nobody* knows the effects of a child's exposure to multiple toxics, and yet no child on earth is being exposed to only one toxic chemical or pollutant at a time. Similarly, nobody knows how a given toxic behaves in a child who is deficient in particular nutrients; or who is genetically incapable of handling a particular chemical; or who is on medications. From these perspectives, the idea of estimating a "safe" dose of a toxic chemical is absurd.

What is *not* absurd is changing from the current "innocent until proven guilty" approach of risk-assessment that favors the moneyed interests of large corporations to the more humanely focused approach, guided by the precautionary principle, called "alternatives-assessment." This newer model advises taking precautionary measures and considering all safer alternatives when science cannot conclusively prove whether something is harmful or not. Industries often take blatant advantage of these interim periods of uncertainty to keep dangerous products on the market and

> We must do more. The evidence is incontrovertible. We must move quickly to phase out those toxic chemicals that are known to pose a danger to human health. And we must institute a system of regulation that tests new synthetic chemicals and proves them safe before they are allowed to be sold, before our children are exposed. Isn't that the system you thought we already had?[1]

> "Those who have the privilege to know also have a duty to warn."
> — Albert Einstein

Sandra Steingraber paints a vivid picture in *Living Downstream*: "Suppose we assume for a moment that the most conservative estimate concerning the proportion of cancer deaths due to environmental causes is absolutely accurate. This estimate, put forth by those who dismiss environmental carcinogens as negligible, is 2 percent. Though others have placed this number far higher, let's assume for the sake of argument that this lowest value is absolutely correct. Two percent means that 10,940 people in the United States die each year from environmentally caused cancers. This is more than the number of women who die each year from hereditary breast cancer – an issue that has launched multi-million-dollar research initiatives. This is more than the number of children and teenagers killed each year by firearms – an issue that is considered a matter of national shame. It is more than three times the number of nonsmokers estimated to die each year of lung cancer caused by exposure to secondhand smoke – a problem so serious it warranted sweeping changes in laws governing air quality in public spaces. It is the annual equivalent of wiping out a whole city. It is thirty funerals a day."[2]

"The obligation to endure gives us the right to know"
— Jean Rostand, writer.

Where chemicals are found in elevated concentrations in biological fluids such as breast milk, they should be removed from the market immediately.[3]

---

continue to act destructively, stopping only when enough damage has been done to force a halt to these practices. But what if your child is injured in this indecisive cross fire? What if your child gets cancer, or suffers neurological, immune, or developmental damage as a result of someone else's risk assessment calculations that this is acceptable? Why are we placing such heavy burdens of proof on our children? Who can be held responsible for these decisions?

The alternatives assessment approach recommends that all decision-making processes must include all the potentially affected parties. How else can decisions be made that are both wise and just? This is a human rights issue. Yet our current climate of risk assessment and special interest groups places almost impenetrable barriers before common citizens who wish to either voice an opinion or know what chemical contaminants and other pollutants they or their family are being subjected to without their consent. Even with the advent of federal right-to-know laws that now make information about the ongoing contamination of our environment publicly available, there are still many loopholes that keep us from the real truth. Many of these laws are currently being unraveled. In *Silent Spring*, Rachel Carson spoke of this predicament 40 years earlier saying that "the full knowledge of this situation would lead us to reject the counsel of those who claim there is simply no choice but to go on filling the world with poisons."

In response to this situation, concerned and irate citizens have gathered together forming several excellent non-governmental organizations. These groups, such as the Natural Resources Defense Council; the Center for Health, Environment and Justice; the Children's Environmental Health Network; and others are savvy in their research and interpretative capabilities and provide us with much-needed information and common-sense guidance (see Appendix C for more organizations).

The Many Things You Can Do

The first place to exercise your decision-making power is within your own home. Here, you can affect great change, both short- and long-term, to protect your family's health and wellbeing. At last, some good news! Hopefully, this book has shown you multiple ways to make better choices. Let's review a few of them.

If you are interested in building a home, put this new knowledge into action and require that your architect and builder use proven healthy materials and systems; introduce them to the complementary science of Building Biology. Give them a copy of this book to read so you can all speak the same language. Coordinating such an effort will increase awareness and involvement and over time will help to change the way we currently build to ensure healthier and more humane living environments for everyone.

The same goes if you are looking to buy a new home that has already been built, if you are planning a remodel, or are planning to bring some other professionals, such as a decorator, into your home. You have more power than you may realize. This is your home, you are the one paying these professionals for their services, therefore you call the shots!

Then there is the world of consumer products. Let your buying power speak loud and clear. Stop buying and using toxic products. This includes toxic cleaning and laundry products, personal care products, home furnishings, art and craft supplies, yard and lawn products, and pet products. If you want to reclaim your power, here is a massive arena in which to make yourself heard. If we all rally together and use these bite-sized pieces of power, sooner or later manufacturers (the ones that want to stay in business) will have to change their practices to meet these consumer demands for healthier products. Together our actions can direct a spirit of urgency, inventiveness, and ingenuity toward the development of better approaches to help restore our children's health. That's where the bigger solution will be found.

Clearly not an institution of power, children don't vote and they don't pay taxes. They have no money, and they don't buy newspapers or watch the news on television. Consequently, children are one of the most neglected segments of society in the news. Children are in serious trouble in this society, which means the foundation of our society is in trouble, which means the future is in trouble, and that is news.
— Joan Konner, former dean,
Columbia School of Journalism.

The purpose of education is action, not knowledge.

The challenge for humanity is to develop human design processes which enable us to remain in the natural context. Almost every phase of the design, manufacturing, and construction processes requires reconsideration. Linear systems of thought, or short-term programs which justify ignorant, indifferent, or arrogant means are not farsighted enough to serve the future of the interaction between humanity and nature. We must employ both current knowledge and ancient wisdom in our efforts to conceive and realize the physical transformation, care and maintenance of the Earth.[4]

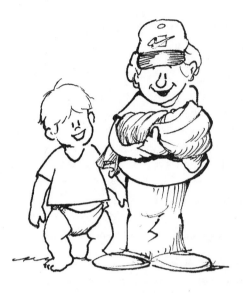

Our Most Precious Resource

Have you noticed how quickly each day passes? I know I am not alone in experiencing this phenomenon. I watch my son growing up at a breathtaking pace. Living happily ever after requires that we experience it mixed within the fabric of a busy everyday life. Pivotal decisions are made between loads of laundry, answering the phone, and dashing out to the grocery store to get home in time to cook dinner for everyone. But as busy as we are as parents, we must never forget one important fact. The world's most precious resource is our children (not oil!) and raising them is our most important work. While it is still not generally recognized as the quintessential human right, our children's health and well-being must be better protected. By eliminating poisons from their world at home you will have given society an incredible gift, the promise of a healthy, unencumbered, vital member of society and in exchange you will have proven yourself to be worthy of such trust.

Think with your heart and see life through the eyes of a child.

Glossary

Absorption: The uptake of substances by the skin, respiratory, and gastrointestinal tract.

Acute: One-time or short-term exposure. Used to describe brief exposures and effects that appear promptly after exposure (usually within 24 hours).

Acute toxicity: The rapid onset of an adverse effect from a single exposure. Acute toxicity of a compound is not an indicator of its chronic effects.

Aerosol: A suspension of extremely small particles or liquid in air.

Aerosol Product: A pressurized, self-dispensing product used for a wide variety of chemical specialty products.

Allergen: Anything that causes an allergic reaction.

Asbestos: A naturally occurring mineral that exists in several forms. Asbestos has been used in thousands of products including insulation and construction composites. It is carcinogenic.

Backdrafting: Complete reversal of flow in a chimney, usually due to negative pressures indoors.

Bau-biologie: Used interchangeably with "Building Biology." It is the study of how buildings affect our health. This knowledge is applied to the design and construction of new buildings, renovations, or remediation (fixing sick buildings).

Blood-brain barrier: A filtering mechanism of the capillaries that carry blood to the brain and spinal cord tissue, blocking the passage of certain substances. Prevents accumulation of toxins and amino acids that cause brain damage. Not fully formed in the unborn and young child.

Body burden: Process in which a substance (or multiple substances) builds up in the body faster than the body can eliminate it. Also known as "bioaccumulation" or "chemical load."

Breathing walls: Breathing walls do two things: 1. They take in air. 2. They can take in large amounts of humidity without damaging the wall material and quickly release it as conditions change. See "Hygroscopic."

Building Biology: See "Bau-Biologie."

Carbon monoxide: A colorless, odorless, poisonous gas formed by incomplete burning of coal, oil, wood, and gas. In low concentrations causes headaches and nausea and in high concentrations can cause coma and death.

Carcinogen: A substance or agent capable of producing cancer in living tissue.

Caustic: A chemical that will burn skin on contact (corrosive effect on living tissue).

Caution: Indicates a moderate hazard when placed on product labeling.

Chemical sensitivity: An increased sensitivity to chemicals and other irritants found in the environment. Symptoms may include respiratory distress, muscle pain, headache, dizziness, eye and throat irritation, fatigue, neurological problems, and cognitive difficulties. Also called Multiple Chemical Sensitivity (MCS) and Environmental Illness (EI).

Chronic: Occurring over a long period of time, either continuously or intermittently. Used to describe ongoing exposures and effects that develop only after a long exposure.

Chronic toxicity: The slow or delayed onset of an adverse effect, usually from multiple, long-term exposures. Chronic toxicity of a compound is not an indicator of its acute effects.

Combustible: Substance that can easily be set on fire and that will burn readily or quickly. Flammable.

Condensation: A change of state from gas (vapor) to liquid; the opposite of evaporation. In a bathroom after someone has showered, the haze on a mirror is formed by condensation of water vapor onto a surface.

Corrosive: Having the power to dissolve. Can burn and destroy living tissue.

Cumulative: Often the effects of repeated exposures to chemicals are greater than single exposures. The cumulative effect is what occurs from repeated exposures over time. This can include exposures to one chemical over time, or exposures to multiple chemicals in a short amount of time.

Danger: Warning label placed on products meaning extremely flammable, corrosive, or highly toxic.

Dioxins: Pollutant byproducts of PVC production, industrial bleaching, and incineration. Causes cancer. Persist for decades in the environment. Very toxic to developing endocrine (hormone) system.

Dose: The quantity of chemical administered at one time.

Dust Mites: Tiny members of the arachnid family. Dust mites, found in pillows, mattresses, and carpets, subsist on skin scales and can cause asthma and other allergic symptoms.

EMFs: Electromagnetic fields. The more accurate term is electromagnetic radiation (EMR). When people say EMF they are usually refering only to AC magnetic fields, whereas EMR refers to both AC electric and AC magnetic fields, both of which have health effects. These fields are created by the flow of electricity and the space surrounding that flow. The most common sources include high-tension power lines, house wiring, and household appliances.

EMR: Electromagnetic radiation. See "EMFs."

Exposure: Contact of an organism with a chemical, physical, or geological agent.

Fiberglass: A non-woven mixture of threadlike fibers made from molten glass and often held together by microscopic droplets of glue (often formaldehyde).

Flammable: Substance that can easily be set on fire and that will burn readily or quickly.

Formaldehyde: An extremely irritating, strong-smelling gas. Very soluble in water. Formaldehyde is widely used in many products including building materials such as particleboard and insulation, and synthetic materials such as carpet, fibers, and cosmetics as a preservative. Formaldehyde offgasses from many materials. It can be inhaled, ingested, or absorbed and is linked to many health problems such as cancer and nervous system damage.

Fumes: Small particles created in high heat operations such as welding or soldering that become airborne when exposed to heat. Fume particles are very small and tend to remain airborne for long periods of time. Metals, some organic chemicals, plastics, and silica can produce fume particles.

Fungus: A plantlike life form that lacks chlorophyll and thus depends on other living or dead organisms for its nourishment. Fungi (plural of fungus) include mushrooms and microscopic molds.

Gases: Substances that become airborne at room temperature. They may or may not mix with air.

Hazard: The potential that using a product will result in an adverse effect on a person or the environment.

HEPA filter: A high efficiency particulate arrestance filter. A HEPA filter is supposed to remove 99.97 percent of 0.3 micron particulates from the air flowing through it and 100 percent of the particulates larger than 1 micron. It is capable of capturing all mold spores and almost all bacteria, as well as construction dust.

Hygroscopic: The ability of a material to absorb humidity and release it again when conditions change until a balance of air humidity is established.

IAQ: Indoor air quality. The quality of the air found inside buildings. Quality is defined by the absence of toxic chemicals and substances.

Ignitable: Substance capable of being set on fire.

Immunotoxic: Toxic substances that reduce the body's own defenses against disease.

Inert Ingredient: A substance contained in a product that will not, by itself, add materially to the effectiveness of the product. Many inert ingredients are poisonous and/or hazardous.

Ingestion: When a substance is taken into the body through swallowing.

Inhale: To take into the lungs by breathing.

IPM: Integrated Pest Management. A system of pest control utilizing the least toxic materials.

Irritant: An agent that produces chafing, soreness, or inflammation, especially to the skin.

Lethal: Products with this label are capable of causing death.

Mildew: A plant pathogen. This is often misused as a generic term to describe microbial growth. Mildew is a type of mold; most molds are not mildew.

Mold: A term used synonymously with "fungal growth." Often used to describe visible microbial growth on surfaces. Molds require oxygen and moisture to flourish, but they also need a source of nutrients such as wood or other plant material (cellulose).

Mold spore: The reproductive cell (or cells) of fungi. They are microscopic and dispersed into the air. Some spores may be allergens or toxigenic.

MSDS: Material Safety Data Sheets. Manufacturers are required by law to publish the hazards and safety precautions for chemicals used in their manufacturing process. These are made available to the general public upon request. Many companies now have them available on their websites.

Multiple chemical sensitivity: For MCS, see chemical sensitivity.

Mutagen: A chemical or substance that can permanently change the genetic content of the mother or father's cells (usually their reproductive cells), which in turn can then affect all their offspring.

Mycotoxin: Metabolic byproducts of certain molds that are known to increase health risks.

Neurotoxic: Term describing substances that are toxic to the nervous system.

Offgassing: Emission of a solvent or other chemical from the surface of a solid into the air; generally produced by volatile organic compounds. Also referred to as outgassing

Organic: 1. Containing carbon, as in organic chemistry. 2. Grown without synthetic or other toxic chemical pesticides, as in organically grown food.

Ozone: Pale-blue gas. An unstable form of oxygen with a sharp smell. At ground level is the main component of smog. The thin later of ozone in the stratosphere absorbs the sun's ultraviolet radiation, protecting plants and animals from its adverse effects. Closer to the earth, ozone is a powerful lung irritant.

Particulate: A microscopic fragment of a solid or droplet of a liquid that is suspended in air. Particulates vary in size. If large, they may settle on surfaces; if small, they may remain suspended.

PCB: Polychlorinated biphenyls. Invented in the 1930s and added to oil inside electrical devices to protect oil breakdown at high temperatures. They conduct electricity and resist heat. Most PCBs made are still in the environment, despite being banned in the U.S. in the 1970s as toxic and causing cancer. Found in water, soil, fish, crops, animals, and humans today.

Pesticide: A chemical or biological agent that kills pests. A pest can be an animal, fungi, insect, plant, or any unwanted species.

Petroleum distillates: Mixtures of chemical compounds derived from the distillation of petroleum. Most are highly toxic if ingested.

Phthalates: Plasticizers used to soften plastics such as PVC. Have reproductive and developmental toxicity. Cause birth defects of male reproductive organs. Found in a wide range of foods, cosmetic, and personal care products.

Poison: Any toxic substance that upsets normal functions in living organisms by surface absorption, injection, or ingestion; eventually leading to death if the dosage is sufficiently strong. When "poison" is on a product label it means that the chemical or substance inside is highly toxic.

Pressure-treated wood: Wood containing a preservative (pesticide) that permeates much of the wood structure rather than simply coating the surface. Copper chromated arsenate (CCA) is the most commonly used treatment making wood resistant to decay caused by bacteria, mold, and insects

PVC: Polyvinyl chloride. Plastic used in many products including floor tiles, pipes, and shower curtains to name but a few. Releases vinyl chloride that causes cancer and birth defects. PVC manufacture and disposal via incineration produces deadly dioxins.

Radiant heat: Radiant heat home heating systems most commonly include in-floorwater filled heating tubes and radiators (fluid-filled heating elements). It is generally considered a more comfortable form of heating because it heats objects and people directly, while forced air or convection heating heats the air by blowing warm air into a space.

Radiation: The emission of energy. There is an entire spectrum (from low to high energy), called the electromagnetic spectrum, which includes extra-low frequencies, radio waves, microwaves, infrared, visible light, ultraviolet light, X rays, and gamma rays.

Radioactive: Substance capable of giving off radiant energy in the form of particles or rays by the spontaneous disintegration of atomic nuclei. Can damage and destroy cells and chromosomal material.

Radon: A naturally occurring, radioactive gas released from soils containing uranium. Can build up in homes and basements that are not properly vented. Second leading cause of lung cancer in the U.S.

Reactive: Tendency of a substance to undergo chemical change. May occur when exposed to other substances or through exposure to heat, sudden shock, or pressure.

Remediation: The action of remedying something. Reversing or stopping environmental damage such as mold growth.

Risk: The probability of injury, disease, or death under specific circumstances.

Sick building syndrome (SBS): Caused by any structure in which the quality of the air is so poor that the health of the occupants is in jeopardy.

Synthetic: A synthetic chemical is one that has been formulated in a chemical laboratory, usually by combining smaller substances into larger ones. Most synthetic organic compounds are derived from either petroleum or coal.

Smoke: Formed from burning organic matter. Contains a mixture of many gases, particulates, vapors, and fumes.

Solvent: A liquid that will dissolve a substance, forming a solution.

Teratogen: A substance that causes permanent changes to a baby's cells, thereby producing birth defects, but does not necessarily harm the mother.

Toxic: Harmful. Poisonous. Substances with this warning label are capable of causing injury or death through ingestion, inhalation, or absorption.

Toxicology: The study of poisons, their effects and cures.

Toxin: Poisonous substance, whether in solid, liquid, or gas form. It harms life.

Vapors: The gaseous form of any substance that is usually a liquid or a solid. Most liquids vaporize continually. The rate of evaporation increases as the temperature rises. Vapors are easily inhaled.

Ventilation rate: The amount of fresh air supplied to a space. The ventilation rate is commonly expressed as cubic feet of air per minute (cfm) or air exchanges per hour (ACH).

Volatile: A substance that evaporates quickly, such as alcohol.

Volatile and Semi-volatile organic chemicals (VOC and SVOC): An easily vaporizing substance. Usually a combination of chemical elements such as xylene and ethyl benzene. Found in industrial solvents, gasoline ingredients, and various construction and maintenance operations. Toxic to nervous system, some heavily used VOCs (benzene) cause cancer.

Warning: When placed on a product label, indicative of a moderate hazard. When no warning label is present, the product is among the least hazardous products to use.

Acronyms and Abbreviations

The following acronyms and abbreviations are listed as helpful reminders:

AAEM	The American Academy of Environmental Medicine
AAP	American Academy of Pediatrics
ACMI	Art and Creative Materials Institute
ALA	American Lung Association
AMA	American Medical Association
APHA	American Public Health Association
ASHRAE	American Society of Heating, Refrigerating, and Air-Conditioning Engineers
ATSDR	Agency for Toxic Substances and Disease Registry, part of the Public Health Service
CDC	Centers for Disease Control and Prevention
CMA	Chemical Manufacturers Association
CPSC	Consumer Product Safety Commission
CSPI	Center for Science in the Public Interest
EPA	Environmental Protection Agency
FDA	Food and Drug Administration
FTC	Federal Trade Commission
HHS	Health and Human Services
HUD	Housing and Urban Development
JAMA	Journal of the American Medical Association
NAS	National Academy of Sciences
NASA	National Aeronautics and Space Administration
NCAMP	National Coalition Against the Misuse of Pesticides (now named Beyond Pesticides)
NCAP	Northwest Coalition for Alternatives to Pesticides
NCEHS	National Center for Environmental Health Studies

NCHS   National Center for Health Statistics

NCI   National Cancer Institute

NIH   National Institute of Health

NIOSH   National Institute for Occupational Safety and Health

NPL   National Priorities List

NRC   National Research Council (NAS's research arm)

NRDC   Natural Resources Defense Council

NTP   National Toxicology Program (part of Health and Human Service)

NYCAP   New York Coalition for Alternatives to Pesticides

OSHA   Occupational Safety and Health Administration

SEER   Surveillance, Epidemiology, and End Results Program of U.S. National Cancer Institute

SVTC   Silicone Valley Toxics Coalition

TRI   Toxics Release Inventory

USDA   United States Department of Agriculture

WHO   World Health Organization

Sources and Resources

Books to Build a Healthy Home Library

An Alternative Approach to Allergies, Revised Edition, Theron G. Randolph, M.D. and Ralph W. Moss, Ph.D., Harper & Row, 1990.

Are You Poisoning Your Pets? Nina Anderson and Howard Peiper, Avery Publishing Group, 1998.

Artist Beware, Michael McCann, Lyons Press, 1992.

Basic Guide to Pesticides, Shirley A. Briggs and Rachel Carson Council, Taylor & Francis, 1992.

Better Basics for the Home, Annie Berthold-Bond, Three Rivers Press, 1999.

The Body Electric, Robert O. Becker M.D., and Gary Selden, William Morrow and Company, 1985.

Cell Phones: Invisible Hazards in the Wireless Age, Dr. George Carlo and Martin Schram, Carroll and Graf, 2001.

Chemical Exposures: Low Levels and High Stakes, Nicholas Ashford and Claudia Miller, John Wiley & Sons, 1998.

Child Health and the Environment, Donald T. Wigle, Oxford Press, 2003.

Clean House, Clean Planet, Karen Logan, Pocket Books, 1997.

Common Sense Pest Control, William Olkowski, Sheila Daar, and Helga Olkowski, Taunton Press, 1991.

The Cot Death Cover-Up, Jim Sprott OBE, Ph.D., Penguin Books, 1996.

Designer Poisons, Marion Moses, M.D., Pesticide Education Center, 1995.

Electromagnetic Fields, B. Blake Levitt, Harcourt Brace, 1995.

The Fluoride Deception, Christopher Bryson, Seven Stories Press, 2004.

Generations at Risk: Reproductive Health and the Environment, Ted Schettler, M.D., Gina Solomon, M.D., Maria Valenti, and Annette Huddle, MIT Press, 2000.

Green Remodeling, Davis Johnston, New Society Publishers, 2004.

The Healthy Household, Lynn Marie Bower, The Healthy House Institute, 2000.

Mothers and Others for a Livable Planet Guide to Natural Baby Care, Mindy Pennybacker and Aisha Ikramuddin, John Wiley & Sons, 1999.

Having Faith, Sandra Steingraber, Perseus, 2001.

Healing Environments, Carol Venolia, Celestial Arts, 1988.

Health and Light, John Ott, Ariel Press, 2000.

Home Safe Home, Debra Lynn Dadd, Tarcher Putnam, 1997.

Household, Yard and Office Chemicals, Ruth Winter, Crown, 1992.

How to Grow Fresh Air, B.C. Wolverton, Penguin, 1991.

Is This Your Child? Discovering and Treating Unrecognized Allergies in Children and Adults, Doris J. Rapp, M.D., William Morrow and Company, 1996.

Living Downstream, Sandra Steingraber, Vintage Books, 1997.

Living Healthy in a Toxic World, David Steinman and R. Michael Wisner, The Berkley Publishing Group, 1996.

Making Better Environmental Decisions, Mary O'Brien, MIT Press, 2001.

Multiple Chemical Sensitivity, Pamela Reed Gibson, New Harbinger, 2000.

My House is Killing Me, Jeffrey C. May, John Hopkins University Press, 2001.

Natural Family Living, Peggy O'Mara, Mothering Magazine, Atria Books, 2000.

The New Natural House Book, David Pearson, Fireside, 1998.

The New Organic Grower, Eliot Coleman, Chelsea Green, 1995.

Our Children's Toxic Legacy, John Wargo, Yale University Press, 1998.

Our Stolen Future, Theo Colborn, Dianne Dumanoski, and John Peterson Myers, Penguin Group, 1997.

Preparing For Pregnancy, Suzanne Gail Bradley and Nicholas Bennett, Argyll, 1997, see Foresight UK in next section.

Prescriptions for a Healthy House, Paula Baker-Laporte, Erica Elliot, and John Banta, New Society Publishers, 2001.

Protecting Public Health and the Environment: Implementing the Precautionary Principle, edited by Carolyn Raffensperger and Joel Tickner, Island Press, 1999.

The Rodale Book of Composting, edited by Deborah L. Martin and Grace Gershuny, Rodale Press, 1992.

The Safe Shoppers Bible, David Steinman and Samuel S. Epstein, M.D., Macmillan, 1995.

Silent Scourge: Children, Pollution and Why Scientists Disagree, Colleen Moore, Oxford Press, 2003.

Silent Spring, Rachel Carson, Houghton Mifflin, 1962.

Staying Well in a Toxic World, Lynn Lawson, Lynnword Press, 1993.

Synthetic Planet: Chemical Politics and the Hazards of Modern Life, edited by Monica J. Casper, Routledge, 2003.

Toxic Deception: How the Chemical Industry Manipulates Science, Bends the Law, and Endangers Your Health, Dan Fagin, Marianne Lavelle, and the Center for Public Integrity, Birch Lane Press, 1996.

Toxics A to Z, John Harte, Cheryl Holdren, Richard Schneider, and Christine Shirley, University of California Press, 1991

Raising Healthy Children in a Toxic World, Philip J. Landrigan, M.D., Herbert L. Needleman, M.D., and Mary Landrigan, Rodale, 2001.

Warning: The Electricity Around You May Be Hazardous To Your Health, Ellen Sugarman, Miriam Press, 1992.

What Every Home Owner Needs to Know About Mold, Vicki Lankarge, McGraw-Hill, 2003.

Your Home, Your Health and Your Well-Being, David Rousseau, W.J. Rea, M.D., and Jean Enwright, Ten Speed Press, 1988.

Staying Current Through Websites, Newsletters, and More

American Academy of Pediatrics (AAP)

141 Northwest Point Boulevard, Elk Grove Village, IL 60007-1098 Telephone: 874-434-4000 Web: <www.aap.org/healthtopics/environmentalhealth.cfm> Referrals for Environmental Pediatricians. Publishers of *Pediatric Environmental Health 2nd Edition*, Edited by Ruth A. Etzel M.D., PhD, and Associate Editor: Sophie J. Balk, M.D., written for health professionals but suitable for parents looking for more in-depth information about pediatric environmental health hazards.

American Academy of Environmental Medicine (AAEM)

7701 East Kellogg, Suite 625, Wichita, Kansas 67207 Telephone: 316-684-5500 Web: <www.aaem.com> Referrals for Environmental Health Physicians

Art and Creative Materials Institute (ACMI)

P.O. Box 479, Hanson, MA 02341-0479 Telephone: 781-293-4100 Web: <www.acminet.org> ACMI publishes a list of art and craft products that have been certified through its program. This list is updated approximately two times a year and is available for free upon request.

Beyond Pesticides

701 E Street SE #200, Washington, DC 20003 Telephone: 202-543-5450 Web: <www.beyondpesticides.org> A national network focused on pesticide safety and the adoption of alternative pest management strategies that reduce or eliminate a dependency on toxic chemicals. Beyond Pesticides produces two informative newsletters. *Pesticides and You* (PAY), published quarterly, and *Technical Report* published monthly.

Building Green

122 Birge St, Suite 30, Brattleboro, VT 05301 Telephone: 802-257-7300 Web: <www.buildinggreen.com> Publishers of *Environmental Building News,* available electronically and in paper version, to help building industry professionals and policy makers improve the environmental performance, and reduce the adverse impacts, of buildings.

Center for Children's Health and the Environment (CCHE) of the Mount Sinai School of Medicine

P.O. Box 1043, One Gustave Levy Place, New York, NY 10029 Telephone: 212-241-7840 Web: <www.childrenvironment.org> The Center for Children's Health and the Environment is the nation's first academic research and policy center to examine the links between exposure to toxic pollutants and childhood illness. Comprehensive coverage on how chemicals can affect children's health.

Center for Health, Environment and Justice

P.O. Box 6806, Falls Church, VA 22040 Telephone: 703-237-2249 Web: <www.chej.org> Founded by Lois Gibbs, the Love Canal community leader, CHEJ helps local citizens and organizations take an organized, unified stand in order to hold industry and government accountable and work toward a healthy, sustainable future. See their "Be Safe" campaign and "GreenFlag" healthy schools program. A quarterly journal, *Everyone's Backyard* and an e-mail service, *CHEJ's E-Action Bulletin,* to keep you updated.

Children's Environmental Health Network (CHEN)

5900 Hollis Street, Suite R3, Emeryville, CA 94608 Telephone: 510-597-1393 Web: <www.cehn.org> Focuses on protecting the fetus and child from environmental health hazards and promoting a healthy environment. Good information and resources.

Children's Health Environmental Coalition (CHEC)

P.O. Box 1540, Princeton, NJ 08542 Telephone: 609-252-1915 Web: <www.checnet.org>
Public education about environmental toxins that affect children's health. Has a quarterly print newsletter, *The CHEC Report,* and two electronic newsletters, *HealtheNews,* and *First Steps,* for pregnant or new parents. Website also has HealtheHouse, a virtual tour to show where toxins lurk in the home. Many good articles and lots of information.

Environmental Defense

1875 Connecticut Ave NW, P.O. Box 96969, Washington, DC 20077-7254
Telephone: 800-591-1919 Web: <www.scorecard.org>
Environmental Defense evaluates environmental problems. Enter your zip code and find out what pollutants are being released into your community, and who is responsible. Very informative.

Environmental Health News delivers a daily e-mail of compiled links to news, reports, and new scientific discoveries about environmental links to health in the US and around the world. A simple way to be plugged in globally. Web: <www.EnvironmentalHealthNews.org>

Environmental Protection Agency (US EPA)

Ariel Rios Building, 1200 Pennsylvania Avenue, Washington, DC 20460
Telephone: 202-272-0167 Web: <www.epa.gov> Resources for mold, lead, asbestos, radon, IAQ and more. Fact sheets and downloadable pdf's such as *Mold, Moisture and Your Home.* Many hard copies available via mail for free. Call 1-800-490-9198 to order publications. Referrals for asbestos professionals and lead inspectors. Specialized services such as the InfoLine for the National Lead Information Center at 1-800-424-LEAD (5323).

Environmental Research Foundation (ERF)

P.O. Box 160, New Brunswick, NJ 08903-0160 Telephone: 732-828- 9995 or toll-free 888-272-2435 Web: <www.rachel.org> Information about the influence of toxic substances on human health and the environment. Weekly online newsletter, *Rachel's Environment and Health News.*

Environmental Working Group (EWG)

1436 U Street NW, Suite 100, Washington, DC 20009 Telephone: 202-667-6982
Web: <www.ewg.org> EWG conducts research on a variety of environmental issues. Their website is full of many excellent reports including *Body Burden: Pollution in People, Not Too Pretty* and more.

Foresight

28 The Paddock, Godalming, Surrey, GU7 1XD, England
Telephone: 01483-427839 Web: <www.foresight-preconception.org.uk>
A British association focused on promoting preconceptual care. They offer programs, books, and other information to help couples prepare for pregnancy and conceive a healthy child.

Fragranced Products Information Network

No address or phone number currently available. Web: <www.fpinva.org>
A comprehensive web site on health, environmental, and regulatory aspects related to fragrance. Many helpful articles about chemicals in fragrance and health.

Greenpeace USA

702 H Street, NW, Washington, DC 20001 Telephone: 800-326-0959
Web: <www.greenpeaceusa.org> Focuses on global environmental problems and promotes solutions for a green and peaceful future. See article *Toxic Toy Story* and more.

Healthy Building Network

Institute for Local Self Reliance, 2425 18th Street, Washington, DC 20009-2096
Telephone: 202-232-4108 Web: <www.healthybuilding.net> Focuses on promoting healthier building materials as a means of improving public health and preserving the global environment. Fact sheets and PDFs on CCA-treated wood, arsenic, PVC. Free newsletter.

Human Ecology Action League (HEAL)

P.O. Box 29629, Atlanta, GA 30359-0629
Telephone: 404-248-1898 Web: <http://members.aol.com/HEALNatnl/>
Publishes the quarterly magazine *The Human Ecologist*. Helpful information for those concerned about sensitivities, allergies, asthma, and other conditions responsive to environmental conditions. HEAL offers many other specialized publications.

Natural Resources Defense Council (NRDC)

40 West 20th Street, New York, NY 10011 Telephone: 212-727-2700 Web: <www.nrdc.org>
Focuses on law and science to protect the planet's wildlife and wild places, and to ensure a safe and healthy environment for all living beings. Many downloadable reports and studies. Hard copies available for a fee. See *The Five Worst Threats to Children's Health* and more.

Northwest Coalition for Alternatives to Pesticides (NCAP)

P.O. Box 1393, Eugene, OR 97440 Telephone: 541-344- 5044 Web: <www.pesticide.org>
NCAP focuses on protecting people and the environment by advancing healthy solutions to pest problems. Website has many fact sheets and pdf's. Helpful with right-to-know information about pesticides. Publishes the quarterly magazine, *Journal of Pesticide Reform*.

Physicians for Social Responsibility (PSR)

1875 Connecticut Ave, Suite 1012, Washington, DC 20009 Telephone: 202-667-4260
Web: <www.psr.org> Physicians for Social Responsibility represents medical and public health professions and concerned citizens, working together for nuclear disarmament, a healthful environment, and an end to the epidemic of gun violence. See Greater Boston PSR for a copy of *In Harm's Way: Toxic Threats to Child Development,* <www.psr.igc.org>

The Green Guide Institute

Prince Street Station, P.O. Box 567, New York, NY 10012 Telephone: 212-598-4910
Web: <www.thegreenguide.com> Publishes *The Green Guide,* an environmental lifestyle newsletter and website providing information on environmental and health issues of immediate importance to consumers, as well as hands-on, practical solutions that include everything from product reports that will help you make shopping choices to responsible consumer and citizen actions.

Washington Toxics Coalition

4649 Sunnyside Ave N, Suite 540, Seattle, WA, 98103 Telephone: 206-632- 1545
Web: <www.watoxics.org> Promotes alternatives, advocates policies, empowers communities, and educates people to create a healthy environment by eliminating toxic pollution. See *Researching Household Products,* and "Pesticide-Free Zone" signs.

Working Group on Community Right-To-Know

218 D Street SE, Washington, DC 20003 Telephone: 202-544- 2714 Web: <www.crtk.org>
The Working Group on Community Right-to-Know helps people defend and improve our right-to-know about environmental and public health concerns. See *My Environment* to find out more about where you live.

Resources for Products and Services Mentioned in This Book

American Formulating and Manufacture (AFM)
3251 3rd Ave, San Diego, CA 92103 Telephone: 619-239-0321, 800-239-0321
Web: <www.afmsafecoat.com> Paints, stains, sealants, and carpet cleaning products developed specifically for chemically sensitive people in consultation with environmental medicine physicians. See Safe Seal, a product to seal particleboard and more.

AirCheck, Inc.
1936 Butler Bridge, Fletcher, NC 28732-9365 Telephone: 800-247-2435, 828-684-0893
Web: <www.radon.com> Home radon test kits and radon information.

Anderson Laboratories
P.O. Box 323, West Hartford, Vermont 05084 Telephone: 802-295-7344
Web: <www.andersonlaboratories.com> Testing for IAQ affected by carpets, mattresses, perfume. Order copies of their published research and articles. Phone consultations available.

Bi-O-Kleen
P.O. Box 820689, Vancouver, WA 98682 Telephone: 360-576-0064, 800-477-0188
Web: <www.bi-o-kleen.com> A family owned and operated company providing cleaning products that are environmentally safe, non-toxic, high quality, affordable, easy to use with great cleaning results. Available at many natural product and grocery stores.

Chemically Sensitive Living
377 Wilbur Ave, Suite 213, Swansea, MA 02777 Telephone: 888-891-7293
Web: <www.chemsenlvng.com> Organic products for the home including mattresses, bedding, pillows, and more.

Cot Life 2000
10 Combes Road, Auckland 5, New Zealand Telephone: 64-9-5231150
Web: <www.cotlife2000.co.nz> Website of Jim Sprott, OBE, author of *The Cot Death Cover-Up*. Many good articles on SIDS. Purchase Baby Safe products including special plastic covers to wrap new baby mattresses in.

EcoBaby Organics
332 Coogan Way, El Cajon, CA 92020 Telephone: 800-596-7450 Web: <www.ecobaby.com>
Mail order company supplying organic baby and toddler clothes, diapers, wooden toys, solid wood cribs, child-sized beds, and other bedroom pieces finished with beeswax and tung oil.

Essential Aura Aromatics
3688 Glen Oaks Drive, Nanaimo, BC, Canada V9T 5A1 Telephone: 250-758-9464
Web: <www.essentialaura.com> An artisan distiller of organic essential oils from an eco-agricultural system.

Frontier Natural Products Co-Op
P.O. Box 299, 3021 78th St. Norway, IA 52318 Telephone: 800-669-3275
Web: <www.frontiercoop.com> Suppliers of certified organic essential oils. Not all their products are organic so read descriptions carefully. Look for Aura Cacia organic essential oils in your health food store.

GAIAM
360 Interlocken Blvd., Suite 300, Broomfield, CO 80021-3440 Telephone: 877-989-6321

Web: <www.gaiam.com> Mail order catalogue with extensive selection of household products including microfiber cleaning cloths, cellulose sponges, laundry sorters, some furniture, and much more.

Gardens Alive!

5100 Schenley Place, Lawrenceburg, Indiana 47025 Telephone: 513-656-1482
Web: <www.gardensalive.com> Mail order company dedicated to biological control of garden pests. Beneficial insects for pest control, organic plant foods, and more.

Green Home

850 24th Ave, San Francisco, CA 94121 Telephone: 877-282-6400
Web: <www.greenhome.com> Mail order company for environmental home products including cellulose bags, organic clothing, all natural hardwood beds and furniture, and more.

Healthy Building Network

Institute for Local Self Reliance, 2425 18th Street, Washington, DC 20009-2096
Telephone: 202-232-4108 Web: <www.healthybuilding.net>
Home test kits for arsenic. Test your deck, play set, or other wooden structures.

HealthyHome.com

2435 Dr. MLK Jr. St. N., Saint Petersburg, FL 33704 Telephone: 800-583-9523
Web: <www.healthyhome.com> Mail order catalogue of healthy home supplies including IQ Aire air filters, low- and no-VOC paints, full spectrum lighting, some furniture, and more.

Healthy Home Designs

180 Harbor Drive, Suite 231, Sausalito, CA 94965 Telephone: 415-331-3383
Web: <www.healthyhomedesigns.com> Healthy Home Designs offers detailed floor plans that incorporate healthy design, passive solar, energy efficiency, mold prevention, and the use of non-toxic building materials.

Homes that Heal

16869 SW 65th Ave #335, Lake Oswego, OR 97035 Telephone: 503-699-0052
Web: <www.homesthatheal.com> Homes that Heal offers a study and discussion course designed to provide an enjoyable and supportive setting that helps people explore lifestlye habits, engage in stimulating discussion, and make personal changes towards creating a healthy home. For information on how to start a course on your area, visit the website or call. Other products include Athena's healthy home maintenance and laundry charts, and the quarterly newsletter *Homes that Heal*.

Humabuilt Healthy Building Systems

16869 SW 65th Ave #335, Lake Oswego, OR 97035 Telephone: 503-699- 0052
Web: <www.humabuilt.com> Consults with architects, builders, developers and homeowners on healthy design and new construction using Building Biology principles. Supplier of key healthy building materials and systems such as breathing block walls, whole house water filtration systems, two stage shower filters, healthy doors and kitchen cabinetry, ERVs and more.

HybriVet Systems

17 Erie Drive, Natick, MA 01760 Telephone: 800-262-5323 Web: <www.leadcheck.com>
Home test kits for lead.

International Institute for Bau-biologie and Ecology (IBE)

1401 A Cleveland St, Clearwater, FL 33755 Telephone: 727-461-4371
Web: <www.buildingbiology.net> U.S. training programs in Building Biology. Correspondence

courses, Internet courses, seminars. Referals for certified Building Biology Environmental Inspectors (BBEIs) for home inspections including water quality, mold, IAQ, dust mites, EMRs, chemicals. Supplier of Gaussmeters, body voltage meters, and more. Quarterly newsletter *EcoDwell*.

Janice Corporation

198 Route 46, Budd Lake, NJ 07828 Telephone: 800-526-4237 Web: <www.janices.com> Mail order company providing bed, bath, kitchen and personal care items that are free of harmful additives. Suppliers of 100 percent untreated cotton ironing board covers and pads.

Less EMF

26 Valley View Lane, Ghent, NY 12075 Telephone: 888-537-7363 Web: <www.lessemf.com> Suppliers of Gaussmeters, microwave oven testers, computer shielding, and more.

Lifekind Products

P.O. Box 1774, Grass Valley, CA 95945 Telephone: 800-284-4983 Web: <www.lifekind.com> This company has their own "Eco" factory where they hand make their own organic beds and bedding, guaranteeing their purity. Many other organic and healthy home products.

MCS Referral and Resources

508 Westgate Rd, Baltimore, MD 21229 Telephone: 410-362-6400 Web: <www.mcsrr.org> Carbon monoxide monitors and non-radioactive smoke detectors.

National Testing Laboratories

6555 Wilson Mills Road, Suite 102, Cleveland, OH 44143 Telephone: 440-449-2525, 800-458-3330 Web: <www.ntllabs.com> Homeowner water testing kits.

Naturlich

7120 Keating Ave, Sebastopol, CA 95472 Telephone: 707-829-3959 Web: <www.floorguy411.com> Specializes in floor coverings that are environmentally safe and made from durable materials. Large selection of area rugs and more.

Rawganique

9000 Rayelyn Lane, Denman Island, BC, Canada, V0R 1T0 Telephone: 866-729-4367, 250-335-0050 Web: <www.rawganique.com> Hemp and organic cotton clothes for women, men, and children, shower curtains and other household items.

Safe Effective Alternatives

P.O. Box 528, Belleville, IL 62222 Telephone: 877-730-2727 Web: <www.licebgone.com> Lice B Gone is a non-toxic alternative to toxic pesticides for flea and tick control on pets. Recommended by environmental physician Dr. Marion Moses of the Pesticide Education Center, <www.pesticides.org>

Seventh Generation

212 Battery Street, Suite A, Burlington, VT 05401-5281 Telephone: 802-658-3773, 800-456-1191 Web: <www.seventhgeneration.com> Complete line of non-toxic household products. Products use renewable, non-toxic, phosphate-free, and biodegradable ingredients, and are never tested on animals. Includes household cleaning products, bathroom tissue, paper towels, trash bags, and more. Available at many natural product and grocery stores.

Terressentials

2650 Old National Pike, Middletown, MD 21769 Telephone: 301-371-7333 Web: <www.terressentials.com> Handcrafted natural and organic personal care products including skin care, shampoo, soap, and body products with no synthetic petrochemical or oleochemical ingredients of any kind.

The 25 Principles of Building Biology

1. Site buildings on geologically undisturbed land.

2. Residential homes are best located away from industrial centers and main traffic routes.

3. Housing shall be developed in a decentralized and loose manner interlaced with sufficient green space.

4. Housing and developments shall be personalized, in harmony with nature, fit for human habitation and family oriented.

5. Use natural and unadulterated building materials.

6. Use wall, floor, and ceiling materials that allow air diffusion and are hygroscopic.

7. Indoor air humidity shall be regulated naturally.

8. Filter and neutralize air pollutants.

9. An appropriate balance of thermal insulation and heat retention is needed.

10. The air and surface temperatures of a given room need to be optimized.

11. Use radiant heat and as much passive solar heat as possible for the heating system.

12. The total moisture content of a new building shall be low and dry out quickly.

13. A building shall have a pleasant or neutral smell.

14. Light, lighting, and color shall be in harmony with natural conditions.

15. Protective measures against noise pollution as well as infrasonic and ultrasonic vibrations need to be human oriented.

16. Use building materials with little or preferably no radioactivity.

17. Maintain the natural balance of atmospheric electricity and ion concentration.

18. The Earth's natural magnetic field shall not be altered or distorted.

19. Eliminate or reduce man-made electromagnetic radiation (EMR) as much as possible.

20. Cosmic and terrestrial radiation is essential and shall be interfered with as little as possible.

21. Interior and furniture design shall be based upon physiological findings.

22. Harmonic measures, proportions, and shapes need to be taken into consideration.

23. Produce, install, and dispose of building materials in a way that does not contribute to environmental pollution and high energy costs.

24. Building activities shall not contribute to the exploitation of non-renewable and rare resources.

25. Building activities shall not cause a rise in social and medical costs.

Endnotes

Chapter 1: The Basics

1. Center for Health, Environment and Justice, "Poisoned Schools: Invisible Threats, Visible Actions," A report of the Childproofing Our Communities: Poisoned School Campaign, March, 2001, p. 9.
2. Jane Houlihan, *Body Burden; The Pollution in People* [online], [Cited September, 2003], Environmental Working Group, January 31, 2003, <www.ewg.org/reports/bodyburden/es.php>
3. Rachel Carson, *Silent Spring,* Houghton Mifflin, 1962.
4. Carolyn Raffensperger and Joel Tickner, *Protecting Public Health and the Environment: Implementing the Precautionary Principle,* Island Press, 1999.
5. Richard Gullickson, *Reference Data Sheet on Formaldehyde* [online], [Cited January, 2003], Meridian Engineering & Technology, January 1994, <www.meridianeng.com/formalde.html>

Chapter 2: The Healthy versus the Unhealthy Home

1. American Lung Association, "Indoor Air May Be a Source of Allergy Attacks," March 24, 1999.
2. Paula Baker-Laporte, *Bau-Biologie and the Healthy House* [online], [Cited January, 2002], 2001, <www.bakerlaporte.com/articles/baubiologie>
3. Canada Mortgage and Housing Corporation (CMHC), *Evaluation of Pollutant Source Strengths and Control Strategies in Conventional and R - 2000 Houses* 1997, p. 35.
4. Paula Baker-Laporte, Erica Elliot and John Banta, *Prescriptions for a Healthy House,* New Society Publishers, 2001, p. 288.
5. *Asthma Statistics* [online], [Cited July, 2002], Asthma in America, <www.asthmainamerica.com/statistics.htm>
6. Environmental Protection Agency, Office of Air and Radiation, "Healthy Buildings, Healthy People: A Vision for the 21st Century," (6609J) Document 402-K-01-003, October, 2001.

Chapter 3: The Conventionally Built New Home

1. Paulin Moszczynski, "Organic solvents and T lymphocytes," *Lancet,* February 21, 1981, p. 438, as cited by Ronald Finn, "Organic Solvent Sensitivity," *Clinical Ecology,* Vol. V, No. 4, 1987/88.

2. Paula Baker-Laporte, Erica Elliot and John Banta, *Prescriptions for a Healthy House,* New Society Publishers, 2001, p. 125.

3. Wolfgang Maes, *Recommendations of Bau-Biological Standard Values for Sleeping Areas,* (IBN, 1998) International Institute for Bau-biologie and Ecology, Indoor Air, Materials and Water Quality Seminar 1B/2

4. U.S. Department of Health and Human Services, *NIOSH Pocket Guide to Chemical Hazards,* NIOSH Publications, June, 1997, p. 22.

5. Baker-Laporte, Elliot and Banta, *Prescriptions for a Healthy House,* p. 175.

6. P.W. McRandle, *Carpets: Think Small* [online], [Cited November, 2003], The Green Guide, November/December 2003, #99 <www.thegreenguide.com>

7. The Carpet and Rug Institute, *Who is CRI* [online], [Cited November, 2003], <www.carpet-rug.com>

8. Cindy Duehring, "Carpet Part One: EPA Stalls and Industry Hedges While Consumers Remain at Risk," *Informed Consent,* November/December, 1993, p. 8.

9. Baker-Laporte, Elliot and Banta, *Prescriptions for a Healthy House,* p. 171

10. *Toxic Toy Story* [online], [Cited March, 2001], Greenpeace, 1998, <www.greenpeaceusa.org>

11. *PVC Fact Sheet* [online], [Cited April, 2003], Healthy Building Network, 2003, <www.healthybuilding.net/pvc/index.html>

12. Institute for Bau-biologie and Ecology, Professional Course, Course Pack 5/6, p. 13.

13. Institute for Bau-biologie and Ecology, Professional Course, Course Pack 15, pp. 6-10.

14. "Both Electric and Magnetic Fields Seen as Critical to Cancer Risk," *Microwave News,* July-August, 1996, pp. 1, 5-7.

15. "Strong Electric Fields Implicated in Major Leukemia Risk for Workers," *Microwave News,* May-June, 2000, pp.1-3.

16. Baker-Laporte, Elliot and Banta, *Prescriptions for a Healthy House,* p. 270.

17. *PVC Fact Sheet* [online], [Cited April, 2003], Healthy Building Network, 2003. <www.healthybuilding.net/pvc/index.html>

18. *What's On Tap? Grading Drinking Water in U.S. Cities* [online], [Cited August, 2003], Natural Resource Defense Council, June 2003, <www.nrdc.org>

19. *Arsenic and Old Laws: A Scientific and Public Health Analysis of Arsenic Occurrence in Drinking Water, Its Health Effect and EPA's Outdated Tap Water Standard* [online] [Cited August, 2003], National Resource Defense Council, Executive Summary, February, 2000, <www.nrdc.org/water/arsenic/execsum.asp>

20. Rep. Glenn Donnelson, *Statement on Opposition to Fluoridation* [online], [Cited December, 2003], National Conference of State Legislators, 2003, www.ncsl.org/programs/health/forum/shld/32c2.htm>

21. Baker-Laporte, Elliot and Banta, *Prescriptions for a Healthy House,* pp. 152-153.

22. "The Dirt On Diesel," Report by Oregon Environmental Council, February, 2003, p. 9.

Chapter 4: The Remodeled Home

1. Environmental Protection Agency, Office of Air and Radiation, Indoor Environments Division, *Mold Remediation in Schools and Commercial Buildings,* March, 2001, p. 37.

2. Ibid., p. 41.

3. Environmental Protection Agency, Office of Air and Radiation, Indoor Environments Division, *A Brief Guide to Mold, Moisture and Your Home.* July, 2002, p. 2.

4. T. A. Oxley and E. G. Gobert, *Dampness in Buildings,* Butterworth-Heinemann, 1983, p. 79.

5. Will Spates, Indoor Environmental Technologies, Clearwater, Florida, E-mail correspondence, 2002-2203,

6. Ibid.

7. Environmental Protection Agency, *A Brief Guide to Mold, Moisture and Your Home,* July, 2002, p. 2.

8. Environmental Protection Agency, *Mold Remediation in Schools and Commercial Buildings,* p. 40.

9. International Institute for Bau-biologie and Ecology, Indoor Air, Materials, Water Quality, 2002, seminar notes, p. 040103.

10. Ruth A. Etzel, M.D., PhDl, "Mycotoxins" *Journal of the American Medical Association,* January 23/30, 2002, pp. 425-427.
    Ruth A. Etzel, M.C., PhD., Eduardo Montana, M.D., William G. Sorenson, PhD. et al. "Acute pulmonary hemorrhage in infants associated with exposure to *Stachybotrys atra* and other fungi." *Archives of Pediatrics and Adolescent Medicine,* 1998; 152: pp. 757-762.

11. Chin S.Yang, Ph.D., "Toxic Effects of Some Common Indoor Fungi," *Enviros: The Healthy Building Newsletter,* Volume 4, Number 9, September, 1994.

12. Environmental Protection Agency, *Mold Remediation in Schools and Commercial Buildings,* p. 18.

13. Philip J. Landrigan, M.D., Herbert L. Needleman, M. D. and Mary Landrigan, M.P.A., *Raising Healthy Children in a Toxic World: 101 Smart Solutions for Every Family,* Rodale, 2001, p. 131.

14. Lyn Marie Bower, *Creating a Healthy Household,* The Healthy House Institute, 2000, pp. 538-539.

15. Ibid., p. 537.

16. Landrigan, Needleman and Landrigan, *Raising Healthy Children in a Toxic World: 101 Smart Solutions for Every Family,* p. 104.

17. Baker-Laporte, Paula, Erica Elliott and John Banta, *Prescriptions for a Healthy House,* New Society Publishers, 2001, p. 130.

Chapter 5: The Healthy New Home

1. "Insulation Materials: Environmental Comparison," *Environmental Building News,* January/February, 1995, Volume 4, No. 1.

2. Ibid.

3. Pamela O'Malley Chang, *Natural Linoleum Makes A Comeback* [online],

[Cited September, 2003], Healthy Home Designs, March 2001, <www.healthyhomedesigns.com/articles/information8.php>

4. Theron G. Randolph, M.D. and Ralph W. Moss, Ph.D., *An Alternative Approach to Allergies,* Revised ed. Harper and Row, 1990, p. 99.

5. Baker-Laporte, Paula, Erica Elliot and John Banta, *Prescriptions for a Healthy House,* New Society Publishers, 2001, p. 1.

6. Linda Mason Hunter, *The Healthy Home: An Attic to Basement Guide to Toxin-Free Living,* iUniverse.com, 2000, p. 175.

7. Ibid.

8. Ibid.

9. David Pearson, *The Natural House Catalogue,* Fireside, 1996, p. 98.

10. Institute for Bau-biologie and Ecology, *Light, Illumination and Color,* Professional Correspondence Course, 1989, Course Pack 15, p. 15,

11. Spark Burmaster, *Electrical Wiring Specifications for New Construction for Minimizing Electro Magnetic Exposure,* Institute for Bau-biologie and Ecology, 2002, p. 5.

12. Baker-Laporte, Elliot and Banta, *Prescriptions for a Healthy House,* p. 275.

13. Ibid., p. 279.

14. David Pearson, *The New Natural House Book,* Fireside, 1998, p. 97.

15. Ibid.

16. "Leading Epidemiologists See Childhood Leukemia Risk at 4mG." *Microwave News.* September/October, 2000, pp. 1, 11-13.

17. International Institute for Bau-biologie and Ecology, *House Technique-Interior Design,* Profesional Correspondence Course, 1988, Course Pack 10, p. 7.

18. Pearson, *The New Natural House Book,* p. 108.

Chapter 6: Environmental Health at Home

1. *A Primer on Solid Waste* [online], [Cited August, 2003], Energy Information Administration, <www.eia.doe.gov/kids/recycling/solidwaste/primer.html>

Chapter 7: Bedrooms

1. National Sleep Foundation, *Most Common Sleep Problems in Women,* [online], [Cited September, 2003], August, 2003, <www.sleepfoundation.org/publications/women.cfc#6>

2. "Are There More Chemicals in Your Mattress or a Barrel of Oil?" *Lifekind Bulletin* Volume IV-1, 2001, p. 1.

3. Jack Thrasher, Ph.D. and Alan Broughton, M.D. *The Poisoning of Our Homes and Work Places,* Seadora Publishing and Research, 1989, p. 12.

4. Debra Lynn Dadd, *Home Safe Home,* Tarcher/Putnam, 1997, p. 269.

5. Life Kind, *Mattress Materials* [online], [Cited November, 2003], <www.lifekind.com/catalog/mattress_materials.php>

6. Oregon Environmental Council, *Bad Fashion Sense: A Hazard for the Environment* [online],

[Cited August, 2003], Aug 26, 2003. <www.orcouncil.org>

7. Sonya Lunder and Renee Sharp, *Tainted Catch: Toxic Fire Retardants Building Up in San Francisco Bay Fish* [online], [Cited August, 2003], Environmental Working Group, July, 2003. <www.ewg.org/reports/taintedcatch/es.php>

8. Michael Saunders, FRCS., *War On Dust Mites* [online], [Cited November, 2003], University of Bristol, <www.bris.ac.uk/Depts/ENT/war%20on%20dust%20mites.htm>

9. Annie Berthold Bond, *Better Basics for the Home,* Three Rivers Press, 1999, p. 88.

10. Baker-Laporte, Paula, Erica Elliot and John Banta, *Prescriptions for a Healthy House,* New Society Publishers, 2001, p. 172.

11. Philip J. Landrigan, M.D., Herbert L. Needleman, M.D., and Mary Landrigan, M.P.A, *Raising Healthy Children in a Toxic World,* Rodale, 2001, p. 68.

12. David Steinman and R. Michael Wisner, *Living Healthy in a Toxic World,* Perigree, 1996, p. 13.

13. Athena Thompson, *Answer #2 ; Chapter 5, Section E: Energy,* International Institute for Bau-biologie and Ecology, Mini-Correspondence Course, 2001.

14. International Institute for Bau-biologie, *Energy* Mini Correspondence Course, 1995, E11.

15. Environmental Protection Agency, *Facts About Americium-241* [online], [Cited September, 2003], July, 2003, <www.epa.gov/superfund/resources/radiation/pdf/americium.pdf>

16. Baker-Laporte, Elliot and Banta, *Prescriptions for a Healthy House,* p. 29.

17. Betty Bridges, *Fragrances By Design* [online], [Cited July, 2003], Fragranced Product Information Network, March, 2003, <www.fpinva.org>

18. Ibid.

19. Baker-Laporte, Elliot and Banta, *Prescriptions for a Healthy House,* p. 29.

20. Landrigan, Needleman and Landrigan, *Raising Healthy Children in a Toxic World,* p. 41.

21. Lynn Marie Bower, *Creating a Healthy Household.* Healthy House Institute, 2000, p. 557.

22. Environmental Protection Agency, *Ozone: Good Up High, Bad Nearby* [online], [Cited July, 2003], June, 2003, <www.epa.gov/oar/oaqps/gooduphigh/>

23. National Sleep Foundation, *Children, Obesity and Sleep* [online], [Cited September, 2003], August, 2003, <www.sleepfoundation.org/PressArchives/kidsandobesity.cfm>

24. The Green Guide, *Mattresses and Box Springs* [online], [Cited October, 2003], The Green Guide Institute Product Report, <www.greenguide.com/reports/product.mhtml?id=1>

25. Greenpeace, *Toxic Toy Story* [online], [Cited September, 2003], 1998. <www.greenpeaceusa.org/index.fpl?article=532&object_id=8270>

26. Greenpeace, *Determination of the Composition and Quantities of Phthalate Ester Additives in PVC Children's Toys* [online], [Cited September, 2003], <www.greenpeaceusa.org/index.fpl?article=534&object_id=8270>

27. George Carlo and Martin Schram, *Cell Phones: Invisible Hazards in the Wireless Age,* Carroll and Graf, 2001, Photo Section between pp. 142-143.

28. Landrigan, Needleman, and Landrigan, *Raising Healthy Children in a Toxic World,* p. 6.

29. "Disposable Diapers Linked To Asthma," *Mothering Magazine,* Issue 98, January/February, 2000.

30. Mindy Pennybacker and Aisha Ikramuddin, *Mothers and Others Guide To Natural Baby*

     Care, John Wiley and Sons, 1999, p. 160.

31. Ibid., p. 155.

32. John Wargo, Ph.D. and Linda Evenson Wargo, *The State of Children's Health and Environment 2002,* Children's Health Environment Coalition, February, 2002, p. 8.

Chapter 8: Bathrooms

1. Theron G. Randolph, M.D. and Ralph W. Moss, Ph.D., *An Alternative Approach to Allergies,* Harper Perennial, 1990, p. 50.

2. Cynthia Wilson, *Chemical Exposure and Human Health,* MacFarland, 1993, p. 148.

3. Houston Tomasz, National Sales Director, Sun Water Systems, e-mail correspondence, February, 2004.

4. Ibid.

5. Charles Strand, "Editorial," *The Aquasonic Delux Shower Filtration System,* Sun Water Systems, p. 2.

6. Debra Lynn Dadd, *Home Safe Home,* Tarcher/Putnam, 1997, p. 56.

7. Pamela Lundquist and Aisha Ikramuddin, *PVC: The Most Toxic Plastic* [online], [Cited July, 2003], Children's Health Environment Coalition, September 1998, <www.checnet.org/healthehouse/education/articles- detail.asp?Main_ID=185>

8. John Bower, *Understanding Ventilation,* The Healthy House Institute, 1995, p. 55.

9. United States Department of Agriculture, *Definitions-Regulatory Text* [online], [Cited November, 2003], Agricultural Marketing Service, The National Organic Program, <www.ams.usda.gov/nop?NOP/standards/DefineReg.htmll>

10. Sharon Kirtey, *Deodorants Might be Linked to Cancer* [online], [Cited January, 2004], CanWest News Service, January 16, 2004, <www.canada.com>

11. Institute for Children's Environmental Health, *Children's Environmental Health Basics>* [online], [Cited September, 2003], <www.iceh.org/Pages/basics.html>

12. David Steinman and Samuel S. Epstein, M.D., *The Safe Shoppers Bible,* Macmillan, 1995, p. 181.

13. Ibid., p. 263.

14. Samuel S. Epstein M.D., *Cancer Prevention Alert No. 9, Cosmetic and Personal Care Products: Questions and Answers* [online], [Cited July, 2003], <www.preventcancer.com>

15. Steinman and Epstein, *The Safe Shoppers Bible,* p. 265.

16. Epstein, *Cancer Prevention Alert No. 9, Cosmetic and Personal Care Products: Questions and Answers* <www.preventcancer.com>

17. The Green Guide, *From Gray to "Green"* [online].[Cited September, 2003] The Green Guide Institute, September 30, 2003, <www.greenguide.com>

18. Lynn Marie Bower, *Creating a Healthy Household,* The Healthy House Institute, 2000, p. 198.

19. Seventh Generation, *How Much Chlorine Is In My Home?* [online], [Cited October, 2003], <www.seventhgeneration.com/page.asp?id=1295>

20. Dadd, *Home Safe Home,* p. 275.

21. Seventh Generation, *Bathroom Tissue-400 Sheet, 12 pack:You Are Making a Difference*

[online], [Cited September, 2003], <www.seventhgeneration.com>

22. Mindy Pennybacker, *Healthier Home Cleaning* [online], [Cited October, 2003], The Green Guide Institute, Online Newsletter, September/October, 2003 #98, <www.thegreenguide.com>

23. Mary O'Brien, *Making Better Environmental Decisions: An Alternative to Risk Assessment,* MIT Press, 2000, back cover.

Chapter 9: Kitchens

1. Sharon Cadwallader, *The Living Kitchen,* Sierra Club Books, 1983, p. 10.

2. Barry Forbes, *Prominent Researcher Apologizes for Pushing Fluoride,* "The Tribune," Mesa, AZ., December 5, 1999.

3. Rep. Glenn Donnelson, *Statement on Opposition to Fluoride* [online], [Cited February, 2004], 2003 State Health Lawmaker's Digest: Community Water Fluoridation (Vol. 3, No. 2), <www.ncsl.org/programs/health/forum/shld/32c2.htm>

4. Natural Resources Defense Council, *Bottled Water: Pure Drink or Pure Hype?* [online], [Cited October, 2003], March, 1999, <nrdc.org/water/drinking/bw/bwinx.asp>

5. Sandra Steingraber, *Living Downstream,* Vintage Books, 1998, p. 76.

6. Environmental Protection Agency, *Safe Drinking Water Act,* [online], [Cited May, 2004], EPA Office of Water, List of Contaminants and Their MCLs, Pdf version "National Primary Drinking Water Standards," June, 2003, <www.epa.government/safewater/mcl.html>

7. Kurt Kleiner, "Safe lead levels still damage children's I.Q." *New Scientist,* April 16, 2003.

8. Environmental Protection Agency, *Chloroform* [online], [Cited December, 2003], October, 2003. <www.epa.gov/region1/eco/airtox/chloroform.html>

9. David Goldbeck, *The Smart Kitchen,* Ceres Press, 1994, p. 45.

10. Paula Baker, John Banta and Erica Elliot, *Prescriptions for a Healthy House,* New Society Publishers, 2001, p. 6.

11. Annie Berthold Bond and Mothers and Others for a Livable Planet, *Green Kitchen Handbook,*> Harper Perennial, 1997, p. 248.

12. William P. Kopp, *The Proven Dangers of Microwaves* [online], [Cited October, 2003], LessEMF, <www.lessemf.com/mwstnds.html#AREC>

13. Ibid.

14. International Institute for Bau-biologie and Ecology, *The Climate of Radiation in the Living Spaces of Civilized People,* 1989, Professional Correspondence Course Pack 17, p. 35.

15. B. Blake Levitt, *Electromagnetic Fields,* Harcourt Brace, 1995, p. 263.

16. The Green Guide, *Is it Safe to Microwave Food in Plastics?* [online], [Cited July, 2003], The Green Guide Institute, March/April 2001 (#88-89), <www.thegreenguide.com/doc.mhtml?I=88-89&s=lundquist4>

17. Goldbeck, *The Smart Kitchen,* p. 58.

18. Debra Lynn Dadd, *Home Safe Home,* Tarcher/Putnam, 1997, p. 100.

19. Pamela Lundquist and Aisha Ikramuddin, *PVC: The Most Toxic Plastic* [online], [Cited July, 2003], Children's Health Environment Coalition, September, 1998,

<www.checnet.org/healthehouse/education/articles-detail.asp?Main_ID=185>

20. P.W. McRandle and Andreea Matei, *Paint>* [online], [Cited June, 2003], The Green Guide Institute, May/June, 2003 # 96, <www.thegreenguide.com/doc.mhtml?I=96&s=paint>

21. Berthold Bond and Mothers and Others for a Livable Planet, *Green Kitchen Handbook,* p. 15.

22. Lundquist and Ikramuddin, *PVC: The Most Toxic Plastic*
<www.checnet.org/healthehouse/education/articles-detail.asp?Main_ID=185>

23. Environmental Working Group, *PFC's: Global Contaminents* [online], [Cited June, 2003], April, 2003, <www.ewg.org/reports/pfcworld/es.php>

24. Ibid.

Chapter 10: Laundry

1. Theo Colburn, Dianne Dumanoski and John Peterson-Myers, *Our Stolen Future: Book Basics: The Bottom Line,* [online], [Cited October, 2003], <www.ourstolenfuture.org/Basics/bottomline.htm>

2. Theo Colburn, Dianne Dumanoski and John Peterson-Myers, *Our Stolen Future,* Plume, 1997, p. 264-265.

3. Phyllis G. Tortora, *Understanding Textiles,* Prentice Hall, 2001, p. 195.

4. Angela Hobbs, *The Sick House Survival Guide,* New Society Publishers, 2003, p. 29.

5. Ibid., p. 97, and John Harte et al., *Toxics A to Z: A Guide to Everyday Pollution Hazards,* University of California Press, 1991, p. 308.

6. Debra Lynn Dadd, *Home Safe Home,* Tarcher/Putnam, 1997, p. 291.

7. Jim Rimer, President of Bi-O-Kleen Products, personal conversation, 10/20/03.

8. Hobbs, *The Sick House Survival Guide,* p. 97.

9. Seventh Generation, *How Much Chlorine is in my Home?* [online], [Cited Septemeber, 2003], <www.seventhgeneration.com/page.asp?id=1295>

10. Mindy Pennybacker, *Healthier Home Cleaning,* September/October, 2003 #98, [online], [Cited November, 2003], <www.thegreenguide.com/doc.mhtml?I=98&s=clean>

11. Oregon Environmental Council, *Dry Cleaning Clothes Without Toxics,* [online], [Cited September, 2003], Online Newsletter, Aug. 26, 2003, <www.orcouncil.org>

Chapter 11: Home Offices

1. Reinhard Kanuka-Fuchs, *Healthy Home and Healthy Office,* Harald W. Tietze Publishing, 2001, p. 47.

2. International Institute for Bau-biologie and Ecology, *Air Ions,* Mini-Correspondence Course, 1995, p. E61.

3. EMF Bioshield, *Are Computer Monitors Harmful to Your Health?* [online], [Cited October, 2003], <www.emf-bioshield.com/emf/arecrt.html>

4. Doris J. Rapp, M.D., *Is This Your Child's World?,* Bantam Books, 1996, p. 232.

5. B. Blake Levitt, *Electromagnetic Fields,* Harcourt Brace, 1995, p. 282.

6. Allison Sloan, *Conscientious Computing,* [online], [Cited August, 2003], The Green Guide Institute, November/December, 2000, #84/85,

<www.thegreenguide.com/dec.mhtml?I=84-85&s=sloan1>

7. Levitt, *Electromagnetic Fields,* p.272.

8. Ibid.

9. George Carlo and Martin Schram, *Cell Phones: Invisible Hazards in the Wireless Age,* Carroll & Graf , 2001, p. 244.

10. Department of Health, U.K., *Mobile Phones and Health,* [online], [Cited October, 2003], October, 2002, <www.doh.gov.uk/mobilephones.htm>

11. Levitt, *Electromagnetic Fields,* p. 285.

12. Michelle Conlin, "Is Your Office Killing You?", *Business Week,* June 5, 2000.

13. Ibid.

14. Rapp, *Is This Your Child's World?,* p. 230.

15. Carlo and Schram, *Cell Phones: Invisible Hazards in the Wireless Age,* p. 216.

Chapter 12: Other Rooms

1. Vicki Lankarge, *What Every Home Owner Needs To Know About Mold,* McGraw Hill, 2003, p. 30.

2. American Academy of Pediatrics Committee on Environmental Health. "Toxic Effects of indoor molds." *Pediatrics.* April, 1998; 101: pp. 712-714. Available online at <http://aappolicy.aappublications.org/cgi/reprint/pediatrics;101/4/712.pdf>.

3. Environmental Protection Agency, *EPA Administrator Whitman Urges Home Testing for Radon* [online], [Cited August, 2003], EPA Newsroom, January, 2003, <www.epa.gov/epahome/headline_011403.htm>

4. Wolfgang Maes, *Recommendations of Bau-Biological Standard Values for Sleeping Areas,* 1998, International Institute for Bau-biology and Ecology, Indoor Air, Materials and Water Quality Seminar 1B/2.

5. John Bower and Lynn Marie Bower, *The Healthy House Answer Book,* The Healthy House Institute, 1997, p. 92.

6. Paula Baker-Laporte, Erica Elliot and John Banta, *Prescriptions for a Healthy Home,* New Society Publishers, 2001, p. 6.

7. B. Blake Levitt, *Electromagnetic Fields,* Harcourt Brace, 1995, p. 269.

8. Allison Sloan, *Conscientious Computing,* [online], [Cited August, 2003], The Green Guide Institute, November/December, 2000, #84/85, <www.thegreenguide.com/dec.mhtml?I=84-85&s=sloan1>

9. State of Washington Department of Ecology, *Health Effects of Wood Smoke,* [online], [Cited October, 2003], March 1997, <www.ecy.wa.gov/biblio/92046.html>

10. Linda Mason Hunter, *The Healthy Home,* iUniverse.com, 2000, p. 90.

11. Environmental Protection Agency, *Respiratory Health Effects of Passive Smoking: Lung Cancer and Other Disorders* [online], [Cited October 2003]; 1992, <www.cfpub1.epa.gov/ncea/cfm/recordisplay.cfm?deid=2835>

12. Natural Resources Defense Council, *Our Children at Risk: The 5 Worst Environmental Threats to Their Health* [online], [Cited October, 2003], November, 1997,

<www.nrdc.org/health/kids/ocar/ocarinx.asp>

13. Ibid.

14. Michael McCann, Ph.D., C.I.H., *Artist Beware,* The Lyons Press, 1992, pp. 532-533.
American Academy of Pediatrics Committee on Environmental Health. Pediatric Environmental Health. 2nd Ed. Etzel, RA, ed. Elk Grove Village, IL: American Academy of Pediatrics; 2003, pp. 9-20.

15. California Office of Environmental Health Hazard Assessment, *Guidelines For The Safe Use of Art and Craft Materials,* [online], [Cited August, 2003], August, 2002, <www.oehha.org/education/art/artguide.html>

16. Ibid.

Chapter 13: Garages

1. Bill Baue, *Traffic Congestion: The Chemicals in Your Car*> [online], [Cited August, 2003], Children's Health Environment Coalition, HealtheHouse, Garage, October 2001, <www.checnet.org/healthehouse/education/articles-detail.asp?Main_ID=96>

2. Andrew Schneider, *U.S. Imports Of Asbestos Brake Material Are On Rise,* St. Louis Post-Dispatch, October 25, 2003.

3. Baue, *Traffic Congestion: The Chemicals in Your Car* <www.checnet.org/healthehouse/education/articles-detail.asp?Main_ID=96>

4. Environmental Protection Agency, *What is Household Hazardous Waste?* [online], [Cited November, 2003], April, 1993, <www.epa.government/epaoswer/non-hw/household/hhw.htm>

Chapter 14: Yards, Plants, and Pests

1. Peter Montague, *Common Weed Killer Now Linked to Cancer Deaths in New Study* [online], [Cited August, 2003], Environmental Research Foundation, Rachel's Environment and News, December 15, 1986, <www.rachel.org/search/index.cfm?St=1>

2. Sandra Steingraber, *Living Downstream,* Vintage, 1998, p. 53.

3. Caroline Cox, *2,4-D: Toxicology, Part 1* [online], [Cited November, 2003], Northwest Coalition for Alternatives to Pesticides, Journal of Pesticide Reform, Spring 1999, Vol.19, No.1, <www.pesticide.org/factsheets.html#pesticides>

4. Sandra Marquardt, Caroline Cox and Holly Knight, *Toxic Secrets: "Inert" Ingredients in Pesticides 1987- 1997* [online], [Cited October, 2002], Northwest Coalition for Alternatives to Pesticides and Californians for Pesticide Reform, Report 1998, www.pesticide.org/inertspage.html>

5. Caroline Cox, *Are Pesticides Hazardous To Our Health?*, Northwest Coalition for Alternatives to Pesticides, Journal of Pesticide Reform, Summer 1999, Vol.19, No 2.

6. Center for Children's Health and the Environment of the Mount Sinai School of Medicine, *More Kid's Are Getting Brain Cancer. Why?* [online], [Cited October, 2003], 2002, Advertisement published in the NY Times, <www.childenvironment.org>

7. Macia Nishioka, et al., "Measuring Transport of Lawn-applied Herbicides from Turf to Home: Correlation of Dislodgeable 2,4-D Turf Residues with Carpet Dust and Carpet

Surfaces Residues," *Environmental Science Technology* 30:1, pp. 3313-3320.

8. Paula Baker-Laporte, Erica Elliot and John Banta, *Prescriptions for a Healthy Home,* New Society Publishers, 2001, p. 11.

9. Institute for Children's Environmental Health, *Children's Environmental Health Basics* [online], [Cited October, 2003], <www.iceh.org/Pages/basics.html>

10. D. Donaldson, T. Kiely, A. Grube, *Pesticides industry sales and usage: 1998 and 1999 market estimates* [online], [Cited November, 2003], US EPA OPPTS Office of Pesticide Programs, Biological and Economic Analysis Division, August 2002, www.epa.gov/oppbead1/pestsales/99pestsales/market_estimates1999.pdf>

11. R. W. Whitmore, J. E. Kelly and P. L. Reading, *National home and garden pesticide use survey. Final report, Vol.1: Executive summary, results, and recommendations,* Research Triangle Institute, 1992.

12. Baker-Laporte, Elliot and Banta, *Prescriptions for a Healthy Home,* p. 7.

13. Northwest Coalition for Alternatives to Pesticides, *Pesticides and Breast Cancer* [online], [Cited August, 2002], April 1996, <www.pesticide.org/factsheets.html>

14. Steven Arnold et al., "Synergistic Activation of Estrogen Receptor with Combinations of Environmental Chemicals," *Science* 272, June 7, 1996, pp. 1489-1492.

15. Jack Leiss and David Savitz, "Home Pesticide Use and Childhood Cancer: A Case Control Study," *American Journal of Public Health,* February, 1995, pp. 249-252.

16. E. Gold et al., "Risk Factors for Brain Tumors in Children," *American Journal of Epidemiology* 109, 1979, pp. 309-319.

17. American Cancer Society, *Drug-free Lawns,* Pamphlet, 1993.

18. National Research Council, *Arsenic in Drinking Water,* The National Academies Press, 1999, pp. 83-149.

19. Environmental Working Group, *Healthy Building Network, Environmental Working Group Petition Consumer Product Safety Commission to Ban Sale of Arsenic-Treated Lumber for Playgrounds* [online], [Cited October, 2003], May 23, 2003, <www.ewg.org/reports/poisonedplaygrounds>

20. Healthy Building Network, *Arsenic Wood Fact Sheet* [online], [Cited October, 2003], 2002, <www.healthybuilding.net>

21. Ibid.

22. Jan Williams, *The Household Detective,* Children's Health Environment Coalition, 2003, p. 35.

Chapter 15: Pets

1. J. R. Davis et al., "Family Pesticide Use and Childhood Brain Cancer," *Archives of Environmental Contamination and Toxicology,* 1993, pp. 87-92.

2. M. Hansen, *Pest Control for Home and Garden,* Consumers Union, 1993, p. 293.

3. R.G. Ames et al., "Health Symptoms and Occupational Exposure to Flea Control Products Among California Pet Handlers," *Journal of the American Industrial Hygiene Association,* 1989, pp. 466-472.

4. Ibid.

5. S. A. Briggs and Rachel Carson Council, *Basic Guide to Pesticides: Their Characteristics and*

Hazards, Taylor and Francis, 1992, p. 211.

6. Ibid., p. 158.

7. Ibid., p. 210.

8. Davis et al., "Family Pesticide Use and Childhood Brain Cancer," pp. 87-92.

9. H. Hayes et al., "Case-Control Study of Canine Malignant Lymphoma: Positive Association With Dog Owner's Use of 2,4, Dichlorophenoxyacetic Acid Herbicides," *Journal of the National Cancer Institute,* 83, 1991, pp. 1226-1231.

10. David Wallinger, M.D. and Linda Greer, Ph.D., *Poisons On Pets, Health Hazards From Flea and Tick Products* [online], [Cited October, 2003], Natural Resource Defense Council, November, 2000, <www.nrdc.org/health/effects/execsum.asp>

11. Natural Resources Defense Council, *Harmful Pet Products FAQ* [online]. [Cited October, 2003], Based on the November, 2000 report *Poisons on Pets: Health Hazards from Flea and Tick Products* <www.nrdc.org/health/effects/qpets.asp>

12. Jan Williams, *The Household Detective,* Children's Health Environment Coalition, 2003, Appendix E, p. 3.

13. C. J. Puotinen, *The Encyclopedia of Natural Pet Care,* Keats Publishing, 2000, p. 260.

14. Williams, *The Household Detective,* Appendix E, p. 4.

Chapter 16: Cleaning

1. Jacob Lieberman, O.D., Ph.D., *Light: Medicine of the Future,* Bear and Company, 1991, p. 140.

2. David Steinman and R. Michael Wisner, *Living Healthy in a Toxic World,* Perigree, 1996, pp. 12-13.

3. Seventh Generation, *Dish Liquid, the Inside Scoop: You are Making a Difference* [online], [Cited March,

4. On Your Side, *Doctors Believe Household Cleaners Linked to Rise in Asthma* [online], [Cited November, 2003], Wavy.com, 2003, <www.wavy.com/Global/story.asp?S=1154097>

Chapter 17: Home Maintenance

1. Lynn Lawson, *Staying Well in a Toxic World,* Lynnword Press, 1993, p. 113.

Chapter 18: Living Happily Ever After ...

1. Center for Children's Health and the Environment of the Mount Sinai School of Medicine, *She's The Test Subject For Thousands Of Toxic Chemicals. Why?* [online], [Cited October, 2003], 2002, Advertisement published in the N.Y. Times, <www.childenvironment.org>

2. Sandra Steingraber, *Living Downstream,* Vintage, 1998, p. 269.

3. Royal Commission on Environmental Pollution U.K., *Chemicals in Products* [online], [Cited November, 2003], June, 2003, <www.rcep.org.uk>

4. William McDonough and Michael Braungart, *The Hanover Principles Design For Sustainability,* William McDonough+Partners, 1999, p. 6.

Index

About the Author

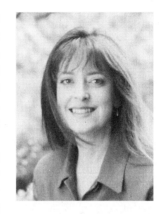

ATHENA THOMPSON has over 18 years experience as a Natural Health Specialist with undergraduate and graduate degrees in Natural and Environmental Health Sciences. She is currently engaged in post-graduate studies. Athena previously established and managed her own Natural Health Clinic in England before moving to the United States. A mother herself, she specializes in environmental health relating to children's issues.

As a certified Bau-biologist (Building Biologist), Athena is considered a leading proponent in this internationally recognized approach to healthy building design and construction. She co-founded Humabuilt™, Healthy Building Systems (www.humabuilt.com). Humabuilt consults with architects, builders, developers and individuals to create healthier built environments, as well as providing affordable, high-performance products and solutions to the building community worldwide.

For ongoing and updated information about healthy home issues, visit (www.homesthatheal.com) where you can subscribe to Athena's newsletter, the *Homes That Heal News*. Athena currently lives in Lake Oswego, Oregon with her husband and son.

If you have enjoyed *Homes that Heal*, you might also enjoy other

BOOKS TO BUILD A NEW SOCIETY

Our books provide positive solutions for people who want to make a difference. We specialize in:

Sustainable Living ◆ Ecological Design and Planning ◆ Natural Building & Appropriate Technology

New Forestry ◆ Environment and Justice ◆ Conscientious Commerce ◆ Progressive Leadership

Educational and Parenting Resources ◆ Resistance and Community ◆ Nonviolence

For a full list of NSP's titles, please call 1-800-567-6772 or check out our web site at:

www.newsociety.com

New Society Publishers

ENVIRONMENTAL BENEFITS STATEMENT

New Society Publishers has chosen to produce this book on Rolland Enviro 100, recycled paper made with 100% post consumer waste, processed chlorine free, and old growth free.

For every 5,000 books printed, New Society saves the following resources:[1]

47	Trees
4,239	Pounds of Solid Waste
4,664	Gallons of Water
6,084	Kilowatt Hours of Electricity
7,706	Pounds of Greenhouse Gases
33	Pounds of HAPs, VOCs, and AOX Combined
12	Cubic Yards of Landfill Space

[1]Environmental benefits are calculated based on research done by the Environmental Defense Fund and other members of the Paper Task Force who study the environmental impacts of the paper industry.

NEW SOCIETY PUBLISHERS